Population Health

Population Health

Concepts and Methods

Second Edition

T. Kue Young
M.D., M.Sc., FRCPC, D.Phil.

Professor of Public Health Sciences
Faculty of Medicine
University of Toronto

OXFORD
UNIVERSITY PRESS
2005

OXFORD
UNIVERSITY PRESS

Oxford   New York
Auckland   Bangkok   Buenos Aires   Cape Town   Chennai
Dar es Salaam   Delhi   Hong Kong   Istanbul   Karachi   Kolkata
Kuala Lumpur   Madrid   Melbourne   Mexico City   Mumbai   Nairobi
São Paulo   Shanghai   Taipei   Tokyo   Toronto

Library of Congress Cataloging-in-Publication Data
Young, T. Kue.
Population health : concepts and methods / T. Kue Young.—2nd ed.
p. cm.
Includes bibliographical references and index.
ISBN-13 978-0-19-515854-0
1. Public health. 2. Epidemiology. I. Title.
RA425.Y68 2004
614.4—dc22   2004050095

3 4 5 6 7 8 9

Printed in the United States of America
on acid-free paper

Preface

Why the term *population health* was chosen as the title of this textbook is explained in some detail in Chapter 1. The book is intended for introductory and intermediate courses in epidemiology, community health, or related course work given primarily in schools or graduate programs of public health. It arose from a graduate course on the principles of epidemiology that I have taught for over 10 years, first at the University of Manitoba, and more recently at the University of Toronto. Despite the proliferation of epidemiology texts, I have had surprising difficulty finding one that suits the needs of students who intend to work in public health, health planning, or program management. These students should be exposed to the excitement of both research and practice. Numerous editorials and articles in recent years have lamented the "drifting away" of epidemiology from its roots in public health. Indeed, there are books on epidemiology where "population" does not matter, and where "health" is not even a focus. It is also increasingly evident that epidemiology as a quantitative science alone is an inadequate tool to understand or to investigate the full complexities of the health of populations.

In writing this book, I have had an ambitious aim: to spark the development of a new type of interdisciplinary, broadly based *foundation* course in population health. Such a course would, for sure, have epidemiology as its core, but this would be integrated with the methods and concepts of relevant social sciences and the humanities, including demography, sociology, anthropology, history, and ethics. The course would focus on defining and measuring population health status, determining health risks and inferring causation, and planning and evaluating interventions.

This book does not intend to replace the standard encyclopedic texts in public health. It is not meant to be a reference text, and I would actually recommend that it be read from cover to cover. Doing so is not to indulge the author in his delusion, but to enable students to take a guided tour of the entire field (with some detours) and to get a good grasp of its key features.

Extensive use is made of boxes throughout the text. These provide explanations of technical terms—etymology, nuance, and usage; worked examples of computations using actual data; supplementary information to illustrate the text; and useful lists, figures, and tables. At the end of each chapter are case studies, which provide short summaries of the methods and results of published studies relevant to the concepts discussed in the chapter. Many of these cases are historical. This represents a deliberate attempt to impress on students entering the field that what we know today has accumulated from what others have learned in the past, and that what we see as "new" issues often are actually recycled old ideas.

The chapters also contain exercises, which mainly involve numerical computations but also deal with the interpretation of graphical and tabular data. Actual data from the published literature are used whenever possible, with examples from the full spectrum of health problems—infectious diseases, chronic diseases, environmental and occupational health, injuries, mental health, dental health, and more. While there is a North American bias, a conscious effort has been made to choose examples from around the world.

Since the first edition was published in 1998, the term population health has become much more widely accepted and the field has advanced. For this second edition much new material has been added to the text, boxes, and exercises reflecting changes in contemporary public health concerns and our response to them, as well as new research directions. In addition, many sections have been expanded, reorganized, or clarified, and I am grateful to the many readers, students, and colleagues who have pointed out errors and weaknesses in the first edition.

The topics that are new to this edition or are discussed in greater depth include: achievements of public health in the twentieth century (Chapter 1); confidence intervals for commonly used rates, and the impact of population aging on mortality trends (Chapter 2); health survey questionnaires, summary measures of population health, the new International Classification of Functioning, Disability and Health, and the epidemiological investigation of bioterrorism (Chapter 3); migrant studies, race and ethnicity, health in the life course, psychoneuroendocrine pathways, and more extensive coverage of genetics and social epidemiology (Chapter 4); expanded coverage of risk perception, and communicating the SARS epidemic (Chapter 5); expanded discussions of ecologic studies, the odds ratio and interactions, participatory research, and Durkheim's classic studies on suicide (Chapter 6); evidence-based community interventions (Chapter 7); and more detailed coverage of evaluation methods and health economics, the Cochrane Collaboration, and systematic reviews (Chapter 8). Chapter 9 is still a student project, but with additional guidance and examples from existing populations.

In writing this book, I have ventured far afield into areas in which I am not expert. There is no better way to understand a subject than to try to explain it to others, and I hope the readers will share my enthusiasm for learning and exploring new ideas about population health.

Jeffrey House of Oxford University Press has actively supported and encouraged the development of this book and its second edition. The highly competent editorial staff (Nancy Wolitzer and Bruce Cleary for the first edition, and Lynda Crawford and Gail Cooper for the second edition) guided the book through its production process. They made the task of the author almost enjoyable. The continuing demand for this book is cause for some optimism for a broad-based multidisciplinary approach to studying population health.

Toronto   T.K.Y.

Contents

Population Health

1

Introduction

Defining Health, Population, and Population Health

This is a book about the health of populations. *Health* and *population* are fundamental concepts that need to be clearly defined. While most people seem to know when they are healthy or when they are not, there is no universal consensus on the definition of health. The World Health Organization's (WHO) definition of health—that health is *a state of complete physical, mental and social well-being, and not merely the absence of disease or infirmity*—first appeared in the preamble to its constitution, which was signed in 1946 and ratified in 1948.[1] It reflected the yearning for a world full of peace and harmony after the global catastrophes of World War II. The definition has been quoted innumerable times and is hailed for its comprehensiveness and emphasis on the broader, "positive," and psychosocial aspects of health, beyond the traditional "biomedical," "negative" aspects such as *death, disease,* and *disability.* (Together with *discomfort* and *dissatisfaction* these constitute the so-called five Ds). The European Region of WHO provided an update of the definition of health in a 1984 document on health promotion:

> [Health] is the extent to which an individual or group is able on the one hand to realize aspirations and satisfy needs, and, on the other hand, to change and cope with the environment. Health is therefore seen as a resource for everyday life, not the objective of living; it is a positive concept emphasizing social and personal resources as well as physical capacities.

There have been numerous other attempts at a definition.[2] Certain recurrent themes and key words can be found in these definitions; for example, coping with and managing stress, achieving functional capacity and structural integrity, ability to make valued contributions to the community, and maintaining equilibrium.

Writers on health issues, such as René Dubos (1901–1982) and Ivan Illich (1926–2002), have also offered their views on the matter. These are generally more forceful and less convoluted than those composed by

committees. Dubos, a distinguished microbiologist, championed the ecological view of the relationship between microbes and humans. A rarity
among scientists, he wrote several books for the general public and even
won the Pulitzer Prize in 1969. In his 1968 book *Man, Medicine and Environment*, Dubos called health

> a modus vivendi enabling imperfect men to achieve a rewarding and
> not too painful existence while they cope with an imperfect world. . . .
> Health and vigor can be achieved in the absence of modern sanitation
> and without the help of western medicine. Man has in his nature the po-
> tentiality to reach a high level of physical and mental well-being with-
> out nutritional abundance or physical comfort.[3]

Illich, a theologian by training, was a noted critic of advanced industrial societies and their social institutions, such as medicine and education. In 1975, he published his highly provocative *Medical Nemesis* in draft
form, a book that was circulated worldwide in nine languages and created
a heated debate in medical circles. In it, he described health as

> an autonomous yet culturally shaped reaction to reality. It designates
> the ability to adapt to a changing environment, to growing up and to ag-
> ing, to healing when damaged, to suffering and to the peaceful expecta-
> tion of death. Health embraces the future as well, and therefore includes
> anguish and the inner resources to live with it.[4]

The U.S. Surgeon General's landmark 1979 report on health promotion,
Healthy People, did not offer a definition of health. Yet its first sentence declared, "The health of the American people has never been better." This
and subsequent updates established detailed health goals and age-related
objectives for Americans. (Devotees of "positive health" may find the
overall tone and approach still too "disease-oriented").[5]

In 1986, the Canadian Department of National Health and Welfare published a report titled *Achieving Health for All*, in which "a new vision of
health" was proposed:

> a concept which portrays health as a part of everyday living, an essen-
> tial dimension of the quality of our lives . . . the opportunity to make
> choices and to gain satisfaction from living. Health is thus envisaged as
> a resource which gives people the ability to manage and even to change
> their surroundings. This view of health recognizes freedom of choice
> and emphasizes the role of individuals and communities in defining
> what health means to them.

While a broad and "positive" definition of health serves to orient
health professionals to think in terms of health promotion and not just the

---

BOX 1.1.   Words and Origins

That health is more than just physical health but mental/emotional as well is not a modern concept.[6] The Latin word *sanitas* (adj. *sanus*) gave rise to both "sanity/sane" and "sanitation/sanitary." The famous saying by the Roman satirist Juvenal—*mens sana in corpore sano* ("a sound mind in a sound body")—sums it up very well. There is a recent trend towards the use of the word *wellness* in place of health. This is a particular favorite of health ministry bureaucrats, as if "health" were still too disease-oriented and not "positive" enough. The English word *health* is quite old, as one can trace it back to the *hal* of the Anglo-Saxons in the eleventh century, which ultimately gave rise also to *heal, hale,* and *whole*. *Wellness*, despite its trendiness, is in fact also quite old, and can be traced back to the mid–seventeenth century. The word *sick* and its variants have been used since at least the ninth century. Although *ill* and *evil* were not related etymologically, the two have been used synonymously from the twelfth century on—no doubt in people's minds the two were related etiologically. *Disease*, or *dis-ease*, is of Anglo-French origin from the early fourteenth century.

---

treatment of disease, the rhetoric can be carried too far. The WHO definition has its critics and supporters, and indeed has been wryly observed to be "honored in repetition, rarely in application."[7] Health may become so inclusive that all human endeavors, up to and including the pursuit of happiness, are considered within its domain. Ministries of health will then become ministries of everything! In day-to-day population health practice and research, there remains a need for an "operational" definition.

In everyday usage, *population* means the number of people in a given area. This can be defined geographically or politically, as in a country, although physical boundaries are not always necessary, such as when referring to groups of people sharing common characteristics (e.g., ethnicity, religion, etc.) who are scattered throughout a particular geographical or political unit. When counting individuals and deciding on membership, distinction is sometimes made between *de facto* and *de jure* criteria, based on the premise that a person can only be at one place at any one time and should be counted only once. The former category includes individuals who are actually there at the time and place of counting, whereas the latter refers to those who usually belong to a specific locale from which they may be temporarily absent.[8] Temporary visitors such as students, diplomats, military personnel, and tourists may not be counted in the place where they happen to be, but "charged back" to where they came from.

Statisticians use population in a special sense, especially when discussing sampling. It is sometimes referred to as the *universe*, the total number of units (animal, vegetable, or mineral) from which a *sample* is drawn.

Sampling is necessary since obtaining information from all members of the population may be too cumbersome, inefficient, or not feasible. (Sampling is discussed in more detail in Chapter 6.) The characteristics of a universe or population (such as its mean and standard deviation) are referred to as *parameters*. Much of statistics is concerned with estimating population parameters from a sample.

Populations also have specific meaning for geneticists, who define them in terms of the sharing of genes. The collection of genes of all the individuals in a population is referred to its *gene pool*. *Deme* is often used to refer to small and isolated populations. Because small and non-industrialized populations have been the subject of study by anthropologists, the term *anthropological populations* is sometimes also used.

The term *population health* has been used for some time as a less cumbersome substitute for the "health of populations." In the 1990s the phrase took on a new connotation, especially in Canada and the United Kingdom. The Canadian Institute for Advanced Research established a program in population health alongside other leading-edge "hard" sciences. The Canadian Institutes of Health Research, established in 2000, include also an Institute of Population and Public Health among its 13 institutes. *Population health* can be regarded as a conceptual framework for thinking about why some people are healthier than others and the policy development, research agenda, and resource allocation that flow from this. The difference between it and terms such as *community health* and *public health*, which have been around a long time, is subtle.

In North America, *public health* usually refers to the array of programs and services organized primarily, but not exclusively, by various levels of governments to protect, promote, and restore the health of citizens. The Institute of Medicine's 1988 report on the future of public health in the United States defines the mission of public health as:

> fulfilling society's interest in assuring conditions in which people can be healthy. Its aim is to generate organized community effort to address the public interest in health by applying scientific and technical knowledge to prevent disease and promote health. The mission of public health is addressed by private organizations and individuals as well as by public agencies. But the governmental public health agency has a unique function: to see to it that vital elements are in place and that the mission is adequately addressed. The committee finds that the core functions of public health agencies at all levels of government are assessment, policy development, and assurance.

In the same year, the Acheson Report was released in England, and it also pondered the future of public health. It defined public health simply as "the science and art of preventing disease, prolonging life, and promoting health through organized efforts of society."[9]

Terms such as *social medicine* and *preventive medicine* were once popular and are still in use, but the use of medicine rather than health may be viewed by some as too "biomedical" in orientation, locating these fields within the medical profession (albeit often as poor cousins). On the other hand, social medicine is sometimes confused with *socialized* medicine, which is anathema in certain political circles. The British have now adopted the term *public health medicine* to refer to the medical specialty. While not quite an oxymoron, it certainly encompasses within the same term two very different perspectives on health.

Proponents of the concept of population health envision something more than traditional public health. Population health supposedly "increases our understanding of the determinants of health and reaffirms the need for public health professionals to examine critically social inequities and policies that maintain them."[10] In 1994 the Canadian government released a document entitled *Strategies for Population Health*, in which the population health approach is ascribed these characteristics:

1. Addresses the entire range of factors that determine health, rather than focusing on risks and clinical factors related to particular diseases;
2. Affects the entire population rather than only ill or high-risk individuals.

This approach claims to be able to provide benefits in increased prosperity, since a healthy population contributes to a vibrant economy with reduced health and social service expenditures and increased overall social stability and well-being. The term "population health" is still relatively new in the United States but is catching on, and a commentary in a 2003 issue of the *American Journal of Public Health* clarified the distinction between population health as a concept of the health status of a group of people and its distribution within the group, and as a field of study that focuses on both health outcomes and health determinants, as well as the policies and interventions that link them. "Population health" is not without its critics, especially among social scientists of the "critical" school, who consider its analytical framework as flawed in lacking a significant "class" and social structural perspective.[11]

In the United Kingdom, the 1993 Leeds Declaration proposed 10 principles for action on population health research and practice. It urged health authorities to turn away from an exclusive focus on individual risk and toward social structures and processes, and to investigate the causation of health rather than disease. In research, it urged the need for interdisciplinary approaches, integrating qualitative and quantitative methods, and recognition of the importance of lay knowledge and participatory research.[12] It is in the spirit of this new "population health" that this textbook is written.

Objectives and Uses of Population Health Studies

While one is entitled to study any subject for its own sake and for the intellectual challenge it presents, there are four practical reasons why one should engage in studying the health of populations:

1. To describe;
2. To explain;
3. To predict; and
4. To control.

This book is indeed structured around these four objectives. As a first step, one should describe the state of health of the population and identify the prevalent health problems. With a firm foundation of such knowledge, one can then seek explanations of why the state of health is what it is and why certain health problems occur. Based on the results of studies of disease patterns and their determinants, one can offer individuals and communities predictions of health effects and strategies for risk avoidance. Ultimately, knowledge from population health studies must be translated into public health policy (or better still, healthy public policy) to prevent disease and promote health.

The chapter headings of Jerry Morris's influential *Uses of Epidemiology*[13] provide a useful listing:

1. *Community diagnosis*: assessing the health status of a population;
2. *Working of health services*: evaluating health programs;
3. *Individual chances and risks*: practicing clinical preventive medicine;
4. *Completing the clinical picture*: describing the natural history of disease;
5. *In search of causes*: establishing etiology of diseases or associations with risk factors.

There are numerous examples of how our everyday life is increasingly affected by the results of population health studies. Safe sex, electromagnetic fields, pesticides, seatbelts, low-cholesterol foods, cigarette taxes—all are public issues that require some knowledge of the arts and sciences of population health. Scarcely one day goes by without the media informing us of yet another risk factor that is harmful to our health. The public demands to know the safety and health risks of specific industrial and commercial products and processes, and courts are frequently called upon to decide on liability and damages. Epidemiologists have been called in to solve serial murder cases and are indispensable in the investigation of acts of bioterrorism, such as the anthrax outbreak in the United States during 2001.[14]

The Arts and Sciences in Population Health

The core scientific discipline in the study of population health is *epidemiology*. A concern with population phenomena, however, is not unique to epidemiology. Several social sciences, notably *demography, sociology, geography, economics*, and *anthropology*, also study human populations. There are specific branches within these disciplines that have acquired the qualifier "medical" or "health," as in "medical sociology" and "health economics." Not all health phenomena are analyzed at the level of the population, though. Many medical anthropologists, for example, study the cultural aspects of healing, sickness, and medical knowledge at the individual level.[15]

Demographers are concerned with the quantitative analysis of population size, structure, and change, as well as the social, economic, and political factors that affect population trends, processes, and events.

The contribution of the social sciences in applied population health programs has long been recognized and advocated. Milton Terris (1915–2002), an ardent advocate of the important social role of epidemiology, simply stated that epidemiology is "by definition a social science." There has also been a resurgence of social epidemiology in recent years.[16] This book attempts to integrate the social and biological, the quantitative and qualitative, and recognizes the importance of social and cultural factors in assessing health and planning interventions.

The humanities—history, philosophy, ethics, art, and literature—contribute to a broader understanding of the health of populations by inculcating core human values in their practitioners, encouraging non-dogmatism, and developing critical thinking.[17]

The term *epidemiology* reflects the science's earlier preoccupation with epidemics of infectious diseases. As a result of changing disease patterns in the industrialized, developed countries, the scope and definition of epidemiology have also changed. There is, however, no reason why epidemiology should not still be regarded as the study of epidemics and their prevention, if we extend epidemics to not just those caused by microorganisms, but also drugs, diet, workplace, and environmental hazards.[18]

A current definition of epidemiology can be found in every textbook of epidemiology. The *Dictionary of Epidemiology* defines epidemiology as

> The study of the distribution and determinants of health-related states or events in specified populations, and the application of this study to control of health problems.

From this definition one can discern three components to the current understanding of what epidemiology is. There is *descriptive* epidemiology, which describes the distribution of diseases and health conditions; *analytical* epidemiology, which finds out "causes" or determinants; and experimental or interventional epidemiology, which is concerned with the prevention and control of health problems.

David Lilienfeld scoured the literature and found 23 definitions of epidemiology dating from 1927 to 1976. In response to his paper, Alfred Evans (1917–1996) tabulated the different features of these definitions and the frequencies of various key words. The word *disease* appeared in over 90% of the definitions, and the older ones tended to specify "infectious disease." Terms such as *health, physiological condition,* and *injuries* were also used. Other key words used include some sort of group, usually *population,* but also *mass* and *community.* Almost 40% mentioned *distribution,* and less frequently *spread, incidence,* and *occurrence. Etiology* and similar concepts such as *causes, determinants,* and *factors* were used in over one-third of the definitions. Only a few mentioned *natural history* or *prevention and control* at all.

Among the definitions unearthed by Lilienfeld is this amusing portrayal of an epidemiologist, vintage 1942:

> The epidemiologist is the fellow who gets to town at the peak of an epidemic and coasts to glory on the down or eastern leg of the epidemic curve. He goes around town with a sheaf of case cards in his hand and knocks on front doors, asking impertinent questions. When he has drained the community dry of what he calls pertinent information, he then goes into a huddle with a Monroe machine and comes out with a paper for the Epidemiological Society (by invitation!). When he is too old to walk from car to door, he becomes a statistical or armchair epidemiologist, or in extreme cases, a professor.[19]

Few of us know what a "Monroe machine" is, but most of us can recognize a professor when we see one!

As disease ultimately is mediated through biological processes in the human body, population health cannot be isolated from various "basic" biomedical sciences that study disease at the organismic, cellular, and molecular level (e.g., physiology, biochemistry, toxicology). The rapid advances of molecular biology in the second half of the twentieth century, culminating in the Human Genome Project, hold promise for population health. The techniques of molecular epidemiology have proven to be particularly powerful tools in such diverse areas as tracking the origin and spread of epidemics of infectious diseases and in studying genetic susceptibility to chronic diseases. Investigations into the links between the nervous, endocrine, and immune systems offer insights into the biological pathways between social environmental influences and health and disease.[20]

Because they are practical-minded, specialists in population health have not been preoccupied with issues relating to the philosophy and logic of science, although most would consider their own methods as

---

BOX 1.2.   More Words and Origins

It is worth knowing that the word epidemic comes from the Greek roots *epi*, meaning "upon," and *demos*, meaning "people," which conjures up the image of the angel of pestilence knocking on one's door. An epidemic among animals (i.e., animals other than human beings) is more correctly called *epizootic*. Nevertheless, epidemiology of diseases in animals is called *veterinary epidemiology* rather than epizoology. The term *epidemiologist* was first used in the 1860s, shortly after the formation of the London Epidemiological Society.

Variations on the theme of epidemics include *pandemic* and *endemic*. A pandemic is an epidemic that affects large swaths of land and multitudes of people, even the entire world.[21] Examples of pandemics are the Black Death in mid–fourteenth century Europe, caused by bubonic plague, which is believed to have decimated one-fourth to one-half of the population. In the twentieth century the "Spanish flu" pandemic of 1918 killed several times more people than the carnage of World War I that preceded it. A disease is endemic if it is constantly present in an area or population—it is usually when such a "baseline" or "background" level is exceeded that an epidemic is said to occur.

Demos shows up again in *demography*, a sister discipline of epidemiology, both being concerned with human populations. *Anthropology*, of course, is the study of *anthropos*, or man. The word *population* is derived from the Latin *populus*, meaning "people." It was used in French as early as the fourteenth century. In English, philosopher Francis Bacon (1561–1626) is credited with being the first to use both the terms population and depopulation.

"scientific." In epidemiological circles, the work of the philosopher Karl Popper (1902–1994) has evoked considerable debate.[22] His influential *Logic of Scientific Discovery* was originally published in German in 1934. Many scientists believe that science operates by *induction*, which in logic is a process of inferring a general law or principle from the observation of particular instances, according to the *Oxford English Dictionary*. Induction operates on the assumption that if something is true in a few observations, it will be true also in as-yet-unobserved instances, and hence true "in general." This approach can be traced back to the book *Novum Organum*, published in 1620 by philosopher Francis Bacon (1561–1626). Popper argues that science is primarily *deductive*; that is, conclusions are inferred from general premises. Observations are generally made to test a hypothesis that is already in mind, a product often of one's imagination. Knowledge advances only by disproving (or "falsifying") an existing hypothesis.

Historical Antecedents and Future Prospects

Much of current thinking in population health, as well its methods and practices, can be traced back to antiquity. Many contemporary issues have, in fact, old historical roots.[23] History is always instructive and humbling. A few examples are selected for illustration in the case studies at the back of this chapter: James Lind and scurvy, John Snow and cholera, Semmelweis and puerperal fever, and Goldberger and pellagra.

In his *Structure of Scientific Revolution*, first published in 1962 and a major modern work in the philosophy of science, Thomas Kuhn (1922–1996) describes how a scientific paradigm comes to dominate the thinking and approaches to knowledge by prescribing the work that scientists can do, the questions they can ask, and the methods they can use. Paradigms are defined as "universally recognized scientific achievements that for a time provide model problems and solutions to a community of practitioners."[24] When enough unsolved problems under a particular paradigm accumulate, increasing doubts ultimately spark a scientific revolution and the appearance and dominance of a new paradigm.

In their review of the modern development of epidemiology, Mervyn and Ezra Susser identified three major eras, each with its own paradigm.[25] The era of *sanitary statistics* began in the early nineteenth century. This is the era of the Victorian epidemiologists (more about them in Chapter 2) who avidly collected statistics on births and deaths, which allowed them to draw conclusions about disease causation. The major paradigm of that era is *miasma*, that of diseases being caused by the foul emanations from the "airs, waters, and places." This is in fact the title of a book by Hippocrates, who lived in the fourth and fifth centuries BC, an indication of the antiquity of the idea. The word *malaria*, for example, comes from *mal* (meaning "bad") and *aria* (meaning "air").

During the latter part of the nineteenth century, at the dawn of modern bacteriology, the "miasmatists" were challenged by the "contagionists," who believed that diseases were caused by tiny organisms passed from person to person. The miasma school was aligned with political radicals and social reformers of the day, including the noted German pathologist Rudolf Virchow (1821–1902). Virchow's view of the close links between society and health is reflected in his famous saying, "Politics is nothing but medicine on a grand scale."[26] The contagionists, on the other hand, were mostly political conservatives. They eventually won out, as more and more bacteria were discovered—tuberculosis, diphtheria, cholera, and a host of others. The *germ theory* became the dominant paradigm in both clinical medicine and public health during the late nineteenth and first half of the twentieth century. It led to major advances in the development and deployment of vaccines and antibiotics.

While the miasmatists-sanitarians were proven wrong, their conception of social and environmental causation is still valid, and their prescription for control—improving water and sanitation—has been responsible for the major advances in population health in the industrialized countries, and still holds the key in the developing countries today.

While correct for the infectious diseases that dominated much of the world at the time, proponents of the germ theory conceived of diseases as having single causative agents. By the second half of the twentieth century, the disease pattern, at least in the developed countries, has shifted to one dominated by the chronic, noninfectious diseases such as heart disease and cancer. As the germ theory is no longer up to the task, another paradigm shift occurred. From the 1950s onwards, there has been an explosion of knowledge about risk factors for chronic diseases, built on advances in epidemiological and biostatistical methods. The Sussers called the paradigm of the era of chronic disease epidemiology the black box. (Think of a black box as a computer or telephone: we only need to know what goes in and what goes out, and do not need to worry about how the "thing" actually works. Since we know that smoking increases the risk of lung cancer, effective action does not have to wait until all the hundreds of noxious chemicals in cigarette smoke have been isolated.)

A prime example of the contributions of this era is the Framingham Heart Study, launched in 1950 in a community near Boston, which has contributed substantially to our understanding of the causes, incidence, clinical spectrum, and prognosis of cardiovascular diseases. Indeed, it introduced the term *risk factor* into everyday vocabulary and established the significance of smoking, hypertension, plasma cholesterol, and being overweight, among others. The control of such factors has occupied a central place in the health promotion and public policy agenda during the second half of the twentieth century.[27]

While the black box approach has allowed public health action to occur without waiting for disease mechanisms to be fully elucidated, at some point it is useful to know what is inside the box; i.e., the cellular and molecular mechanisms of disease pathogenesis. The black box, indeed, also exists at the "macro" level. To say that "poverty causes disease" is helpful up to a point, but one also needs to delve inside the box to investigate and understand the complex of social interactions and political and economic forces that are at work.

There is no shortage of critics of the direction epidemiology has taken in the latter half of the twentieth century. A major theme is that modern epidemiology has overemphasized methodology and the identification of an ever-increasing number of risk factors in individuals. It lacks credibility among the "hard" scientists and bewilders the impressionable general public with its claims. A special news report in the prestigious journal *Science*, based on interviews with noted scientists in the field, was headlined "Epidemiology Faces Its Limits" and generated considerable controversy.[28]

In an introduction to a conference on the future of epidemiology, Rudolfo Saracci identified four major tensions that permeate contemporary epidemiology: between the focus on methods and substantive issues in health, between biological and social orientations, between specialization and integration, and between curiosity-driven and targeted research. The charge that epidemiology is atheoretical and merely a collection of methods is longstanding, not helped by the penchant of some methodologists to engage in "overindulgence in refinements of little practical impact."[29] The biological/social divide goes beyond the different research interests in "micro" and "macro" determinants of health, to issues of whether population health scientists should concern themselves solely with research or engage in influencing public policy and social change, especially in redressing inequities in health. Sub-specialization has occurred at a rapid pace. We now have "epidemiologies" based on diseases (e.g., cancer, cardiovascular), risk factors (e.g., occupational, genetic), and methods (e.g., molecular, spatial).

Another division within epidemiology is that between practitioners of "classical" population-based epidemiology and the newer species of "clinical" epidemiologists. While there is no doubt that clinical epidemiology has made a major impact on clinical medical practice and research, it is perceived by some to divert attention and resources from population health issues, especially prevention, to individual patient care and treatment. It is indicative of the strength of clinical epidemiology that some see the need to designate a separate term: *public health epidemiology*.[30]

The diversion of epidemiology, the basic science of public health, from a primary concern with the occurrence of disease in populations and population factors as causes of disease, needs to be stemmed and reversed. Perhaps the new "population health," by integrating research and practice, and taking advantage of the full range of tools from molecular biology to the social sciences, will ultimately achieve the aim of improving the health of populations.

Summary

This chapter introduces different definitions and usages of the terms *health, population,* and *population health*. Population health studies serve the objectives of describing the health status of a population, explaining the causes of diseases, predicting health risks in individuals and communities, and offering solutions to prevent and control health problems. To achieve these aims, population health requires collaboration between the core science of epidemiology, several social sciences that are also concerned with population phenomena, the humanities, and laboratory-based biomedical sciences. Several case studies are presented to illustrate the historical roots of many contemporary health issues.

BOX 1.3.   Public Health Achievements of the Twentieth Century and Challenges for the Twenty-first

In a series of *fin-de-siècle* reviews, the *Morbidity and Mortality Weekly Report* (MMWR), published by the Centers for Disease Control (CDC), identified ten great public health achievements in the United States during 1900–1999.[31] These are as follows, not arranged in the order of importance:

- Vaccination—the eradication of smallpox; elimination of polio in the Americas; and control of measles, rubella, tetanus, diphtheria, and *Hemophilus influenzae* type b;
- Motor-vehicle safety—reduction in motor vehicle–related deaths due to engineering improvements in vehicles and highways and change in personal behaviors (use of safety devices and reduction in drinking and driving);
- Safer workplaces—control of pneumoconiosis and silicosis; reduction in fatal occupational injuries;
- Control of infectious diseases—control of typhoid and cholera through improved water and sanitation; and of tuberculosis and sexually transmitted diseases (STDs) by antibiotics;
- Decline in deaths from coronary heart disease and stroke—from risk-factor modification (especially smoking cessation and blood pressure control) and improved access to early detection and treatment;
- Safer and healthier foods—decrease in microbial contamination and increase in nutritional content; nutritional deficiency diseases (rickets, goiter, pellagra) almost eliminated;
- Healthier mothers and babies—from better hygiene and nutrition, availability of antibiotics, access to health care, and technological advances in neonatal and maternal medicine;
- Family planning—altered socioeconomic role of women, reduced family size, increased birth intervals, and improved maternal and child health; barrier contraceptives also reduced unwanted pregnancies and transmission of STDs;
- Fluoridation of drinking water—resulted in reductions in tooth decay and tooth loss;
- Recognition of tobacco use as a health hazard—resulted in changes in social norms, reduced prevalence of smoking and mortality from smoking-related diseases.

During the same period, important changes also occurred in the public health system, which provided the infrastructure necessary for these interventions to succeed. These included advances in epidemiological methods, the systematic collection and analyses of health data at the national and regional levels, establishment of schools of public

(continued)

health and other training programs, and the involvement of both governmental and nongovernmental organizations in program planning and service delivery.

Also looking ahead, the CDC identified 10 challenges for the future:

- Institute a rational health care system;
- Eliminate health disparities;
- Focus on children's emotional and intellectual development;
- Achieve a longer "healthspan";
- Integrate physical activity and healthy eating into daily lives;
- Clean up and protect the environment;
- Prepare to respond to emerging infectious diseases;
- Recognize and address the contributions of mental health to overall well-being;
- Reduce the toll of violence in society; and
- Use new scientific knowledge and technological advances wisely.

Case Study 1.1.   James Lind and Scurvy among Sailors

Scurvy is a disease characterized by bleeding gums, sore limbs, and general debility, which may ultimately be fatal. It once devastated sailors on long sea voyages. James Lind (1716–1794), a British Navy doctor, performed a classic epidemiological study that examined both causation and intervention.[32] He selected 12 patients with similar clinical features, all having been subjected to the typical horrendous Royal Navy diet:

- Breakfast: water gruel sweetened with sugar
- Dinner: fresh mutton broth with pudding, boiled biscuits with sugar
- Supper: barley, raisins, rice, currants, sago, and wine

Lind divided his patients into 6 groups of 2, who received treatment as follows:

Group 1: A quart of cider a day;

Group 2: 25 drops of elixir vitriol (sulfuric acid, diluted!) three times a day, and gargle;

Group 3: Two spoonfuls of vinegar three times a day mixed with food, and gargle;

Group 4: Half a pint of sea water a day;

Group 5: A potion consisting of garlic, mustard seed, balsam of Peru, and purged 3 times a day;

Group 6: Two of the worst cases were given two oranges and one lemon a day, which lasted for only six days.

Group 6 recovered in dramatic fashion, compared to the other treatment groups.

This early example of an experimental study would probably not pass any present-day peer review committee ("sample size too small!" "not double-blind!") or research ethics committee ("where is the informed consent?"). Nevertheless, Lind showed that citrus fruits cured scurvy. He published his findings in 1753 in a book entitled *A Treatise of the Scurvy in Three Parts, Containing an Inquiry into the Nature, Causes and Cure of That Disease*. It took another 40 years before the Royal Navy finally adopted the policy of issuing citrus fruits on its ships and the problem of scurvy disappeared. British seamen, and by extension all Britons, have since been nicknamed "limeys."

Lesson: One can eliminate a health problem without having to know the exact cause first (an example of "black-box" epidemiology). Another lesson: Great ideas do not always get adopted right away!

Vitamin C, or ascorbic acid, is the ingredient in citrus fruits whose deficiency causes scurvy. The crystalline form of ascorbic acid was isolated in 1928 and the substance synthesized in 1933. Research into vitamin C led to the award of the Nobel Prize for medicine to the Hungarian biochemist Albert Szent-Györgyi (1893–1986) in 1937, and for chemistry to the English chemist Walter Haworth (1883–1950) in the same year.

Case Study 1.2.   John Snow, Cholera, and the Broad Street Pump

In the mid–nineteenth century, cholera devastated London and many European cities. Cholera is an infectious disease characterized by severe vomiting and diarrhea, which may result in death from dehydration. The first pandemic began in 1817 in Calcutta. The second pandemic reached Europe in the 1830s and swept through all the major cities, taking civil and medical authorities by surprise. By the twentieth century, cholera had broken out of India and circled the world six times. A seventh pandemic began in the 1960s in Asia, and spread to Europe, Africa, and finally to Latin America in the 1990s. It is still ongoing.

London experienced cholera epidemics in 1831–1832, 1848–1849 and 1854–1855. The Industrial Revolution had resulted in massive rural–urban migration. Many Londoners lived in conditions of squalor, overcrowding, and lack of sanitation. A key figure in the group of Victorian "sanitary physicians" was John Snow (1813–1858), an anesthetist by profession whose other claim to fame was administering chloroform to Queen Victoria during childbirth. Snow suspected a waterborne route of transmission from his experience with the 1849 epidemic and published a monograph entitled *On the Mode of Communication of Cholera.*[33] During the summer of 1854, he was able to test his ideas by calculating the death rates from cholera according to the source of water supply. The cholera death rate in houses supplied by one water company (the Southwark and Vauxhall Co.) that obtained its water from the Thames in central London greatly exceeded that observed in houses supplied by its competitor (the Lambeth Co.), which had earlier moved its water supply further upstream, where the river was visibly less polluted. In this analysis, Snow was assisted by William Farr of the General Register Office (more about him in Chapter 2), who provided him with the raw data.

Snow also investigated a local outbreak in St. James Parish and presented a dot-map showing a heavy clustering of cases around the water pump on Broad Street. Snow concluded that cholera was caused by a contaminated water supply. He persuaded the local authorities to remove the pump handle, although by then the outbreak had already subsided. Snow was a contagionist at a time when miasma was still the dominant theory of disease causation, and his views were not widely accepted in his lifetime. The bacteria responsible for cholera—*Vibrio cholerae*—was not discovered until 1883, by Robert Koch (1843–1910).

Snow recognized, and took advantage of, a "natural experiment" and presented his data in a statistical manner that allowed the appropriate conclusions to be drawn. While the pump has long since gone, Broad Street still stands in central London under a different name. The Broad Street pump has acquired the status of a metaphor (and even myth), and Snow is today revered as a pioneer and hero in public health.

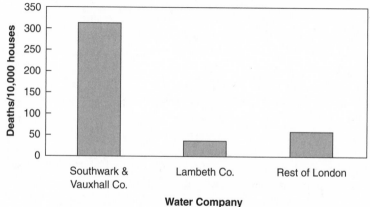

Cholera Mortality in London, 7 Weeks July–August, 1854

Case Study 1.3.   Ignaz Semmelweis and Puerperal Fever

Ignaz Semmelweis (1818–1865), a Viennese obstetrician, attempted to explain and control the devastation of childbed or puerperal fever among patients in the maternity hospital. In 1840, by imperial decree, the hospital was divided into two wards for the purpose of educating health professionals: Klinik 1 (K1 in the graph below) was reserved for medical students (all male), while Klinik 2 (K2) was used for the training of midwives (all female). Admissions to these wards alternated from day to day. On reviewing the records, Semmelweis noted that K1 had consistently higher maternal mortality (graph below) as well as neonatal mortality than K2.

Semmelweis investigated this phenomenon and made several important observations. Women whose cervix had been dilated for more than 24 hours during labor almost invariably developed fever. Such women died if they were on K1, but not on K2. The disease seemed to spread from bed to bed, but again only on K1 and not on K2. Attempts to reduce pelvic examinations by students, and barring foreign students who were believed to be "too rough," did not eliminate the discrepancy between the wards. In 1847, the professor of pathology died after his finger was pricked by a student's knife during an autopsy. What was remarkable was that the clinical features—that of overwhelming sepsis—were very similar to those of puerperal fever. This led Semmelweis to suspect that "cadaverous particles" were responsible. Medical students went directly from the autopsy room in the morning to making rounds on the wards and examining all women in labor. Midwives, on the other hand, were not privileged to learn pathology. Hand-washing was unheard of. Semmelweis instituted an intervention: all students were required to wash their hands with chlorinated lime solution. Mortality rate

Maternal Mortality

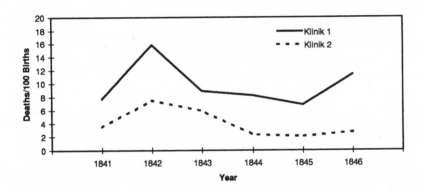

declined dramatically compared to the preintervention period, to a level even slightly below that of K2.

Semmelweis published his observations in a book in 1861, entitled *The Etiology, Concept, and Prophylaxis of Childbed Fever*.[34] Unfortunately for Semmelweis, and especially for Viennese women, his ideas were ridiculed by the medical profession. After years of unequal struggle, Semmelweis was driven mad. He died several days after having been committed to an asylum. The cause of death? A septic wound of the finger, the very disease he had striven so passionately to prevent. A sad day for medicine and public health indeed. It was not until several decades later, with the discovery of staphylococci and streptococci by Louis Pasteur (1822–1895) and the innovations in antiseptic surgery by Joseph Lister (1827–1912) that Semmelweis was vindicated.

Case Study 1.4.   Joseph Goldberger on Diet and Pellagra

Toward the end of the nineteenth century and the beginning of the twentieth century, pellagra was rampant in the southeastern United States. The disease is characterized by dermatitis, diarrhea, and dementia, the last often leading to the victim's being admitted to a mental hospital. The disease has been known in southern Europe since the eighteenth century. The word itself is of Italian origin (*pelle*, skin, and *agra*, sour). Initially pellagra was believed to be an infectious disease. In 1914, Joseph Goldberger (1874–1929), a U.S. Public Health Service medical officer, was assigned to investigate this epidemic. Over the next decade and half, Goldberger conducted a series of observational and experimental studies and concluded that pellagra was not infectious but dietary in origin.[35]

Goldberger observed that while inmates of institutions such as prisons, orphanages, and insane asylums suffered from pellagra, none of their keepers suffered from it. In an early example of social epidemiology, he conducted community surveys and noted that pellagra was primarily a disease of the rural poor. For example, the incidence of the disease in 1916 in seven South Carolina villages varied according to family income.

To prove that pellagra was not infectious, he and his friends injected themselves with, or consumed, preparations containing body fluids of pellagra patients and lived to tell the tale (thankfully it was the pre-AIDS era). He conducted diet experiments in two orphanages and showed that supplementation with milk, eggs, meat, and legumes reduced the disease. He also induced the disease among prisoners in Mississippi by restricting their diet to an unsavory mix of corn, refined carbohydrates, and not much else. (Such studies would be unethical and unthinkable today.)

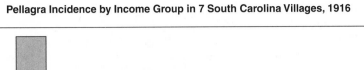

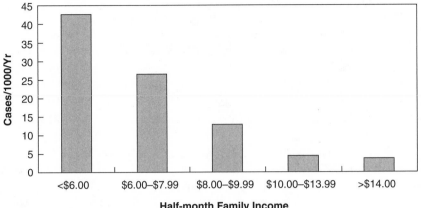

It was not until 1937 that niacin, or vitamin B₃, was identified as the active substance whose deficiency causes pellagra. Among animals, only primates and guinea pigs are unable to synthesize the substance. Supplementation of flour and cereals has all but eliminated this disease. Goldberger reputedly was nominated for the Nobel Prize five times but was never awarded it.

Guide to Resources

Comprehensive, encyclopedic textbooks of public health should be consulted and browsed;* for example, the *Oxford Textbook* (Detels et al., 2002). The *Oxford Handbook* (Pencheon et al., 2001) is a pocket-sized compendium of important tasks and skills required by public health practitioners. Epidemiology must be a growth industry, as there is no shortage of textbooks published in recent years, ranging from the introductory (Lilienfeld and Stolley, 1994), the intermediate (Kahn and Sempos, 1989; Kelsey et al., 1996), to the advanced (Selvin, 1996; Rothman and Greenland, 1998). While not intended to be a textbook, Stolley and Lasky (1995) is a thoroughly enjoyable and richly illustrated book that, when read from cover to cover, will probably give one a better understanding of what epidemiology is all about than many textbooks. There are also self-instruction manuals, such as Norell (1995) and Abramson and Abramson (2001). The *Dictionary of Epidemiology* (Last, 2001), now in its fourth edition, is indispensable. The more rigorous methodologist will want to consult the *Encyclopedia of Epidemiologic Methods* (Gail and Benichou, 2000). For those who want to go to the source, an excellent collection of original reports from classic epidemiological studies is the PAHO reader (Buck

---

*For full references, see the Bibliography.

et al., 1988). Greenland's (1987) selections trace the evolution of key concepts and methods.

For demography texts, there is the condensed edition of Shryock and Siegel (1976), which is a standard classic, and more recent ones such as Weeks (1995) and Preston et al. (2001). Substantial materials relevant to population health can be found in texts in medical sociology, such as Armstrong (1994), Cockerham (1997), and Albrecht et al. (2000); medical anthropology texts such as Helman (2000) and McElroy and Townsend (1996); and medical geography texts such as Meade and Earickson (2000).

Aficionados of Internet surfing should be interested in the following web sites that provide useful information on population health. A good starting-off point is various "virtual libraries" that provide direct links to other relevant web sites in government, academe, and industry. Examples include:

- Epidemiology (http://www.epibiostat.ucsf.edu/epidem/epidem.html) from the University of California School of Medicine at San Francisco
- Demography and population studies (http://demography.anu.edu.au/VirtualLibrary) from the Australian National University in Canberra
- Statistics (http://www.stat.ufl.edu/vlib/statistics.html) from the University of Florida at Gainesville

Useful web sites include the following:

International:
- The Global Health Network (http://www.pitt.edu/~super1)
- World Health Organization (http://www.who.int)
- Pan-American Health Organization (http://paho.org)
- International Agency for Research on Cancer (http://www.iarc.fr)

United States:
- U.S. Bureau of the Census (http://www.census.gov)
- Centers for Disease Control and Prevention (http://www.cdc.gov)
- National Center for Health Statistics (http://www.cdc.gov/nchs)
- National Institutes of Health (http://www.nih.gov)
- National Library of Medicine (http://www.nlm.nih.gov)
- U.S. Environmental Protection Agency (http://www.epa.gov)
- Office of the Surgeon General (http://www.surgeongeneral.gov)
- Institute of Medicine (http://www.iom.edu)
- American Public Health Association (http://www.apha.org)

Canada:
- Statistics Canada (http://www.statcan.ca)
- Health Canada (http://www.hc-sc.gc.ca)
- Canadian Public Health Association (http://www.cpha.ca)

Notes

1. While it is quoted by many, few people have read the original Constitution of the WHO. The definition and relevant historical documents can be found on the WHO web site: www.who.int/about/definition/en.

2. See the entry "Health" in the International Epidemiological Association's *Dictionary of Epidemiology* (Last, 2001:81).

3. This particular quotation is from *Man, Medicine and Environment* (Dubos, 1968:69). His other books include *Mirage of Health* (1959), *Man Adapting* (1965), and *So Human an Animal* (1968).

4. The quotation is from Illich (1975:167). Illich founded the Center for Intercultural Documentation (CIDOC) in Cuernavaca, Mexico, which lasted from 1961–1976. Among his other books are *Deschooling Society* (1970), *Tools for Conviviality* (1973), and *Energy and Equity* (1974). A definitive version of *Medical Nemesis* was published in 1976 under the title *Limits to Medicine*.

5. The latest version is *Healthy People 2010*, available at www.health.gov/healthypeople. It also provides links to other documents such as the *Final Review of Healthy People 2000*, a rich compendium of U.S. health statistics.

6. I am indebted to the weekly column "Word Play" by Robertson Cochrane of the Toronto *Globe and Mail*: "Is 'Health' Unwell?" (11 Feb. 1995); and "A Healthy Choice of Synonyms" (18 Feb. 1995).

7. The quotation is from Evans and Stoddart (1990:1347). Hanslukwa (1985) provided a sampling of various views on the WHO definition expressed by researchers and expert committees. Breslow (1972) defended the WHO definition and quantified it in a health survey in California.

8. The Romans seemed to merge the de jure and de facto methods. It was written in the Gospel According to St. Luke (Chapter II) that Caesar Augustus decreed that all his subjects return to their place of origin to be counted in order to be taxed. Hence Joseph and Mary traveled back to Bethlehem, where the inns were all full, and the rest we know.

9. See Institute of Medicine (1988:7). The definition provided by the Acheson Report can be found in the *Dictionary of Epidemiology* (Last, 2001:145).

10. The quotation is from Frank (1995), who defended the need for such a term. The phrase "population health" appears in the title of several books, such as Dean (1993), Kindig (1997), Kawachi et al. (1999), Green and Ottoson (1999), Tarlov and St. Peter (2000), and Weinstein et al. (2002).

11. See the commentary by Kindig and Stoddart (2003). For a critical social science perspective, see Poland et al. (1998) and Coburn et al. (2003). Among the criticisms is the absence of any mention of capitalism as a root cause of ill health.

12. The Leeds Declaration originated from a conference organized by the Nuffield Institute of Health in Leeds in 1993. An editorial in *Lancet* (19 Feb. 1994) promotes it to a wider audience. "Upstream" refers to the story of the hero who saves one drowning man after another from the river, but never discovers that someone upstream is pushing people into the water!

13. Morris and *Uses of Epidemiology* have had a profound impact on the disciplines of epidemiology and public health. The book was first published in 1957, with new editions in 1964 and 1975. For a celebratory essay on the author, his prescience, and the current relevance of his book, see Davey Smith (2001).

14. See, for example, Lilienfeld and Black (1986) on the epidemiologist in court. The Centers for Disease Control was called in to investigate a series of unexplained deaths at the Toronto Hospital for Sick Children in the 1980s, using the approach and technique of a disease outbreak investigation (Buehler et al., 1985). This study is included as a case study in Exercise 5.2. To date, the case remains unsolved—in the criminal justice sense, if not in the epidemiological sense. During the months of October and November 2001, a total of 22 cases of anthrax—an infection by the bacteria *Bacillus anthracis*—were identified in seven states and the District of Columbia. For an account of the anthrax outbreak, see Jernigan et al. (2002) and Exercise 3.5. The UCLA School of Public Health web site contains a wealth of information on bioterrorism: www.ph.ucla.edu/epi/bioter/bioterroism.html.

15. Hahn (1995), a CDC epidemiologist, provided an anthropological perspective on sickness and healing. The impact of cultural concepts of health and disease on the assessment of population health status is discussed in more detail in Chapter 3.

16. See Terris (1985). For a comprehensive review of the "re-engagement" of epidemiology and social science, see Krieger (2000). The resurgence of "social epidemiology" as a branch of epidemiology is attested to by the appearance of books such as Marmot and Wilkinson (1999), Berkman and Kawachi (2000), and others in recent years. Works by Janes et al. (1986), Swedlund and Armelagos (1990), and Hahn (1999) demonstrate the increasing confluence of anthropology and epidemiology. Elsewhere I have used the term *biocultural epidemiology* to emphasize the need for an integrated approach to the study of population health (see Young, 1994), a view shared by McElroy (1990). Inhorn (1995) noted that studies demonstrating true collaboration and integration between epidemiology and anthropology were rare and pointed out several stereotypes that anthropologists had of epidemiology.

17. See Weed (1995) and editorial comments by Oppenheimer (1995).

18. See Kuller (1991). By concentrating on the study of epidemics—broadly defined—the drifting away of epidemiology from its roots in public health may perhaps be corrected.

19. See Lilienfeld (1978). Evans's addendum appeared as a letter to the editor of the *American Journal of Epidemiology* (1979; 109:379–82). The caricature of the epidemiologist is quoted from an unnamed editorial in the *American Journal of Public Health* (1942; 32:868–69).

20. See Hunter (1999) and the text by Carrington and Hoelzel (2001) on some of the uses of molecular epidemiology. The confluence of interests in the brain, behavior, and hormones can be seen in the title of the journal *Psychoneuroendocrinology*.

21. For an account of the major epidemics in history, see Karlen (1995). Lilienfeld (1979) discussed the development of epidemiology in nineteenth-century England. Bacon spoke of "depopulation of towns and homes of husbandry" (cited in Thomlinson, 1976:5).

22. The Austrian Popper spent the war years in New Zealand and moved to England after World War II, where he was eventually knighted. The German title of his book is *Die Logik der Forschung*. Buck (1975) first introduced Popper in the pages of the *International Journal of Epidemiology*, and the debate has continued ever since:

see, for example, Jacobsen (1976), Maclure (1985), Pearce and Crawford-Brown (1989), Karhausen (1995), and Greenland (1998), and the considerable volume of letters to the editor that they generated. Susser (1986) concluded that there was a need for both induction/deduction and verification/falsification in research and practice. Weed (1986) provided a good general introduction to the logic of science and its relevance to epidemiology. For the scientifically trained, but philosophically challenged, an excellent primer to the philosophy of science is Ladyman (2002).

23. A few histories of public health, as distinct from histories of medicine, do exist; for example, the classic by George Rosen, originally published in 1958 and reprinted in 1993. The book of readings published by the Pan American Health Organization (PAHO) (Buck et al., 1988) provides excerpts from the original reports of many historically significant studies.

24. This quotation is from the preface to the third edition (1996). For an application of Kuhn's ideas to an analysis of epidemiology textbooks, see Bhopal (1999).

25. See Susser and Susser (1996) and the accompanying editorial in the *American Journal of Public Health* (1996; 86:621–22).

26. Rosen (1947) provides the English translation.

27. See Kannel (1995). The Framingham Study has generated numerous research papers. For more background, see the monograph by Dawber (1980).

28. See Taubes (1995), and other critiques by Skrabanek (1992), Pearce (1996), and Krieger (1999). Several of the epidemiologists interviewed by Taubes responded in a letter to correct the impression that "evidence based on epidemiology is not usually credible" (*Science* 1995; 269:1325–28).

29. See Saracci (1999). The views of those against broadening the role of the epidemiologist can be sampled from Rothman et al. (1998), and Savitz et al. (1999).

30. Last (1988) considered the term clinical epidemiology itself an oxymoron, and its effect on health detrimental. Naylor et al. (1990), in response, emphasized the complementarity of the two approaches and urged collaboration. Mackenbach (1995) suggested qualifying epidemiology as "public health epidemiology."

31. For the achievements, see MMWR 1999; 48:241–43; 243–48; 369–74; 461–69; 621–29; 649–56; 849–57; 905–13; 933–40; 986–93; 1073–80; and 1141–47. Koplan and Fleming (2000) discussed the challenges.

32. Excerpts of Lind's book can be found in the PAHO reader (Buck et al., 1988:20–23). Lind was credited with other naval and novel practices such as delousing sailors, the design of hospital ships, and the distillation of sea water.

33. Snow's *Report on the Cholera of 1849* and the second (1855) edition of *On the Mode of Communication of Cholera* were reprinted as *Snow on Cholera: Being a Reprint of Two Papers* in the United States by the Commonwealth Fund in 1936. The editor was Wade Hampton Frost (1880–1938), the first professor of epidemiology at the Johns Hopkins School of Public Health, who was responsible for rescuing Snow from relative obscurity and initiated the tradition of teaching Snow in introductory courses of epidemiology. Excerpts of Snow's writings can be found in the PAHO reader (Buck et al., 1988:42–45; 415–18). For an analysis of the historical context of Snow and other "sanitary physicians" of his era, see Lilienfeld (1979). Ralph Frerichs created a comprehensive web site devoted to the life and work of John Snow, including relevant historical documents, www.ph.ucla.edu/epi/snow.html. Vandenbroucke et al. (1991) traced the revival of Snow to Frost. McLeod (2000) examined the various versions of Snow's map and sets the record straight for much of the myth that has sprung up around the Broad Street pump. A new biography of

Snow was produced by Vinten-Johansen et al. (2003). For an up-to-date report of the current global cholera pandemic, check the WHO web site: www.who.int/ health-topics/cholera.html.

34. An excerpt of Semmelweis's book can be found in the PAHO reader (Buck et al., 1988:46–59). See Rosen (1993:293–94) for an account of his last days. Nuland (2003) provides a biography for the general readers.

35. Goldberger published a series of papers in *Public Health Reports*, the official journal of the U.S. Public Health Service. Three of these, published in 1914, 1920, and 1923 are reprinted in the PAHO reader (Buck et al., 1988:99–102, 584–609, 726–30). Additional background information can be found in Stolley and Lasky (1995:45–49). Roe (1973) has written a social history of pellagra, dubbed "a plague of corn."

2

Measuring Health and Disease in Populations (I)

Measures of Disease Occurrence

The two basic measures of disease occurrence in populations are *incidence* and *prevalence*. They are generally discussed in textbooks of epidemiology within the first two chapters, although the depth of discussion varies considerably. The two are often confused in everyday usage, in the media, and in clinical circles.

Incidence is the rate at which new events occur in a population in a defined time period. The numerator is composed of a count of the events of interest. "Events" may be new episodes of disease or the number of people becoming sick; "mortality rate" is a special kind of incidence where the event is death. The key concept is a *change* in status, from healthy to sick, from alive to dead, over a period of time.

The denominator is the population "at risk" for the event. Ideally, it should consist only of people who do not already have the disease and of those among whom it is possible for the disease to develop (e.g., women who have had hysterectomies are not "at risk" for cancer of the cervix).

There are two kinds of incidence: *cumulative incidence* and *incidence density*. The cumulative incidence is the *proportion* of an initially disease-free group of individuals who develop the disease within a specified period of observation. An example is the so-called *attack rate* used in epidemic investigations. For example, if 100 people attended a wedding reception and 20 of them came down with diarrhea within 24 hours, this is referred to as an attack rate of 20%. According to the definitions in Box 2.1, the correct term should be *attack proportion* rather than *rate*.

It is important to specify the period of observation. The cumulative incidence of death in a cohort of newborn infants is 100% if the period is, say, 130 years—in the long run, we are all dead! Comparing one cumulative incidence with another using a different period of observation is therefore meaningless.

BOX 2.1.   Ratios, Proportions, and Rates

Several basic mathematical terms need to be clarified. These are *rates, ratios,* and *proportions.*[1] They are often used interchangeably. While this practice is acceptable and common even among experts, it is important to note their differences. Indeed, as this chapter proceeds, instances where the distinctions are ignored will surface. It is the intention of this book at least to try to get it straight at the outset.

A *ratio* is simply one number divided by another (x/y or x : y). It is dimensionless; i.e., it has no units. An example is the sex ratio. Note that x and y may be totally unrelated, as in apples and oranges. When x is part of y, the ratio x/y becomes a *proportion* (or *fraction*), a special kind of ratio. Example: the proportion of women among patients in a hospital. Note that a *percentage* is a proportion where the denominator is set at 100. A proportion is dimensionless and it cannot exceed 1 (or 100%). (It is irksome to hear of "percentage points" as if they were units.)

A *rate* is a ratio that measures change in one quantity per unit change of another quantity (usually time). Examples: speed in kilometers/hour (change in distance covered per hour of time). There is no upper limit to a rate, at least theoretically! Rates may be *instantaneous,* denoting a concept of potential for change in status at an instant; or *average,* when measured over an interval of time. (A formal explanation of rates requires an understanding of the mathematical concept of *limits*).

Strictly speaking, the number of new cases of disease in an area per year qualifies as a rate, but such information is of little use since the size of the population from which the cases arise is not specified. In population health studies, rates are usually expressed *relative* to the size of the population per unit of time.

In Chapter 5 the reader will be introduced to a related group of terms—*risk, hazard,* and *odds.*

Cumulative incidence is best used in a *closed* population or cohort, where there are no new additions and people exit from it by dying. Ours being a free country, study subjects can leave a study or region as they please. The term *censoring* is used to refer to stopping the observation at the end of the study, when someone leaves the cohort and becomes lost to followup, or when someone dies from a condition other than the outcome being studied (i.e., a competing cause). One can never be certain if the event of interest occurs or not after the censoring.

If the loss to observation becomes substantial, the cumulative incidence becomes less and less accurate. For such losses and other censored observations, one can apply a correction factor to the cumulative incidence by subtracting half of the number of these losses from the denominator, based on the assumption that the censoring occurred uniformly throughout the period and such individuals were at risk for only half of the period.

Instead of using the number of people at the start of the observation period as the denominator, one could determine for each person the actual time period of risk, from the beginning of the period to the time the disease is detected, or in the case of a person who does not become sick at all, to the end of the period of observation. The total *person-time* becomes the denominator, and this type of incidence is called *incidence density*, which is a true *rate*. Note that the assumption is that 100 persons each followed for one year is the same as 10 persons each followed for 10 years (100 person-years in both cases).

Incidence density is sometimes also called simply *incidence rate*. Other terms include *force of morbidity*. It is best suited for *open* or *dynamic* populations or cohorts, where people come and go. In fact, not everyone needs to start at the same time, and individuals can join the study partly into the observation period, as long as their actual person-time at risk is recorded.

When incidence density (ID) is low and the time period (t) short, the relationship between cumulative incidence (CI) and ID is:

$$CI = ID \times t$$

In public health, one usually deals with large populations such as a city, state/province, or country where it is not feasible to establish a disease-free group to be followed in time or calculate the person-time of observation for each person. While the numerator is still the same, the denominator is usually approximated by the midyear population of the jurisdiction as determined by the census. This is the average population at risk and the assumption is that everybody has been observed for the same time period.

Prevalence differs from *incidence* in that it refers to "status" rather than "change." The numerator is the count of "existing" cases rather than "new" cases. Incidence is about *becoming*, whereas prevalence is about *being* something or *having* something. (Think of prevalence as one's bank balance and incidence the monthly income—the two are certainly different!) Prevalence and incidence represent different concepts of disease occurrence, and have different definitions, units, and ranges of possible values (Table 2.1).

Prevalence refers to the proportion of people who possess a certain attribute either at a certain *point* in time or within a specific time *period*. The period may be the past 12 months or a person's lifetime experience. A "point" in geometry has no physical existence. Thus, even a nanosecond, short though it may be, cannot be considered a "point in time." In practice, and population health is very practical, point prevalence often refers to counts of events or cases in a day (census day, day of survey, or perhaps

Table 2.1. Measures of Disease Frequency

	Incidence		Prevalence	
	Cumulative incidence	Incidence density	Point prevalence	Period prevalence
Synonym	Incidence proportion	Incidence rate, person-time incidence	—	—
Numerator	New cases	New cases	Existing cases	Existing cases
Denominator	Number of individuals at start of period	Sum of individual person-times at risk	Number of individuals at point of observation	Number of individuals at mid-period of observation
Unit	Dimensionless	Per unit of person-time	Dimensionless	Dimensionless
Type of Ratio	Proportion	Rate	Proportion	Proportion

judgment day!). When the type of prevalence is not specified, point prevalence is usually implied.

Note that "a point in time" refers to a fixed point in the experience of an individual. For a group of individuals, a "point" can refer to a specific date that is identical for many people taking part in a survey or a census, or it could be at the point of birth, death, hospital discharge, etc., which may be different for different people in a group being studied and thus staggered over a period of time. Thus the statement "x percent of autopsies show evidence of cancer" refers to prevalence, not incidence, since it refers to the proportion of dead bodies with signs of cancer at the point of death, even though the actual dates of death are not all the same.[2] Similarly, the statement "x in 10,000 infants are born with congenital cleft palate" is also a prevalence, not an incidence, since it refers to the presence of a congenital anomaly at the point of birth.[3] One can speak of birth defects incidence if one can measure the rate of development of defects among all embryos over the period of gestation. This is never known, as many women conceive and abort spontaneously without being aware of it. One can also speak of incidence if one is referring to the rate of new cases of birth defects being added to a population in a year, in which case the denominator should not be per 1,000 live births, but per 1,000 population per year. As long as birth defects are measured in terms of proportion of live births having the characteristic, it is a prevalence.

Prevalence is sometimes referred to as prevalence "rate." Strictly speaking this is incorrect. Prevalence is a proportion (i.e., the numerator is part of the denominator). It does not involve change in disease quantity per unit change in time. But long usage makes it hard for people to stop calling it a rate. The denominator of point prevalence is the actual population at that "point" (e.g., census day); for period prevalence, it is the "average" population during that period, usually taken to be the mid-period population.[4]

Another commonly used indicator is the *case-fatality ratio*. This refers to the proportion of sick people who die of the disease and is thus a measure of the severity of the disease. It is a proportion, but is often incorrectly called a rate.

There is a mathematical relationship between incidence (I) and prevalence (P), expressed as:

$$P/(1-P) = I \times D$$

where D is the average duration of the disease, which is influenced by the success of treatment and mortality.[5] In a stable situation and when P is low (and thus $1-P$ is almost equal to 1), the relationship approximates to

$$P = I \times D$$

BOX 2.2.   Guns and Crime, Incidence or Prevalence?

In a study comparing homicide and guns on both sides of the United States–Canada border, the following statistics were obtained.[6] Decide if the measure is incidence or prevalence.

- There were 5 privately owned handguns per 100 households in the Prairie provinces of Canada, compared to 36 per 100 households in the Prairie states.
- There were 243 privately owned rifles per 1,000 population in British Columbia, compared to 262 per 1,000 population in Washington State.
- There were 0.2 criminal homicides committed with handguns per 100,000 population per year in Ontario, compared to 4.8 per 100,000 in New York State.
- There were 179 aggravated assaults per 100,000 population per year in Manitoba, compared to 42 per 100,000 population in North Dakota.
- There were 2.2 handgun homicides per 10,000 handguns per year in Canada, compared to 2.5 handgun homicides per 10,000 handguns in the United States.

The answers can be found on p. 59 of this text, note 6.

This example shows that the concept of incidence and prevalence can be applied to areas other than health. It also illustrates the importance of the choice of denominator in quantifying the frequency of occurrence of events and attributes. It further shows how statistics can be used to bolster one's argument for or against a particular viewpoint; in this case, the causal relationship between guns and violence, a hotly debated political subject in many countries.

To use an analogy: how much water is in the bathtub at any one moment depends on how much water is being added when the tap is open (incidence) and how much water is being drained out (mortality and cure). Medical treatment that improves a patient's survival but does not offer a cure (e.g., insulin for diabetes) actually increases the prevalence of the disease in a population. Increased detection through screening also increases the prevalence. A vaccine that prevents the occurrence of a disease, on the other hand, reduces the incidence and eventually also the prevalence.

Both incidence and prevalence, and indeed any rate and proportion, can be expressed as x per 100 (i.e., percent), per 1,000, per 10,000, and so on. The choice of the multiplier is entirely arbitrary and has to do with one's "comfort level" with decimals. Many people consider 5% a nice figure but feel uncomfortable with 0.05%, and tend to prefer 5 per 10,000 instead. The rarer the disease, the larger the multiplier tends to be.

While both *incidence* and *prevalence* are used in measuring disease frequency, incidence is more useful in studies of causation, while prevalence is useful for health planning purposes (as a measure of "caseload"). Because of the relationship between P and I, P is often used as a proxy for disease risk.

Population Structure and Dynamics

To describe and understand the pattern of health and disease in a population, knowledge of the size, composition, and growth of the population itself is required. It will furnish the raw data for the computation and estimation of various rates and proportions of epidemiological interest. It also allows the identification of "vulnerable" subgroups in terms of burden of illness, such as the elderly, the young, and women in their reproductive period.

The chief source of data on the various characteristics of a population is the *census*, which in most developed countries is conducted at regular 5- (as in Canada) or 10-year (as in the United States) intervals. Other countries conduct them irregularly, while many developing countries have never had a census. Note that even in developed countries there are still significant problems of under-enumeration, particularly among certain ethnic and socioeconomic groups in the population. The homeless and illegal immigrants have often been "missed" by the census.

The census has become the source of all types of information that is required by governments, businesses, and individuals for a variety of reasons. There is not much direct "health" information, although sometimes questions on disability are added. Many determinants of health (see Chapter 4), however, are available from the census—age, sex, marital status, income, employment, ethnicity, etc. In both the United States and Canada, the census requires all individuals to fill out a "short form" consisting of a small number of questions primarily related to basic demographic information such as age and sex. A "long form" consisting of questions on socioeconomic and housing conditions is administered to a representative sample of respondents, from which national estimates can be derived.

Census information has many uses, but also misuses. Information on the ethnic and religious composition of regions within a country has often been exploited to perpetrate civil wars, ethnic cleansing and genocide, copious examples of which occurred during the twentieth century.

Some countries, notably the Scandinavian countries, maintain central *population registries* which are continuously updated and allow a more accurate determination of the size of the population than interpolations and adjustments of periodic census data. In Canadian provinces, universal health insurance administrations also maintain registries of beneficiaries, which, for practical purposes, cover the entire population.

Conducting censuses regularly and maintaining a population registry are beyond the financial and technical means of most developing countries, and population characteristics can only be determined by special demographic surveys, often conducted under the auspices of international development agencies. Such surveys may ask essentially the same questions that are usually found in a census. Sometimes they are retrospective and collect information on the reproductive history of individuals and families. One should be cautious when perusing United Nations and WHO publications that provide annual "updated" demographic data—the fine print will often indicate that the estimates may have been interpolated and/or extrapolated from surveys and censuses conducted many years ago.

The key events and phenomena that affect the size, structure and growth of populations are deaths (*mortality*), births (*fertility*), marriages (*nuptiality*) and *migration* (both *im*migration and *e*migration). The first three are referred to as *vital* events, meaning "related to life." Most national and subnational jurisdictions in the developed countries have special agencies (not necessarily part of the health care system) that are responsible for the registration and maintenance of *vital statistics*. There are usually legal requirements for obligatory notification of vital events. In less developed countries, such systems often do not exist or are poorly developed.

In the United States the National Center for Health Statistics (NCHS) operates the National Vital Statistics System. Since 1985 all states and the District of Columbia have transmitted computer tapes of their entire birth and death data files to NCHS. In Canada, Statistics Canada is the national agency responsible for collecting and publishing data from all provinces and territories.

The *age-sex structure* of a population is best represented graphically by a *population pyramid*. Conventions require that men stay on the left and women on the right, babies at the bottom, and the elderly on top. As the population "ages" (i.e., the proportion of the elderly increases), the shape of the pyramid changes. Many developing countries still have relatively "wide-based" pyramids typical of the population of the developed countries during the nineteenth century and before (Figure 2.1).[7] As much as half of the population may be under 15 years of age. Detailed examination of a population pyramid can reveal much about the demographic history of a population, where "bulges" and "pinched waists" can be correlated with "baby booms," wars, famines, and economic depressions. The age-sex structure of a population has important implications for the planning of health care, social services, and economic development.

The age structure of a population is affected primarily by fertility. A decline in fertility will narrow the base of the pyramid, and over many years work its way through to affect older ages. Decreasing infant mortality has the opposite effect, by expanding the base. A change in adult mortality has a less dramatic effect, as it is spread over all adult years. Migration tends to affect specific age-sex groups selectively. The large number of

BOX 2.3. Historical Notes

Governments have been conducting some form of census-taking from the days of the ancient civilizations, initially to facilitate taxation and conscription. In the Old Testament Book of Numbers (I, 1-2), Moses was told by God in the Sinai wilderness to take a census of all men age 20 and above. In the Middle Ages, the Domesday Book of 1086 in England was a massive land-use and population survey that has survived and provides a wealth of information for the social historian. (Although sometimes also spelled *Doomsday*, it has nothing to do with doom; the *domes* in *Domesday* refer to houses). The first modern nationwide census in the United States was conducted in 1790, followed by Great Britain and France in the early nineteenth century. The first census in Canada after confederation was held in 1871.

The keeping of vital statistics has a long history in the Western world, dating back to the "Bills of Mortality" in the seventeenth century in London. John Graunt (1620–1674), a haberdasher with a statistical bent, analyzed these Bills and published in 1622 a book entitled *Natural and Political Observations Made upon the Bills of Mortality*, on the strength of which he was admitted a Fellow of the recently founded Royal Society, composed of leading British scientists of the day.[8] Some of the seventeenth-century disease categories include: "falling sickness," "dead in the street," "lunatique," "overlaid and starved," "excessive drinking," and "grief." Data collection was in the hands of elderly women "searchers" who kept track of burials and other happenings in the parish. While there were deficiencies in the quality of the data, Graunt nevertheless made use of what was available and drew important conclusions regarding the incidence of conditions such as plague and murders and, indirectly, the demographic trends and social conditions of his day. Graunt's statistical analyses were known at the time as *political arithmetic*.

Graunt described how the Bills were compiled (note the spelling has not been modernized):

When anyone dies, then, either by tolling, or by ringing of a Bell, or by bespeaking of a Grave of the Sexton, the same is known to the Searchers . . . The Searchers hereupon (who are antient Matrons, sworn to their office) repair to the place, where the dead Corps lies, and by view of the same, and by other enquiries, they examine by what Disease, or Casualty the corps died. Hereupon they make their Report to the Parish-Clerk, and he, every Tuesday night, carries in an Accompt of all the Burials, and Christnings, hapning that Week, to the Clerk of the Hall. On Wednesday the general Accompt is made up, and Printed, and on Thursdays

(continued)

published and dispersed to the several Families, who will pay four shillings per Annum for them.

One must marvel at how up-to-date these bills were and the speed with which they were compiled and distributed more than 350 years ago.

Graunt's assessment of the searchers was most uncharitable: "The Old-women Searchers after the mist of a cup of Ale, and the bribe of a two-groat fee . . . given them, cannot tell whether this emaciation, or leanness were from a Phthisis, or from an Hectic Fever, Atrophy, &c or from an Infection of the Spermatick parts."

Another milestone was the appointment of William Farr (1807–1883), a physician, to the newly established General Register Office in 1839, where he eventually became superintendent. Farr compiled statistical data on births and deaths, and his annual reports provided a wealth of information. He pioneered such concepts as incidence, prevalence, and person-years, and developed a system of disease classification. He assisted and collaborated with other Victorian "epidemiologists" such as John Snow, whose acquaintance we have made in Chapter 1, and nursing pioneer Florence Nightingale (1820–1910). In 1885, a memorial volume of his selected writings was published under the title *Vital Statistics*.

It is not well known that Nightingale was also a pioneer in the use of statistics to assess health status, evaluate health care, and reform medical institutions—in her case, the British Army. In her *Notes on Matters Affecting the Health, Efficiency and Hospital Administration of the British Army*, published in 1858, she demonstrated with ample charts that deaths from infectious diseases among soldiers outnumbered deaths in combat, and that the mortality rate of soldiers in peacetime exceeded that of civilians.

male migrant workers in many developing countries affects the age-sex structure of both the "donor" and "recipient" countries.

The *sex ratio* is usually expressed as the number of males per 100 females. The ratio is slightly less than 100 (females predominate) in most developed countries, and the reverse in most developing countries. The ratio changes throughout life. At birth, males predominate (usually around 105), but as age increases, the sex ratio declines, as male mortality is consistently higher than the female one. Beyond age 45, the proportion of women in the U.S. population overtakes that of men (see Exercise 2.1 for data from the 2000 U.S. Census). The sex ratio can be affected by cultural traditions that favor boys over girls, the most extreme form of which is female infanticide. The availability of prenatal sex determination by ultrasound, often followed by selective abortion of female fetuses, will further exacerbate the relative female deficit.

The ratio of the number (or proportion) of young and elderly people in a population to all people in the other ages is referred to as the *total*

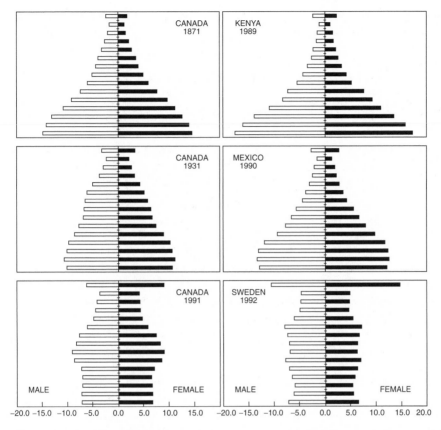

Figure 2.1. Historical change in age-sex structure of the Canadian population and selected age-sex pyramids of several contemporary populations.

dependency ratio. It can be further divided into the *youth dependency ratio* (referring usually to those under 15, or under 18, or under 20) and the *aged dependency ratio* (usually referring to those 65 and older). It supposedly indicates the extent to which the "working" population supports the "non-working" (hence economically dependent) population, an assumption that is not always valid. For example, many seniors continue to work beyond retirement age, or engage in volunteer, unpaid work; on the other hand, many people in the working ages are not gainfully employed. One can conceive of society as being composed of interdependent segments, or alternatively as one in which the generations are in conflict, where the elderly are considered to be a drain on the rest of the population.[9] Thus a simple measure such as the dependency ratio may appear to be neutral, but how it is used often is not.

Several indicators are used to measure the fertility of a population, a major reason for population growth. Commonly used and easily available from existing data is the *crude birth rate* (CBR), which is simply the number of births per 1,000 population per year. The denominator, however, refers to the total population, including men and boys, young girls and old women. The *general fertility rate* (GFR) is more accurate as it restricts inclusion in its denominator only to women in the reproductive age range (generally taken to be 15–44 or 15–49). The number of children born to women in a specific age group constitutes the *age-specific fertility rate* (ASFR; see Figure 2.2). The *total fertility rate* (TFR) is computed by summing all age-specific fertility rates for women in the childbearing ages. It is a hypothetical rate, and can be interpreted as the number of children that would be born to a group of woman who experience each of the ASFRs of a population in a given year as they progress through their reproductive lives (Box 2.4). The disadvantage of the GFR and TFR is that they require more data than the CBR.

A TFR of 2.0 is considered the *replacement* level for the population, since basically a couple will need two children to replace themselves. (When childhood mortality is taken into account, a population will need a TFR of 2.1 or 2.2 to replace itself.) A population at replacement level will eventually stop growing (if there is no immigration). It is clear that many developed countries are now at the stage of zero population growth.

The concept of fertility can be further refined, by only considering daughters being born to women. The *gross reproduction rate* is computed similarly to the TFR, but uses a set of female age-specific fertility rates (where both numerator and denominator are female). But not all daughters survive to reproductive age. By multiplying each ASFR by the probability of surviving from birth to that age (which requires a life table), the *net reproduction rate* (NPR) can be derived. As far as the population is concerned, only the matrilineal matters!

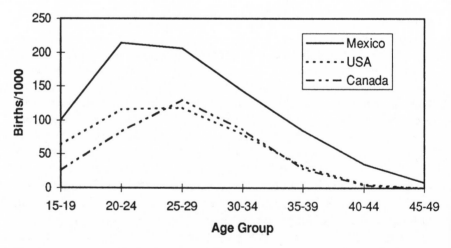

Figure 2.2. Age-specific birth rate among women in Canada, the United States, and Mexico.

BOX 2.4.   Computing the Total Fertility Rate (TFR)

To demonstrate how the TFR is derived, the ASFRs of women in five-year age groups can be used.[10] For the United States, the rates in 2000 (all races combined) were:

    15–19:   48.5/1,000
    20–24:   112.3/1,000
    25–29:   121.4/1,000
    30–34:   94.1/1,000
    35–39:   40.4/1,000
    40–44:   7.9/1,000
    45–49:   0.5/1,000

The sum of these rates is 425/1,000. Since the rate for each five-year age group is in fact the average of the rates for five single years of age, to obtain the sum of all single-year rates for ages 15 to 49, one needs to multiply 425 by 5, which equals 2,125. (It goes without saying that, if actual single-year ASFRs are used, there is no need to multiply by 5). Note that whether the 10–15 and 50–54 age groups (among whom births do occur, albeit rarely) are included, or the 45–49 group is omitted, does not make much difference.

The TFR for American women in the early 1990s was therefore 2,125/1,000, or 2.1/woman. In other words, the average woman in the United States produces about 2.1 babies in her lifetime, which is typical of most developed countries. Canada's TFR is lower, at 1.7. Compare this to rates as high as 7.5 in some sub-Saharan African countries. Note that the TFR is an age-adjusted measure and can be directly compared between populations with different age structures, whereas the CBR is not, and the GFR only partially so, as substantial variation can still occur within the relatively large age group of 15–44 or 15–49.

Fertility should be distinguished from *fecundity*. The former refers to the actual reproductive performance of a population, whereas the latter is the biological potential for childbearing, unhindered by the various biomedical and sociocultural means that human beings use to prevent conception and birth.[11]

Fertility rates vary between ethnic groups and socioeconomic classes in most populations. Many factors can influence the fertility level of a population. There are factors affecting exposure to intercourse, both within and outside marriage (e.g., age of entry into sexual union, coital frequency, duration of abstinence); factors affecting exposure to conception (e.g., diseases causing infecundity, contraception, sterilization); and factors affecting gestation and successful parturition (e.g., fetal mortality, induced abortion).

At the most basic level, mortality can be measured as the total number of deaths per 1,000 population per year, the *crude death rate* (CDR). This can be refined by breaking it down into specific causes and specific age, sex, and other demographic groups. The crude death rate tends to be highest in the least-developed countries, where they may be as high as 20/1,000/year, compared to around 10 in most Western, industrialized countries. At that level, however, the ability of the CDR to discriminate population health status is limited. Mexico, for example, has a CDR lower than that of the United States. This is due to the higher proportion of older people in the latter nation, and old people tend to do most of the dying. While it is possible to compare *age-specific mortality rates* between populations (Figure 2.3) it is often more convenient to "adjust" for the different age structures that may exist between populations using special statistical procedures to produce *standardized mortality ratios* or *rates*.

In all human populations, the age-specific mortality pattern is in the form of a "U" with high mortality at infancy and at old ages. For the developed countries, it is more of a "J" as infant mortality is much less pronounced. Of the three countries in the North American Free Trade zone shown in Figure 2.3, Mexico has infant and child mortality that is five to six times higher than that of Canada. Among the elderly, though, there is a crossover, where the mortality rate in Mexico is in fact lower than that of Canada and the United States.[12]

Populations differ in terms of the relative importance of different causes of death. While *cause-specific mortality rates* can be computed, sometimes the lack of denominator data (population base) precludes such attempts. The percent distribution of the various causes, however, can be compared. The term *proportionate mortality rate* (PMR) is sometimes used, especially in occupational health studies. [For example: x% of workers in Plant A died of cancer compared to only y% in Plant B.] From

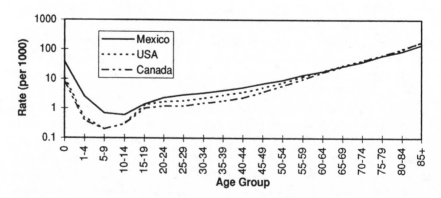

Figure 2.3. Age-specific mortality rate from all causes among men in Canada, the United States, and Mexico.

the discussion at the beginning of this chapter, it is clear that PMR is not a rate but a proportion, and calling it "proportionate rate" is redundant and contradictory. It would be more correct to call it a mortality proportion or fraction. An increase in PMR for a particular cause does not necessarily mean that the incidence of death from that cause has actually increased, only that it has increased relative to all other causes. The mortality rate may actually have declined.

A convenient summary measure of population health status often used in international comparisons is *life expectancy* (LE), which is based entirely on the mortality experience of the population and requires the construction of a *life table* (Box 2.5). LE should not be confused with *life span*, which is the maximum age biologically possible for the human species. LE can be determined for any age, but the one most often used is *life expectancy at birth*, which is heavily influenced by deaths among infants and the very young. Its interpretation is not affected by the different age structures of populations. In the United States in 2001, a newborn male infant can be expected to live to 74 years, and a female to 79 years. LE for Canadians is better, at 77 and 82 years respectively. Japan has the world's highest LE (78 and 85 for male and female respectively), whereas in some of the least-developed countries, life expectancy at birth could be lower than 50 years.[13]

Even if a population has a very low LE at birth, it does not mean that there are no or few old people around, just that a very high proportion of infants and young children die before they reach adulthood. Indeed, the gap in LE between developed and developing countries beyond middle age is remarkably small. Once childhood has been survived, the chance of living to the ripe old age of 70 and above is very good for most populations in the world. In most countries, LE is higher in females than males, with some notable exceptions such as Bangladesh, reflecting the heavy toll on women's health from harsh living conditions, social disadvantages, and excessive maternal mortality and morbidity.

The *infant mortality rate* (IMR) is the number of infant deaths (under one year of age) per 1,000 live births per year. Most industrialized countries have an IMR under 10; in some developing countries it can be as much as 15 times higher. The IMR can be broken down into *neonatal* (under 28 days) and *post-neonatal* (from the beginning of the twenty-eighth day up to the end of the first year of life) mortality rates. The former is generally considered to be more sensitive to medical care measures, while the latter is reflective of socioeconomic conditions. Because infants who are born prematurely are much smaller in size and their survival tends to be poorer, infant and neonatal mortality rates are often stratified according to the birth weight for more meaningful comparisons. Infants born with a birth weight under 2,500 grams are considered to be *low-birth-weight*, while those weighing under 1,500 grams are *very-low-birth-weight*.

BOX 2.5.   Constructing a Life Table and Computing Life Expectancy

The life table has a long history. John Graunt published a life table in 1662 based on his *Bills of Mortality*. Edmund Halley (1656–1742) of comet fame published one on the German city of Breslau (now the Polish city of Wroclaw) in 1693. While used extensively by demographers in computing life expectancy, it can also be used in comparing outcomes of medical treatments and survival from various diseases.

A life table summarizes the mortality experience of a hypothetical generation or cohort that is subjected throughout its lifetime to a set of ASDRs. Starting off with 100,000 newborn infants, the life table provides estimates of how many will survive to each successive age. It should be recognized that the ASDRs used can only be for a point in time. In reality, as the cohort ages, it will experience new age-specific death rates and not the ones that prevailed at the time of birth. A life table based on Canadian male age-specific mortality rates for 1990–1992 is presented here.[14] This is an example of a complete life table, which lists ages in single years. Smaller populations are usually represented by "abridged life tables," with ages in five-year intervals.

Age n	l_n	d_n	p_n	q_n	L_n	T_n	e_n
0	100,000	709	0.99291	0.00709	99,380	7,455,249	74.55
1	99,291	51	0.99949	0.00051	99,263	7,355,869	74.08
2	99,240	41	0.99959	0.00041	99,216	7,256,606	73.12
:	:	:	:	:	:	:	:
10	99,064	14	0.99985	0.00015	99,057	6,463,561	65.25
:	:	:	:	:	:	:	:
30	97,377	120	0.99878	0.00122	97,317	4,495,417	46.17
:	:	:	:	:	:	:	:
50	93,325	419	0.99551	0.00449	93,115	2,580,044	27.65
:	:	:	:	:	:	:	:

l_n number of persons alive at the beginning of age n

d_n number of persons expected to die before reaching age $(n + 1) = l_n \times q_n$

p_n proportion that will survive from age n to age $(n + 1) = 1 - q_n$

q_n proportion that will die from age n to age $(n + 1)$

L_n number of person-years lived by persons from age n to age $(n + 1)$

T_n sum of all remaining years to be lived by all persons at age n

e_n mean number of years to be lived by those surviving to age n

(continued)

Data for column q_n are derived from the ASDR for that age, obtained from vital statistics. (Note that the ASDR is based on the mid year population, whereas q_n uses the population at the beginning of the year. The two quantities are similar but not identical; q_n can be estimated by $ASDR/(1 + 0.5ASDR)$, under the assumption that the midyear population is the population at the start of the year less half the number who died during that year). Data for all other columns are computed from q_n.

Starting off with 100,000 infants at age 0, the proportion who will die within a year (q_n) is 0.00709. The number expected to die before reaching age 1 (d_n) is therefore ($l_n \times q_n$), or 709. At age 1, there will be 100,000 less 709, or 99,291 individuals alive ($l_{n+1} = l_n - d_n$), or alternatively, ($l_n \times p_n$).

For all ages except those under 5, it is assumed that those who died during the interval lived on the average one-half of the interval. The number of person-years contributed by those who are alive between age n and $n + 1$, L_n is estimated to be ($l_n + l_{n+1}$)/2, or ($l_n - 0.5d_n$). For example, at age 10, $L_{10} = 99,064 - 0.5(14) = 99,057$. At younger ages, however, the assumption that deaths occur evenly in the course of a year does not hold. During infancy, for example, the majority of the deaths occur during early infancy and 0.5 would not be appropriate. For Canadian male infants under 1 year of age, the factor has been calculated to be 0.874, and for age 1, it is 0.549. Thus, $L_0 = 100,000 - 0.874$ $(709) = 99,380$, and $L_1 = 99,291 - 0.549 (51) = 99,263$.

The sum of all remaining years to be lived by all persons at age n, T_n, is obtained by adding up ($L_n + L_{n+1} + L_{n+2} \ldots$) until the highest age at the bottom of the table. Thus, $T_0 = (99,380 + 99,263 + 99,216 \ldots)$. It can also be seen that $T_{n+1} = (T_n - L_n)$. Thus $T_1 = (T_0 - L_0) = (7,455,249 - 99,380) = 7,355,869$.

Finally, the mean number of years remaining to be lived by those surviving to age n, e_n, is equal to ($T_n \div l_n$). Thus $e_0 = (7,455,249 \div 100,000) = 74.55$. This is the life expectancy at birth. From the table, it can be readily determined that for Canadian males, life expectancy at age 10 (e_{10}) is 65.25, and at age 50 (e_{50}) is 27.65, etc.

It is worth noting that the concept of infant mortality emerged only during the late nineteenth century. Although William Farr did not coin the term, he used the current definition and calculated the rate in England in 1875 to be 158/1,000.[15]

Note that the infant mortality rate can be easily determined from the vital statistics system, since the number of deaths and number of births are known for each year. The IMR for year X thus consists of infant deaths occurring in year X, some of whom were in fact born in the previous year, X − 1. The denominator consists of live births occurring in year X, some of whom may in fact go on to die in the following year, X + 1, before their first birthday. This method is in used in most countries (those with a vital statistics system), in which case it can be seen (*vide* Box 2.1) that the IMR is neither a rate nor a proportion, but simply a ratio of two quantities: infant deaths and live births. A more accurate assessment of the probability of death during infancy is to actually track all infants born in a given year (a birth cohort) for 12 months and determine the cumulative incidence of death, by linking electronically the birth and death databases, something that is indeed done by the U.S. National Center for Health Statistics, which produces a National Linked File of Live Births and Infant Deaths. The IMR it generates is a proportion, as the numerator (infant deaths) is part of the denominator (live births).

Another indicator, frequently used in WHO/UNICEF publications on international health, is the *under-five mortality rate*. One indicator which combines *stillbirths* (or *fetal deaths*) and *early neonatal* deaths (under seven days of life) is the *perinatal mortality rate*. As the boundary between "stillbirth" and "spontaneous abortion" is not always clear-cut, the perinatal mortality rate is subject to potential recording bias, particularly in remote areas where many births and abortions are not medically supervised. The WHO defines a live birth as "the complete expulsion or extraction from its mother of a product of conception, irrespective of the duration of the pregnancy, which, after such separation, breathes or shows any other evidence of life, such as beating of the heart, pulsation of the umbilical cord, or definite movement of voluntary muscles." A stillbirth or fetal death is death prior to the complete expulsion . . . etc. (the opposite of the definition of "live birth"). The dividing line between stillbirth and abortion is 21 weeks of gestation in some jurisdictions and 28 weeks in others, making international comparisons difficult. The denominator is also inconsistent: it can be live births or the sum of live births and stillbirths. WHO also recommends the recording of fetal deaths with weight under 1,000 grams or length of 25 cm, as gestational age is often difficult to estimate.[16]

A useful index of premature mortality that gives more weight to deaths among younger people (and hence more "valued" by society on the whole) is the *potential years of life lost* (PYLL). It is sometimes also called *years of potential life lost* (YPLL). It sums the number of years of life "lost" by individuals in a population between their ages at death and some arbitrary age such as 65 or 70. PYLL offers a perspective on mortality that has relevance to the allocation of health care resources. Conditions that kill mostly younger people, such as injuries, contribute more to PYLLs than conditions that affect primarily older people, such as circulatory diseases and cancer.[17] Such an index reflects the prevailing social value assigned to different ages at death. Priority is given to young deaths because of the loss of potential future economic contribution to society. As with the dependency ratio, the PYLL is not entirely a philosophically, ethically, or politically neutral mathematical construct.

BOX 2.6. Computing Potential Years of Life Lost (PYLL)

To demonstrate how PYLL is computed for a particular cause, the age-specific mortality rates for cancer and injuries among Canadians are used.[18] Infants are excluded, and the upper limit is arbitrarily set at 70.

Age group at death	(A) Mean age at death	(B) No. deaths Cancer	(B) No. deaths Injuries	(C)= 70−(A)	PYLL=(B)×(C) Cancer	PYLL=(B)×(C) Injuries
1–4	3.0	55	179	67.0	3,685.0	11,993.0
4–9	7.5	66	155	62.5	4,125.0	9,687.5
10–14	12.5	61	185	57.5	3,507.5	10,637.5
15–19	17.5	93	899	52.5	4,882.5	47,197.5
20–24	22.5	105	1,058	47.5	4,987.5	50,255.0
25–29	27.5	192	1,137	42.5	8,160.0	48,322.5
30–35	32.5	368	1,301	37.5	13,800.0	48,787.5
35–39	37.5	668	1,218	32.5	21,710.0	39,585.0
40–44	42.5	1,178	988	27.5	32,395.0	27,170.0
45–49	47.5	1,864	873	22.5	41,940.0	19,642.5
50–54	52.5	2,691	632	17.5	47,092.5	11,060.0
55–59	57.5	3,978	542	12.5	49,725.0	6,775.0
60–64	62.5	6,131	537	7.5	45,982.5	4,027.5
65–69	67.5	8,237	581	2.5	20,592.5	1,452.5
Total		25,687	10,286		302,585.0	336,593.0

Note that the average age at death is the midpoint of the five-year period. In terms of the number of deaths, the ratio of cancer to injuries is 2.5; in terms of PYLL, the ratio is only 0.9. It is also possible to calculate the rate of PYLL by dividing the number of PYLL by the population aged 1–69.

There are different methods of calculating PYLL/YPLL. The differences are subtle, but they can produce different rankings of leading causes of premature death. They can be expressed mathematically as:

1. $\Sigma d_n (L - n)$, where d_n is the number of deaths at age n and L the arbitrary upper limit. Some also set a lower limit of one year, thus excluding infant deaths under one year. An example of this method can be found in Box 2.6.
2. $\Sigma d_n e_n$, where e_n is the life expectancy at age n, rather than the arbitrary upper limit of 70 or whatever.
3. $\Sigma d_n e_n^c$, where e_n^c is the estimated "cohort" life expectancy at age n, which takes into account the changing mortality experience as a cohort ages, and is more realistic than (2), which assumes an unchanging mortality in the future from the one currently observed.

4. $\Sigma d_n e_n^*$, where e_n^* is the life expectancy at age x based on some ideal standard, say Japanese women or one of the model life tables published by the United Nations.

The *maternal mortality rate* in developed countries is now extremely low, typically less than 5/100,000 live births, compared to rates as high as 500–1,000/100,000 in some developing countries. The denominator should ideally be women at risk for pregnancy or childbirth—this is not a readily available piece of information. As a substitute, the number of live births is used. The rate can thus be interpreted as the number of women who have been "sacrificed" to generate 100,000 live births for the population. (It is thus only a *ratio*, not really a *rate* or *proportion*). The numerator is problematic, too. While it refers to events relating to pregnancy, childbirth, and the puerperium (i.e., the period after childbirth), it is not clear how long after a pregnancy has terminated complications can still be attributed to it. The World Health Organization suggests 42 days, with a category of "late maternal deaths" for deaths between 42 days and a year. The distinction is also made between direct obstetric causes (e.g., pre-eclampsia, hemorrhage from a retained placenta), and indirect ones, which include any medical condition related to, or aggravated by, the pregnant state (e.g., anemia of pregnancy) or its management, excluding accidents. Maternal deaths are such rare events that every occurrence is cause for concern and thoroughly investigated to prevent its recurrence.

The size of a population increases when there is an excess of births over deaths (*natural increase*) and when there is an excess of immigrants over emigrants (*net migration*). Demographers are often called upon by health planners to provide *population projections* years into the future. The complexity may vary from a simple total population size, to detailed estimates of age-sex structure and socioeconomic status. The process is in fact "interactive": while population projections help determine future disease burden, disease frequency and severity can have a major impact on population growth.

The basic approach used in population projection is known as the *cohort-component method*. In simple terms, it starts off with a base population and adds to it natural increase and net migration. This basic equation can be applied to different age-sex cohorts of the population, as well as geographical subdivisions, before aggregating to the total population. For each component such as births, deaths, and migrations, assumptions will be needed in terms of the pattern that they will follow. Often, different scenarios—slow, moderate, and fast growth—are produced.

Comparing Health Events in Populations

One of the reasons why we calculate rates and proportions when comparing the frequency of health-related events, rather than simply compare the number of events, is to ensure that differences in population size have been taken into consideration. Yet such *crude* rates may still be misleading if there are substantial qualitative differences between the populations being compared, such as age-sex structure, socioeconomic status, ethnic composition, and so on.

One way to overcome this is to have *category-specific* measures: for example, comparing death rates in each age group. This may become quite cumbersome, and it does not give a "feel" for the overall picture—in other words, which population is "worse off"?

Another way to obtain a summary measure that "adjusts" for the variable of interest is *standardization*. There are two methods: *direct* and *indirect*.[19] To simplify discussion, let us consider age standardization, as age is one of the commonest variables adjusted for when comparing populations. Suppose one would like to compare mortality rates between two health regions, A and B. These constitute the *study* populations. We then select (or create) a population as the *standard* population. Let:

d_i = number of events in the ith age group for the *study* population
n_i = number of persons in the ith age group for the *study* population
r_i = age-specific event rate for the ith age group among the *study* population
D_i = number of events in the ith age group for the *standard* population
N_i = number of persons in the ith age group for the *standard* population
R_i = age-specific event rate for the ith age group among the *standard* population

For each of the study populations A and B, a set of rates can be calculated:

Crude event rate = $\Sigma d_i / \Sigma n_i$
Age-specific event rate = d_i / n_i
Directly age-adjusted event rate = $\Sigma(r_i N_i) / \Sigma N_i$
Indirectly age-adjusted event rate = $(\Sigma d_i / \Sigma R_i n_i) \times (\Sigma D_i / \Sigma N_i)$

The quantity $(\Sigma d_i / \Sigma R_i n_i)$, the ratio of "observed" to "expected" (O/E) is called *standardized mortality ratio* (SMR). The "M" does not have to be mortality, but can be any event of interest.[20]

Whether the direct or indirect procedure is used depends on what types of data are available. Information about the standard population, particularly if it is the national population, is more likely to be available. For smaller local populations, often only the total number of cases is available, which may not be broken down into categories. In such a situation, one has to use the indirect method. The direct method, however, is preferred if the necessary information is available. For very small populations, where the number of cases and the population are small, the category-specific rates may be very unstable. The resulting directly standardized rates could vary

BOX 2.7.   An Example of Direct and Indirect Standardization

In the 1990s Mexico had a crude mortality rate of 5/1,000, compared to a U.S. rate of 8/1,000. Does it mean that Mexicans are generally "healthier" than Americans? It we examine the age-specific mortality rates (all causes combined), it can be seen that at each age group, the Mexican rate is in fact higher than the American one.[21] (The table has been simplified by rounding off to the nearest thousands.)

Age group	Mexico			United States		
	No. deaths ('000s)	Population ('000s)	Death rate	No. deaths ('000s)	Population ('000s)	Death rate
0–14	70	31,147	0.00225	53	53,542	0.00099
15–44	75	37,363	0.00201	184	117,386	0.00157
45–64	86	8,872	0.00969	369	46,587	0.00792
65+	184	3,377	0.05449	1,564	31,195	0.05014
All ages	415	80,759	0.00514	2,170	248,710	0.00873

It can be seen that the Mexican population is a "young" one (with 39% under the age of 15 and 4% over 65), whereas the American one is "older" (22% < 15 and 13% 65+). To make the comparison more meaningful, one should standardize the mortality rates to account for the different age structures. The choice of a standard population is arbitrary— one can use the United States, Mexican, or some third population. Suppose we use the U.S. population as the standard.

(Tip: To avoid confusion, it is best to keep the death rate as a decimal rather than converting it to something per 1,000. Those who know how to use a spreadsheet software will find the calculations quite painless; those who don't—it is high time to learn! With a spreadsheet you don't have to worry about rounding off your numbers until the very end.)

(1) Direct Standardization:
The directly standardized mortality rate for Mexico is $\Sigma(r_i N_i)/\Sigma N_i$, where r is the Mexican rate and N the U.S. population serving as the standard,

$$= [(0.00224 \times 53,542) + (0.00201 \times 117,386) + (0.00969 \times 46,587) + (0.05449 \times 31,195)] / 248,710$$

$$= 0.01008 \text{ or } 10.08 \text{ per } 1,000$$

It can be seen that the Mexican rate has now increased from 5.13 to 10.08 per 1,000, higher than the American rate of 8.72 per 1,000. The comparison is now more meaningful, as the Mexican death rates have been

(continued)

adjusted to the age distribution of the U.S. population. Since the U.S. population serves as its own standard, its rates do not need to be adjusted.

(2) Indirect Standardization:
First the SMR needs to be calculated. The SMR for Mexico is $\Sigma d_i / \Sigma R_i n_i$, where d is the number of deaths in Mexico, R the mortality rate in the United States and n the population of Mexico,

$$= 415 / [\, (0.00099 \times 31{,}147) + (0.00157 \times 37{,}363)$$
$$+ (0.00792 \times 8{,}872) + (0.05014 \times 3{,}377)]$$

$$= 1.261$$

The indirectly standardized mortality rate is obtained by multiplying the SMR by $\Sigma D_i / \Sigma N_i$, which is really the total mortality rate (i.e., total cases / total population) in the United States,

$$= 1.261 \times 0.00873 = 0.01101 \text{ or } 11.01 \text{ per } 1{,}000$$

Again, the indirectly standardized mortality rate for Mexico is higher than the crude rate, and now exceeds the American rate. Note that the two methods do not give identical results. However, the conclusion, that mortality is higher in Mexico than in the United States, after adjusting for the different age structures, is the same.

substantially if cut-off points for the categories are changed slightly or errors occur in misclassifying cases into categories.

The choice of a "standard" affects the rates, ranking of rates, and the ratio of rates if several populations are being compared.[22] It can be an external standard, derived from a population outside the ones that are being compared (such as using the U.S. national population when comparing states). Or it can be an internal one, with one of the study populations serving as a standard (as was done in Box 2.7), or created by aggregating or averaging the study populations. A standardized rate is thus completely arbitrary and artificial—it is computed to aid in making meaningful comparisons and drawing useful conclusions. The directly standardized rate presents the scenario of what would happen if the standard population, instead of experiencing its own mortality pattern, had assumed the age-specific death rates of the study population. The indirectly standardized rate depicts the situation when the study population experiences the mortality pattern of the standard population. The "real" rate is the crude rate and its age- or other category-specific component rates.

The International Agency for Research on Cancer (IARC), which publishes the statistical compendium *Cancer Incidence in Five Continents*, uses a hypothetical "world population" of 100,000 individuals as the standard in computing age-standardized cancer incidence rates for various countries or populations served by regional cancer registries. Although it does not correspond to any real population, it was originally based on the work of Mitsuo Segi, a pioneer in the international comparison of cancer statistics, who pooled the population of 46 countries in the world, and is sometimes referred to in the literature as "Segi's standard population." An example of the use of this hypothetical standard is provided by Exercise 2.4. In 2000, WHO proposed its own standard population, which is based on the estimated world population averaged over a 25-year projection period (2000–2025). The distribution of both standards is shown in Table 2.2. It should be recognized that once a standard population has been changed, newly computed standardized rates are no longer comparable to rates based on the old standard.

An alternative to the age-standardized incidence rate is the *cumulative rate*. By summing the age-specific incidence rates for each year of age from 0–74, one obtains a quantity that can be considered the lifetime risk of developing a disease. This method is comparable to the method for the total fertility rate described earlier, which is a woman's cumulative risk of childbirth during her reproductive period.

Table 2.2. World Standard Populations

Age group	IARC	WHO
0–4	12,000	8,860
5–9	10,000	8,690
10–14	9,000	8,600
15–19	9,000	8,470
20–24	8,000	8,220
25–29	8,000	7,930
30–34	6,000	7,610
35–39	6,000	7,150
40–44	6,000	6,590
45–49	6,000	6,040
50–54	5,000	5,370
55–59	4,000	4,550
60–64	4,000	3,720
65–69	3,000	2,960
70–74	2,000	2,210
75–79	1,000	1,520
80–84	500	910
85+	500	630
Total	100,000	100,000

BOX 2.8.   Computing 95% Confidence Intervals

More advanced students may want to compute 95% confidence intervals (CI) around vital rates such as the IMR.[23]

$$d = \text{number of vital events (births, deaths)}$$
$$n = \text{denominator of rate (population, live births)}$$
$$95\% \text{ CI of the IMR} = (d \pm 1.96\sqrt{d})/n$$

When comparing two rates, r_1 and r_2, with CI_1 and CI_2, the 95% CI of their ratio (r_1/r_2) or R, is:

$$R \pm R\sqrt{[(CI_1/r_1)^2 + (CI_2/r_2)^2]}$$

and the 95% CI of the difference $(r_1 - r_2)$, or D, is:

$$D \pm \sqrt{[CI_1^2 + CI_2^2]}$$

One can also compute 95% CI around the SMR and the directly standardized mortality rate ASMR.

$$95\% \text{ CI of the SMR} = SMR \pm 1.96 \text{ SE,}$$

where SE is the standard error. Using the same symbols d, R, and n in the formula for SMR,

$$SE = \sqrt{\Sigma d_i}/\Sigma R_i n_1$$

The 95% CI of the directly standardized rate ASMR is also ASMR $\pm$ 1.96 SE, where

$$SE = \sqrt{\Sigma(N_i^2 r_i/n_i)}/\Sigma N_i$$

Demographic and Health Transition

The long-term growth in human populations and the factors and processes that influence it have long fascinated scholars. An early theoretical contribution was made by Thomas Malthus (1766–1834), an English economist and clergyman, who published his famous *Essay on the Principles of Population* in 1798.[24] Malthus proposed two postulates:

1. Food is necessary to the existence of man;
2. Passion between the sexes is necessary.

One can hardly argue with that. Malthus further stated that "population, when unchecked, increases in a geometrical ratio. Subsistence increases only in an arithmetical ratio." It is evident that food supply will not be able to sustain the growth of human population. In the second (1803) and subsequent editions, Malthus elaborated on this theme:

1. Population is necessarily limited by the means of subsistence;
2. Population invariably increases when the means of subsistence increases, unless prevented by some powerful and obvious checks;
3. These checks . . . are all resolvable into moral restraint, vice, and misery.

"Vice and misery," referring to manmade and natural calamities respectively, include war, famine, and pestilence, which apply a "positive" check on population by increasing the death rate. "Moral restraint" exercises a "preventive" check by lowering the birth rate, which can be achieved by delaying marriage. Whether Malthus's theory was right has been the subject of much debate and controversy among economists, demographers, political scientists, and theologians.

Changes in fertility and mortality in populations have generally followed certain patterns, often referred to as *demographic transition* by demographers. In essence, populations move from a stage of high fertility and high mortality to one of low fertility and low mortality. During the transition, the mortality rate falls first, to be followed by fertility, as shown in Figure 2.4.

For a country such as England, Stage 2 probably began around the mid–eighteenth century when the death rate began to fall, whereas Stage 3 began about a century later. The low mortality/low fertility of Stage 4 was achieved by the mid–twentieth century. This is clearly a gross simplification

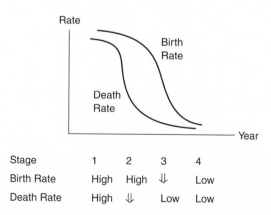

Figure 2.4. Schematic representation of the stages of demographic transition.

of many complex processes and events, and it is not expected that the model would fit all developed countries, at least those with reliable historical data, let alone predict future trends in developing countries, many of which are still at the pre-transition stage. Beyond its utility as a descriptive tool, there is less agreement on the model's ability to explain demographic change in terms of industrialization.[25]

There is a companion theory to that of demographic transition, called *health or epidemiological transition*, which describes and explains the long-term temporal changes in the pattern of health and disease in populations. As originally formulated by the demographer Abdel Omran in the 1970s, there are three stages: the age of pestilence and famines, the age of receding pandemics, and the age of degenerative and manmade diseases. The pace of transition differs between populations: the classical or Western model, exemplified by Western Europe and North America; the accelerated model, characterized by Japan and Eastern Europe; and the delayed model wherein most developing countries would belong. A fourth stage—the age of delayed degenerative diseases—has also been proposed by others to account for the decline in mortality in the industrial countries of such diseases as heart diseases and the postponement of the age of death among the elderly.[26] The concept has gained currency in the population health literature, and a variety of case studies have attempted to fit available health statistics to the models proposed in the theory.

Detailed analyses have shown that there are important variations within these stages. A study from the Netherlands, where excellent historical data are available, used the statistical technique called *cluster analysis* to group causes of death with similar trends in age-sex–standardized mortality rates. Among the infectious diseases, some showed a precipitous decline in the late nineteenth century and early twentieth centuries—for example, typhoid fever and diarrheal diseases—attributable to improvement in water and sanitation. Another group (including diphtheria and tuberculosis) also began their decline in the 1900s, but less sharply, perhaps the result of improvements in housing and working conditions. A third group of infectious diseases (including pneumonia and septicemia) declined slowly at the beginning of the twentieth century, but accelerated after the World War II, probably partly due to the introduction of antibiotics. Similarly, not all degenerative diseases showed the same increasing trend during the twentieth century.[27]

Figure 2.5 shows the change in mortality pattern in the United States between 1900 and 1990. It can be seen that mortality rates from infectious diseases such as tuberculosis, respiratory and intestinal infections, as well as perinatal conditions, declined substantially during the century. Chronic diseases such as cancer and diseases of the heart have become the most important causes of death, although a decline in heart disease mortality can be observed since the 1960s.[28]

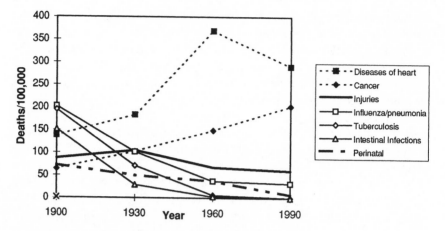

Figure 2.5. Historical trends in crude mortality rate by selected causes in the United States, 1900–1990.

In comparing the mortality rates for selected causes between the three countries of North America (Figure 2.6), Mexico has the highest mortality overall, even after adjusting for the different age-structures. In absolute and proportionate terms, infectious diseases are much more important in Mexico than in either the United States or Canada, whereas cancer and

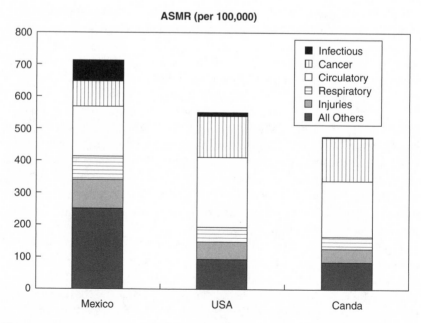

Figure 2.6. Comparison of selected cause-specific mortality rates in Canada, the United States, and Mexico.

circulatory diseases are less important causes of death. The Mexican pattern is typical of many developing countries.[29]

The decline in mortality experienced by most developed countries over the last two centuries has been the subject of much inquiry. Thomas McKeown (1914–1988) tracked the decline in mortality rates from infectious diseases in England and Wales since the late seventeenth century. He attributed this decline primarily to "rising standards of living" and improved nutritional status, and discounted the role of medical care and public health interventions, as the decline generally preceded the introduction of such innovations as antibiotics and vaccines. A decline in the virulence of the pathogens was also deemed unlikely to have played a significant role. The McKeown thesis did not go unchallenged, both for its data analysis and interpretation. It generated considerable controversy at the time of its first publication in the mid-1970s, and continued to do so even 25 years later. For example, historian Simon Sreter reanalyzed McKeown's data and assigned a more prominent role to public health measures such as a clean water and milk supply.[30]

In the United States, John and Sonia McKinlay came to similar conclusions as McKeown, using mortality data from 1900–1973, focusing on 10 specific infectious diseases and their temporal relation to the introduction of specific interventions. With respect to the overall role of medical care, they noted that the precipitate and unrestrained rise in medical care expenditures began when over 90% of the decline in mortality in the twentieth century had already occurred.

Others focused on specific interventions and assessed their contribution to improvement in health status. For example, John Bunker and colleagues provided detailed estimates of the gain in life expectancy for various preventive (screening and immunizations) and curative measures whose efficacy has already been established and for which a mortality decline can be demonstrated. In an analysis of Dutch data from 1875 to 1970, Johan Mackenbach estimated that health care measures contributed between 5% and 19% of the decline in total mortality during this period.[31]

The role of health care does not lie exclusively in reducing mortality, but also in relieving pain and suffering, preventing disability, and improving quality of life, measures of health that are much less amenable to historical trend analyses than mortality. Mere extension of life expectancy is not necessarily a desirable goal, compared to a "collective, full, and vigorous life terminated by a swift and painless decline ending in death."[32] James Fries proposed the concept of *compression of morbidity*, both as a descriptive model and as a health policy goal. By postponing the onset of chronic morbidity among the elderly, against a relatively fixed life expectancy, the period of morbidity associated with a poor quality of life will be reduced or compressed.

No modern society can function without health care, although more health care does not translate into better health status. Health care needs to be seen in the context of the broader determinants of health, which are discussed in Chapter 4.

Summary

Several key concepts in measuring the frequency of occurrence of disease in populations are discussed in this chapter. *Incidence* measures change with new events in the numerator, whereas *prevalence* refers to status, with existing cases in the numerator. Each can be subdivided further: cumulative incidence and incidence density; point and period prevalence.

Populations can be characterized in terms of size, structure, and growth. A population changes through fertility, mortality, and migration. Basic demographic events can be compared between populations using crude, category-specific, and standardized rates. The overall mortality experience of a population can be summarized by indices such as life expectancy and potential years of life lost. Specific stages of the life cycle such as the perinatal period and infancy are often used as general measures of population health because of their sensitivity to the level of medical care and socioeconomic conditions.

Since the time of Malthus, the growth of populations has not been of interest just to those concerned with population health, but has wide social and political implications as well. Theories of demographic and epidemiological transition attempt to categorize populations in terms of stages characterized by the relative magnitude of the birth and death rates and also the predominant causes of mortality and morbidity. The reason for improvement in health status in most populations is also the subject of intense debate. One view, represented by McKeown and the McKinlays among others, de-emphasized the credit claimed by medical care and attributed it to overall improvement in the standard of living and nutritional status.

Case Study 2.1.   Cancer Incidence in Five Continents

The International Agency for Research on Cancer (IARC), an agency of the World Health Organization based in Lyons, France, conducts epidemiological and laboratory research and publishes periodical monographs evaluating various human carcinogens. Since 1966, it has also published *Cancer Incidence in Five Continents*, a compendium of incidence data from a large number of population-based cancer registries in the world. The seventh edition was published in 1997, reporting on data from 150 registries in 50 countries. Some of these registries are national in scope (e.g., Canada, England, Wales, and some European countries). The United States is represented by

SEER (Surveillance, Epidemiology, and End Results program), a collection of regional registries (see Chapter 3). Some registries cover cities or other subnational regions (e.g., Shanghai in China, Myagi Prefecture in Japan, Bas-Rhin in France, Victoria State in Australia, etc.). In some countries, data are also available for specific ethnic groups (e.g., Chinese, Malays, and Indians in Singapore; Maori and non-Maori in New Zealand; Jews and non-Jews in Israel; Black and White in the United States). There are few operational cancer registries in developing countries, and Africa is particularly underrepresented, with only five registries.

These registries provide a description of the burden of cancer in defined populations. The geographical pattern of cancer incidence globally is instructive. In a review of the causes of cancer, Richard Doll and Richard Peto considered geographical differences an important clue to etiology. For some cancers, the highest reported rate may exceed the lowest by several hundredfold. That a certain low rate is achievable in some populations supports the idea that the cancer may be avoidable, if one can elucidate the environmental factors responsible.

In this case study, the age-standardized incidence rates (ASIR) of two cancer sites are presented, using the IARC's hypothetical "world" population as standard.[33] Not all registries included in the IARC report are shown, and in countries where there is more than one registry, the one with the highest rate is selected. Where both national and regional registries from the same country are reported, the national one is used.

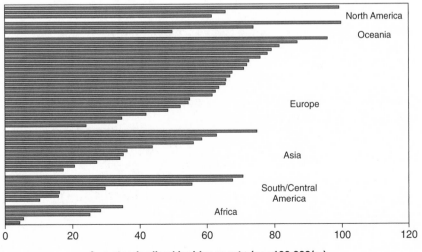

Age-standardized incidence rate (per 100,000/yr)

Lung cancer

Lung cancer incidence is highest in the developed countries of Europe and North America. However, the low rates in African, Latin American, and Asian countries reflect the shorter time since smoking became a widespread practice. Current smoking prevalence is actually higher in these countries where social acceptance is high, taxation is low, and restrictive legislations few. There is also evidence of "dumping" of cheap cigarettes by multinational firms in developing countries, the growth areas for sales. In two or three decades, the geographical pattern of lung cancer will be quite different.

Malignant melanoma of skin

The world's highest incidence of maglignant melanoma is found in Australia and New Zealand, with rates as high as 33/100,000 in New South Wales. Exposure to the ultraviolet rays (especially UVB) in sunlight, particularly in fair-skinned people, is the most important cause, and these two factors are in great abundance in the two antipodean countries. In New Zealand, the non-Maori rate, at 25/100,000, is five times the Maori rate. In Hawaii, the rate is 20/100,000 among whites, compared to <1.0 among Native Hawaiians and those of Chinese, Japanese, and Filipino origin in the same state. While Northern Europe is not known for its hot sun, Scandinavians have a penchant for seeking holidays in more southern climes. The highest rate among Europeans is found among Norwegians, at 14/100,000. Moreover, a study comparing the standardized incidence ratios for malignant melanoma in 19 counties in Norway indicates that the UVB level is positively and independently associated with cancer incidence, independent of foreign vacations and income. The depletion of the ozone layer, which protects the earth's atmosphere from ultraviolet radiation, thus has a potentially serious impact in the northern latitudes even though the UVB levels there are low relative to the tropics.

Case Study 2.2.   Contribution of Population Aging to Changes in Cancer Mortality

When comparing disease frequency between historical periods, geographical areas, or demographic subgroups, it is possible to "partition" a difference in the crude rates into two components: one due to difference in the age structure and the other due to difference in actual disease risk.[34]

Lung cancer mortality has increased among men in France. The following table presents age-specific data for 1970 and 1980:[35]

Age group	Cases		Population		Rate (per 100,000)	
	1970	1980	1970	1980	1970	1980
0–14	4	2	6,199,800	5,904,800	0.06	0.03
15–24	8	4	4,344,700	4,332,600	0.18	0.09
25–34	24	43	3,142,000	4,394,500	0.76	0.98
35–44	309	378	3,383,100	3,115,700	9.13	12.13
45–54	957	2,042	2,643,400	3,204,300	36.20	63.73
55–64	3,094	3,620	2,472,800	2,361,200	125.12	153.31
65–74	3,970	5,431	1,809,100	1,879,400	219.45	288.98
75–84	1,322	3,316	664,800	959,600	198.86	345.56
85+	188	422	129,300	158,000	145.40	267.09
Total	9,876	15,258	24,789,000	26,310,100	39.84	57.99

The crude lung cancer mortality rate is 39.8/100,000 men in 1970 (S_1) and 58.0/100,000 men in 1980 (S_2), with a difference ($S_2 - S_1$) of 18.2/100,000 men. The percent increase, $(S_2 - S_1)/S_1$, is 45.6%.

Since the survival from lung cancer has been (and still is) poor, the increase in mortality reflects an increase in incidence. The increase in incidence is partly due to the aging of the French population, and partly due to changes in disease risk unrelated to aging, such as exposure to smoking and other risk factors. The difference in crude rates can be partitioned into two components by invoking an intermediate rate, S_3:

$$(S_2 - S_1) = (S_3 - S_1) + (S_2 - S_3)$$

S_3 is actually the age-standardized mortality rate for 1970, using the 1980 population as the standard. In other words, S_3 is what the overall lung cancer mortality in 1980 would be if the 1970 age-specific rates had still been in place in 1980—the rates have not changed, but the age distribution has. Thus $(S_3 - S_1)$ is the component of the temporal change due to aging. The difference between the actual rate achieved in 1980 and the age-standardized rate, $(S_2 - S_3)$, can thus be considered the "non-aging" component, over and above that which can be explained by changes in the age distribution.

S_3 can readily be computed according to the procedure described in Box 2.7 and using the notation used in the text. The expected number of cases in each age group ($r_i N_i$) are first summed, where r_i is the age-specific rate of the ith age group of the 1970 population and N_i the number of people in the ith age group of the 1980 population.

$$\Sigma(r_iN_i) = (5{,}904{,}800 \times 0.06/100{,}000) + (4{,}3326{,}000 \times$$
$$0.18/100{,}000) \ldots + (959{,}600 \times 145.5/100{,}000)$$

$$= 3.81 + 7.98 \ldots + 229.73 = 10706.59$$

This is then divided by the total population of 1980 to obtain $S_3 = 10706.59/26{,}310{,}100 = 40.69/100{,}000$

$$(S_3 - S_1) + (S_2 - S_3) = (40.7/100{,}000 - 39.8/100{,}00)$$
$$+ (58.0/100{,}000 - 40.7/100{,}000)$$

$$= 0.9/100{,}000 + 17.3/100{,}000 = 18.2/100{,}000$$

which is the same as $(S_2 - S_1) = 58.0/100{,}000 - 39.8/100{,}000 = 18.2/100{,}000$.

It can be seen that the aging component (0.9) is very small relative to the non-aging component (17.3). The quantities $(S_2 - S_1)$, $(S_3 - S_1)$ and $(S_2 - S_3)$ can each be divided by S_1 to provide the percent change relative to the 1970 baseline. By extending the analyses with data from 1971 to 1993, the following graph can be plotted:

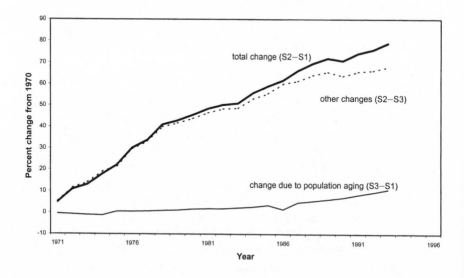

Two observations can be made regarding the temporal changes in lung cancer mortality among French men. The slope between 1980 and 1990 is less steep than that between 1970 and 1980 (i.e., the rate of increase has slowed). Furthermore, the contribution of population aging has increased in more recent years.

Notes

1. More advanced readers may wish to consult Elandt-Johnson (1975) and Morgenstern et al. (1980) for further discussion. Knowledge of calculus would be useful.

2. See the debate in the *American Journal of Public Health* between Flanders and O'Brien (1989) and Feinstein et al. (1989); and subsequent letters to the editor (1990; 80:622–624).

3. For a definitive discussion, see Hook (1982) and related correspondence in the *American Journal of Epidemiology* (1983; 118:608–10; 1984; 119:141–44).

4. Further discussion of period prevalence as applied to drug utilization studies can be found in McFarland (1996).

5. Freeman and Hutchison (1980) provide a comprehensive review of the various relationships among prevalence, incidence, and duration.

6. The data are taken from Centerwall (1991). The answers to the quiz are: P-P-I-I-I [p = prevalence, I = incidence]. See also the commentaries and spirited editorial correspondence in the *American Journal of Epidemiology* (1991; 134:1261–65; and 1992; 136:617–21).

7. Data are from UN *Demographic Yearbook 1993* and relevant Statistics Canada census publications.

8. King Charles II proposed Graunt for admission over the objection of the Fellows, who considered Graunt a mere tradesman. Rothman (1996) reminded members of the Society for Epidemiologic Research of Graunt's important contributions. There is a web site devoted to Graunt, which also reproduces the text of Bills of Mortality (www.ac.wwu.edu/~stephan/Graunt/graunt.html). For a historical review of the social and political context of the General Register Office in its early years, see Goldman (1991) and Sreter (1991). A biography of Farr and his place in Victorian "social medicine" is provided by Eyler (1979). There is also a Farr web site, which is an offshoot of the John Snow web site in the UCLA School of Public Health site www.ph.ucla.edu/epi/snow.html.

9. For a critique of the dependency ratio, see Gee (2002).

10. The age-specific fertility rates are obtained from *Health, United States 2002*, available from the NCHS web site, www.cdc.gov/nchs/hus.htm. Total fertility rates of all the member states of WHO can be found in Annex Table 1 of *The World Health Report 2002*, available from the WHO web site (www.who.int/whr/2002/en).

11. Just to confuse matters, in some European languages the meanings of *fertility* and *fecundity* are the reverse of the English terms. "Fertility" in English is *fécondité* in French, *fecondità* in Italian, and *fecundidade* in Portuguese, but *fertilidad* in Spanish and *Fertilität* in German! For the English term "fecundity," it is *fertilité* in French, *fertilità* in Italian, and *fertilidade* in Portuguese, but *fecundidad* in Spanish and *Fekundität* in German. I am indebted to *EPILEX: A Multilingual Lexicon of Epidemiological Terms*, edited by C. duV Florey and produced by the Department of Epidemiology and Public Health of the University of Dundee in Scotland. It contains lists in English, French, German, Italian, Spanish, Portuguese, Dutch, and Catalan.

12. The data in Figures 2.2 and 2.3 are obtained from the UN *Demographic Yearbook 1993*. The graph in Figure 2.3 is "semi-logarithmic"; i.e., the x-axis is in regular and the y-axis in logarithmic scale (each gradation increases by a multiple of 10). A semi-log graph is particularly useful in accommodating a large range of values without obscuring the details at the lower end of the scale.

13. "Life expectancy at birth" data for all the member states of WHO can be found in Annex Table 1 of *The World Health Report 2002*, available from the WHO web site (www.who.int/whr/2002/en).

14. The data were abstracted from Statistics Canada, *Life Tables: Canada and Provinces, 1990–1992*, Ottawa, 1995 [Cat. No. 84-537].

15. See Armstrong (1986) and the entry "Infant and Perinatal Mortality" (MacFarlane, 2000) in the *Encyclopedia of Epidemiologic Methods*.

16. The WHO definition of live birth dates back to the Third World Health Assembly in 1950 and was reconfirmed for adoption by the tenth revision of the International Classification of Diseases. See WHO (1990) and Last (2001:107).

17. See the review by Murray (1994) and the critique by Gardner and Sanborn (1990).

18. The method described in Box 2.6 is derived from Romeder and McWhinnie (1977). The data are obtained from: Statistics Canada, *Causes of Death 1993*, Ottawa, 1995 [Cat. No. 84-208].

19. One should only compare a study population with the standard population. It is inappropriate to compare multiple SMRs from different areas, even though the same "standard" has ostensibly been used. See Armstrong BG (1995) and more advanced epidemiology texts such as Szklo and Nieto (2000:272–73). For a statistical discussion on testing a null hypothesis of the equality of standardized rates, see Carriere and Roos (1994).

20. There are other, less commonly used, age-adjusted mortality indices, such as the *comparative mortality figure* (CMF) and the *relative mortality index* (RMI). See Kleinman (1977) for a description. Note that the PYLL mentioned earlier in this chapter is also an age-adjusted index.

21. The data are derived from the *UN Demographic Yearbook 1993*.

22. Before 2000, a profusion of standards was used in U.S. government publications when presenting trends in age-adjusted mortality rates. For example, in the annual *Health, United States* report, the 1940 American population was used. In comparing regions in national surveys such as the NHIS, the 1970 population was used, whereas for NHES and NHANES, the 1980 population was used. Now, the DHHS has decreed that the 2000 population be used consistently throughout all NCHS and CDC publications. The new WHO standard population is presented in Ahmad et al. (2001), which also provides a history of direct standardization.

23. The formula for 95% CI of the IMR is provided in *Statistical Notes for Health Planners* No. 3, Feb. 1977, and those for the SMR and ASMR in Morris and Gardner (1988). Alternatively, the "O" in the O/E ratio can be considered a Poisson variable and its 95% CI can be looked up in statistical tables of the Poisson distribution.

24. For a biography of Malthus and a commentary on his work, see Petersen (1979). The first edition of *Essay* is often referred to as *First Essay*, to be distinguished from the second (1803) to the seventh (1872), posthumous edition, which is almost a totally different book and commonly referred to as *Second Essay*. Malthus was grossly misunderstood. Karl Marx (1818–1883) was particularly vituperative in his attacks, calling him "the contemptible Malthus, a shameless sycophant of the ruling classes," and "libel on the human race" (cited in Petersen, 1979:75). Malthus influenced the thinking of Charles Darwin (1809–1882) in the development of his theory of evolution.

25. For a comprehensive cross-national survey of demographic transition patterns, see Chesnai (1992). It is difficult to pinpoint the origin of the "theory" to

a specific individual or publication, although a 1929 paper by Warren Thompson in the *American Journal of Sociology* referred to three different types of countries in terms of the decline of the birth and death rates. The term *demographic transition* was not specifically used. For a recent critique, see Sreter (2003).

26. See Omran (1971). The "fourth stage" was suggested by Olshansky and Ault (1986). Rogers and Hackenberg (1987) conceived of a "hybristic stage," after "hybris" (more commonly spelled "hubris"), a feeling of invincibility, to describe the current disease pattern that is largely determined by personal lifestyles and behaviors. The U.S. Agency for International Development and the National Academy of Sciences sponsored a conference on the planning and policy implications of the epidemiological transition in developing countries (Gribble and Preston, 1993). Epidemiological transition is also given considerable attention in the World Bank's handbook on health care strategies (Jamison et al., 1993). Phillips (1994) argued that the theory can be useful in health planning over the medium and long term, not just in service delivery, but also in medical education and the development of health-related industries.

27. See Wollesinkel-van den Bosch et al. (1997). This study actually used two aggregation levels of the causes of deaths—27 causes for the period from 1875–1992, and 65 causes for 1901–1992.

28. Data for 1900, 1930, and 1960 are obtained from Grove and Hetzel (1968); data for 1990 are from *Vital Statistics of the United States 1990*, vol. II, "Mortality," Part A. The decline in cardiovascular mortality since the 1960s has been observed in several other industrialized countries. The causes of this decline are not well understood, and the role of improved medical care in contributing to this decline is particularly contentious. See Higgins and Luepker (1988).

29. The grouping of diseases in Figures 2.5 and 2.6 is based on the International Classification of Disease, or ICD, discussed more fully in Chapter 3. One must exercise caution when comparing diagnostic rubrics over a period as long as 90 years. The fourth, seventh, and ninth revisions of the ICD were used by the U.S. vital statistics agency in 1930, 1960, and 1990, respectively. Mortality data for the three countries were obtained from the *UN Demographic Yearbook 1993*. The IARC "world population" was used in calculating the age-standardized mortality rates in Figure 2.6.

30. McKeown published a series of seminal papers in the demography journal *Population Studies* in the 1960s and 1970s. His ideas can be found in his two books. *The Modern Rise of Population* (1976) and *The Role of Medicine: Dream, Mirage or Nemesis* (2nd ed., 1979). His last work, published in the year of his death, *The Origins of Human Disease* (1988), is a sweeping view of the history, origins, and control of diseases in human populations from prehistoric times to the present. See Sreter (1988) and Colgrove (2002) for critiques and reinterpretation.

31. See McKinlay and McKinlay (1977), Bunker et al. (1994), and Mackenbach (1996).

32. The concept of compression of morbidity was first introduced in Fries (1980) and updated in Fries (2000). Leibson et al. (1992) attempted to test the validity of the hypothesis in a defined population (Olmstead County, Minnesota) using linked health care data to assess secular trends in mortality and morbidity.

33. The lung cancer data are from Parkin et al. (1999). Doll and Peto's original paper in the *Journal of the National Cancer Institute* was republished as a monograph (1981). The melanoma data are from Bentham and Aase (1996). In the

absence of UVB monitoring data, a UVB index was created for each county based on mathematical modeling of latitude and the hours of sunshine. For a review of ultraviolet radiation and skin cancer, see de Gruijl (1999). For a comprehensive review of cancer epidemiology and prevention, see Schottenfeld and Fraumeni (1996).

34. The procedure and sample data are based on Bashir and Estève (2000).

EXERCISE 2.1. State of the Population

In the 2000 census, the total population of the United States was 281,423,000, with the following age-sex distribution (note the numbers have been rounded off to the nearest thousand):

Age group	Male	Female	Total
0–1	1,949,000	1,857,000	3,806,000
1–4	7,862,000	7,508,000	15,370,000
5–14	21,044,000	20,034,000	41,078,000
15–44	62,647,000	61,577,000	124,224,000
45–64	30,143,000	31,810,000	61,953,000
65+	14,410,000	20,582,000	34,992,000
Total	138,055,000	143,368,000	281,423,000

Compute:

(a) The proportion of the elderly (aged 65+) in the population: _____

(b) The proportion of the young (aged 0–14) in the population: _____

(c) The sex ratio in age group 0–14 expressed as 100 males : _____ females

(d) The sex ratio in age group 65+ expressed as _____ males : 100 females

During that year, 4,059,000 babies were born alive and 2,403,000 people died. Compute:

(e) The crude birth rate: _____

(f) The crude death rate: _____

(g) The rate of natural increase: _____

There were 28,035 infant deaths, of which 18,776 occurred during the neonatal period, and 9,259 during the post-neonatal period. Compute:

(h) The infant mortality rate: _____

(i) The age-specific mortality rate for the under-1 age group: _____

(j)   The neonatal mortality rate: _____

(k)   The postneonatal mortality rate: _____

Among deaths in all ages, 1,226,000 were women. Among women's deaths from all causes, 41,872 were from cancer of the breast. Compute:

(l)   The crude death rate from all causes for women: _____

(m)   The crude death rate from breast cancer among women:

_____

(n)   The proportion of all deaths among women due to breast cancer: _____

Source: 2000 Census data are available from the U.S. Census Bureau web site (www.census.gov), and vital statistics from the National Center for Health Statistics (www.cdc.gov/nchs).

EXERCISE 2.2. Cancer Incidence and Mortality

Inspect the following cancer statistics for Canada in the mid-1990s.

- Crude mortality rate: 195/100,000 per year
- Crude incidence rate: 400/100,000 per year
- Hospital separation rate: 580/100,000 per year

(a)   Explain why the incidence rate is higher than the mortality rate.

(b)   Explain why the hospital separation rate is higher than the incidence rate. (Note: one "separates" from a hospital either by being discharged from it or dying in it; the hospital separation rate for cancer refers to the number of separations with a diagnosis of cancer divided by the population.)

Source: These rounded and averaged data are dervied from the web sites of Statistics Canada (www.statcan.ca), the Canadian Cancer Society (www.cancer.ca), and the Canadian Institute of Health Information (www.cihi.ca).

EXERCISE 2.3. Pattern of Mortality by Cause

The following table provides some data on causes of death in the United States in 2000:

Cause	Number of deaths	PYLLs/100,000
All causes	2,403,000	7,709
Cancer	553,000	1,699
Diseases of heart	711,000	1,271
Unintentional injuries	98,000	1,055

(a) Compute the percent distribution and crude death rates for the three causes of death (Note: the population of the United States in 2000 was 281,423,000).

(b) Why are unintentional injuries so much more important as a cause of death (relative to cancer and heart disease) when PYLL is used as the indicator?

Source: *Health, United States 2002* (available from the National Center for Health Statistics web site: www.cdc.gov/nchs)

EXERCISE 2.4. Prevalence of Diagnosed Diabetes

In a study comparing the prevalence of diagnosed cases of diabetes in several indigenous populations in the circumpolar region, the following data relating to Athapaskan Indians (Dene) in the Northwest Territories, Canada (NWT), and in Alaska, United States, were obtained:

	Alaska Indians		NWT Indians	
Age group	Population	No. cases	Population	No. cases
< 25	14,840	3	6,553	9
25–44	7,304	43	2,782	30
45–64	3,293	156	1,307	16
65 +	1,234	133	552	9

(a) Calculate the crude prevalence of diabetes among Alaskan Indians and NWT Indians.

(b) Calculate the age-standardized prevalence of diabetes among Alaskan and NWT Indians, using the information already given and with the IARC "world" population as standard.
(The age distribution of this population is: < 25: 48,000; 25–44: 26,000; 45–64: 19,000; 65+: 7,000)

(c) What kind of standardization (direct or indirect) has just been done?

(d) To do the other kind of standardization, what additional pieces of information are required? Suggest an appropriate "standard."

Source: Young et al. (1992)

EXERCISE 2.5. Gallbladder Disease and Rate of Cholecystectomy

In a study to compare cholecystectomy rates between Native and non-Native women in the Canadian province of Manitoba, the following data were obtained from the health insurance plan's hospital utilization database:

	Non-Native		Native	
Year	Cases	Rate (per 1,000)	Cases	Rate (per 1,000)
1972	2,970	6.03	72	4.65
1973	2,702	5.43	85	5.23
1974	2,437	4.78	77	4.59
1975	2,114	4.15	67	3.99
1976	1,957	3.79	76	3.87
1977	1,725	3.28	69	3.41
1978	1,680	3.18	76	3.71
1979	1,574	2.96	88	4.16
1980	1,459	2.77	76	3.51
1981	1,467	2.80	71	3.20
1982	1,363	2.60	99	4.41
1983	1,511	2.86	101	4.34
1984	1,520	2.85	119	4.95

(a) Plot the cholecystectomy rate of the two populations on a graph. What comments can you make on the two trends?

The following table compares the age distribution of the Native and non-Native female population in 1981:

Age group	Non-Native	Native	Total
0–9	73,458	6,455	79,913
10–19	85,290	6,154	91,444
20–29	94,243	4,124	98,367
30–39	72,852	2,142	74,994
40–49	50,479	1,344	51,823
50–59	52,755	872	53,627
60–69	46,944	597	47,541
70–79	30,517	337	30,854
80+	16,021	139	16,160
Total	522,559	22,164	544,723

(b) Graph the age distributions of the Native and non-Native populations. How would you characterize these two populations? Would knowledge of the age composition of these populations affect your answer to Question **(a)**?

The following table shows the age-specific rates of cholecystectomy among women in Manitoba in 1972.

Age group	Non-Native	Native
0–9	0.00	0.00
10–19	0.01	0.00
20–29	8.41	10.10
30–39	9.62	14.77
40–49	9.71	18.80
50–59	11.46	13.01
60–69	11.39	11.16
70–79	8.27	4.05
80+	4.73	8.77

(c) Graph the age-specific rates. What observations can be made?

(d) Compute the age-standardized cholecystectomy rate for Native and non-Native women in 1972, using the *combined* population of Manitoba in 1981 as the standard. Use the *direct* method.

The following table provides the necessary information to compute the age-standardized cholecystectomy rates using the *indirect* method, using the surgical experience of all Manitobans in 1981 as the standard. Recall from the first table that the total number of cases in the non-Native population in 1972 was 2,970, and in the Native population, 72.

	1972 Population		1981 Rates
Age group	Non-Native	Native	All Manitobans
0–9	84,354	5,708	0.00
10–19	97,133	4,035	0.00
20–29	77,444	2,178	2.03
30–39	52,885	1,286	4.20
40–49	54,874	851	4.61
50–59	52,007	615	5.58
60–69	37,478	448	6.10
70–79	23,100	247	4.52
80+	13,101	114	3.30
All ages	492,376	15,482	2.82

(e) Compute first the SMRs (M = cholecystectomy rather than mortality) and then the indirectly standardized rates.

Source: Cohen et al. (1989)

3

Measuring Health and Disease in Populations (II)

Health Indicators and Indices

The various demographic indicators discussed in Chapter 2 are often used to characterize the health of a population. They involve only births and deaths, however, and there is more to life than just birth and death. The measurement of the health status of populations has preoccupied planners and researchers for a long time, and a large literature covering various theoretical and technical aspects now exists.[1]

The *Dictionary of Epidemiology* defines a *health indicator* as "a variable, susceptible to direct measurement, that reflects the state of health of persons in a community," the infant mortality rate being a prime example. Several indicators may be further combined into a *health index* based on a specified mathematical formula, such as the *health expectancy index* (see below). At the individual level, a *health index* is sometimes also used to refer to one constructed from responses to survey questionnaires, examples of which can be found in Box 3.3. An index can also transcend health to incorporate other spheres of human activity; for example, the *human development index* produced by the United Nations Development Program, which combines life expectancy, literacy, school enrollment, and per capita gross domestic product. While the terms *indicator* and *index* are often used interchangeably, it is useful to maintain the distinction.

It is also useful to distinguish *health data*, which refers to unprocessed numbers or observations, from *health information*, which results from an appropriate analysis of data. When the information has been interpreted, it becomes *health intelligence*, upon which informed decisions can be made.[2]

When the term *health indicator* is used, "health" can mean health *status*, health *determinants*, or health *care*. Other terms such as health *resources, capacities, consequences, systems, services*, and *programs* are also used but can ultimately be slotted into one of the three broad categories. There are, of course, many ways to classify and categorize health indicators.

BOX 3.1.   Health Indicators: A List of Lists

At the international conference on Primary Health Care at Alma Ata, USSR, in 1978, WHO declared the objective of "Health for all by the year 2000" (HFA2000 for short). To monitor and evaluate the impact of this global strategy, WHO compiled a core list of 20 "indicators of progress."[3] The year 2000 had come and gone, and clearly HFA2000 was far from being achieved, although much progress was made in terms of specific indicators in many countries.

In the United States, the CDC developed in 1991 a consensus set of 18 health indicators suitable for use by state and local health departments. In Canada, Statistics Canada and the Canadian Institute of Health Information (CIHI) collaborate in the production of a regularly updated compilation of health indicators, available on the web. Such indicators are grouped under:

1. Health status: well-being, health conditions, human function, deaths;
2. Non-medical determinants of health: health behaviors, living/working conditions, personal resources, environmental factors;
3. Health system performance: accessibility, appropriateness, effectiveness, efficiency, safety;
4. Community and health system characteristics: population, use of health services, health care resources.

The U.S. Department of Health and Human Services has embarked on the Healthy People initiative since 1979, which sets health objectives for the coming decade. It has now launched Healthy People 2010. To monitor progress, a set of 10 leading health indicators was chosen on the basis of their ability to motivate action, the availability of data, and their importance as public health issues:

1. Physical activity:
   —Proportion of adolescents who engage in vigorous physical activity that promotes cardiorespiratory fitness three or more days per week for 20 or more minutes per occasion;
   —Proportion of adults who engage regularly in moderate physical activity for at least 30 minutes per day.
2. Overweight and obesity:
   —Proportion of adults who are obese (body mass index $\geq 30\,kg/m^2$);
   —Proportion of children and adolescents who are overweight or obese (at or above the age- and sex-specific 95th percentile of BMI based on the CDC growth charts).
3. Tobacco use:
   —Proportion of adults who smoked >100 cigarettes in their lifetime and smoked on some or all days in the past month;

(continued)

—Proportion of adolescents who smoked one or more cigarettes in the past 30 days.
4. Substance abuse:
—Proportion of adolescents who reported no use of alcohol or illicit drugs in past 30 days;
—Proportion of adults who reported binge drinking in past 30 days' use;
—Proportion of adults who reported illicit drug use in past 30 days.
5. Responsible sexual behavior:
—Proportion of adolescents who abstain from sexual intercourse or use condoms if currently sexually active;
—Proportion of sexually active adults who use condoms.
6. Mental health:
—Proportion of adults with recognized depression who received treatment.
7. Injury and violence:
—Mortality rates from motor vehicle crashes and homicides.
8. Environmental quality:
—Proportion of persons exposed to air that does not meet the Environmental Protection Agency's health-based standards for ozone;
—Proportion of non-smokers exposed to environmental tobacco smoke.
9. Immunization:
—Proportion of young children aged 19–35 months who received all vaccines recommended for universal administration for at least five years (diphtheria/tetanus/pertussis; polio; measles/mumps/rubella; Haemophilus influenzae type b, and hepatitis B);
—Proportion of non-institutionalized adults aged 65 and above who received influenza vaccine in the past 12 months and who ever received pneumoncoccal vaccine.
10. Access to care:
—Proportion of persons under age 65 with health insurance coverage;
—Proportion of persons of all ages with a specific source of ongoing primary care;
—Proportion of pregnant women who received prenatal care in the first trimester.

(1)–(5), (8), and (9) can be considered indicators of health determinants; (2), (4), (6), and (7) are health status indicators; and (6), (9), and (10) are health care indicators. Some indicators belong to more than one category; for example, obesity, which is both a health condition and risk factor for other diseases; and immunization as a preventive health service is also a protective factor for infectious diseases.

Health indicators are used by health agencies, whether international, national, or regional, to monitor progress in the implementation of health programs or policies (see Box 3.1). To be useful, a health indicator should possess several characteristics. The Committee on Summary Measures of Population Health of the U.S. Institute of Medicine suggested the following:[4]

1. Reliability/reproducibility—i.e., repeated measurement under similar circumstances by the same or different individuals should produce the same results. For example, in administering a health survey, there should be no change in the proportion of the population who are smokers if the questionnaire is repeated after a week.
2. Validity—i.e., the indicator measures those properties, qualities, or characteristics it is intended to measure. For example, the death certificate should identify the most responsible cause of death, and not a disease that was present at the time of death but did not contribute to the death.
3. Sensitivity—i.e., it can detect differences or changes at a sufficiently fine level to be of interest to the users. The maternal mortality ratio (discussed in Chapter 2) is no longer a sensitive measure of the health status of pregnant women in developed countries because it is now so low.
4. Acceptability—i.e., the intended users should find the indicator understandable, credible and useful. Life expectancy is widely accepted because it is conceptually easily understandable even though its computation is complicated (see Box 2.5 in Chapter 2).
5. Feasibility—i.e., the data can be collected without undue administrative or financial burdens on the health system. Vital statistics are the barebones data source for several health indicators affordable by many governments. To go beyond it—for example, mounting longitudinal health surveys—would require substantial resources dedicated to the purpose.
6. Universality—i.e., it is adaptable to different populations/settings. Time-honored health indicators such as the infant mortality rate are understood universally and often used in international comparisons. Many measures of health determinants (such as education and income), are context and locality-specific.

Most health indicators are measured at the individual level—information is acquired from individuals, which is then aggregated upwards to the community and region. For example, the prevalence of smoking in a region is established by surveying individuals about their smoking habits. It is also possible to assess the extent of smoking, especially in making temporal or spatial comparisons, by using data collected at the aggregate or ecological level—in this case, the total number of cigarettes sold in a geographic area.

How much an individual actually smokes is not known. Sometimes data obtainable at one level are used at another level. For example, if direct inquiry as to individual income is impractical or too sensitive in a survey, the average income of all residents in one area as determined from the census is sometimes used to represent the income of individuals living in that area. On the other hand, while suicides are committed by individuals, the suicide rate of a community can be used as an indicator of social well-being, an ecological variable. It is then possible to compare individuals living in a high-suicide community with those in another community with a low rate, to determine the impact of living in such a social environment on their health, even though such individuals themselves did not commit suicide. Increasingly in population health studies, attention is directed towards multilevel analyses in order to obtain a fuller understanding of the scope of health problems and their determinants.

Health indicators have two primary functions—descriptive and evaluative—which are not always explicitly distinguished. For example, the traffic injury mortality rate as an indicator can simply be used to establish the scope of the problem and identify the need for special prevention strategies. The same indicator becomes a performance measure when it is used before and after an intervention program to evaluate how effective it has been.

Sources and Quality of Health Data

The health status of a population can be represented by a pyramid or iceberg (perhaps even a hippopotamus submerged in water). On the very top, representing the severest consequences of ill health, is mortality. The source of mortality data is usually death certificates maintained by the vital statistics system. Many developed countries also operate computerized mortality databases (e.g., the U.S. National Death Index and the Canadian Mortality Database), which allow the tracking of individuals over time (until death) using suitable identifiers. Each jurisdiction designs its death certificates; a prototype is the WHO's International Form of Medical Certificate of Cause of Death. The type of information captured tends to vary—race is de rigueur in the United States but verboten in Canada. Rules for assigning causes of death are laid down in the International Classification of Diseases (see below), and distinction is made between underlying, antecedent, and contributing causes. The mode of death (e.g., cardiac arrest) is not a cause of death; otherwise most deaths will be attributed to diseases of the heart. While time-honored, the quality of the information contained in death certificates is highly variable (see Case Study 3.1).

As most sicknesses do not result in death, it is evident that the pattern of mortality can only provide a partial picture. There is, however, no overall measure of morbidity. Some measures depend on contact with the health care system, such as hospital separations (departure from a hospital, either dead or alive) or ambulatory care visits; others are based on self reports in a survey setting.

The major sources of data from which health indicators can be compiled are shown in Table 3.1.

The various sources of data differ in terms of whether they obtain their information from individuals (a, b, e) or health care providers (b, c, d); and whether they are *active* [i.e., require special efforts to solicit and collect the information (a, c, e)] or *passive* [i.e., routinely submitted by other individuals or agencies (b, d)]. Some of these data sources are considered *primary*; i.e., new information collected specifically for the purpose of health monitoring (c, e), or *secondary*; i.e., designed originally for different purposes (a, b, d), such as the payment of hospitals and physicians. Finally, most data systems cover the entire population (a, b, c, d) while surveys (e) are conducted only on samples of the population.

The disparate sources of health data collectively constitute a *health information system* (HIS). HIS has been defined as "an organized set of activities

Table 3.1. Sources of Data Used in Compiling Health Indicators

Indicator	(a) Census	(b) Vital statistics	(c) Disease registries	(d) Health care admin databases	(e) Health survey
Health status					
Population/fertility	X	X			
Mortality		X	X		
Disease incidence/ prevalence			X	X	X
Disability/activity limitation					X
Perceived health					X
Health determinants					
Social/cultural/ economic factors	X				X
Personal lifestyles/ practices					X
Physical environment				X	
Human biological factors					X
Health care					
Utilization of services			X	X	
Perception of services				X	

and programs whose purpose is to gather, maintain, and provide health-related information in order to improve individual or population health." HIS can be quite complex and involves multiple agencies and jurisdictions.[5]

The estimation of disease incidence/prevalence requires the establishment of disease *registries*, based on health care records or special surveys of individuals involving clinical examination or laboratory tests. (Note: A register is the actual document, while *registry* is the system of ongoing registration.) Examples include registries for cancer, tuberculosis, other communicable diseases, birth defects, etc. Registries exist not just for diseases, but also for "at risk" behaviors and environmental hazards.

The incidence of various communicable diseases is more readily available as they are legally *notifiable* to the local health authorities, which can be aggregated nationally, although the completeness varies according to disease. In the United States, the National Notifiable Disease Surveillance System is operated by the Epidemiology Program Office of the CDC in partnership with the Council of State and Territorial Epidemiologists. Weekly reports on cases of various diseases notified appear in *Mortality and Morbidity Weekly Report* (MMWR) and annually as the *Summary of Notifiable Diseases*. In 1912, when the system's forerunner was instituted, there were only 10 notifiable diseases. The number had tripled by the 1930s, and surpassed 70 by 2001. Diseases were dropped (typhus in 1994; amebiasis, leptospirosis, granuloma inguinale, and nine others in 1995—a bumper year) and added (enterohemorrhagic *Escherichia coli* O157:H7 in 1994; hantavirus pulmonary syndrome and *Chlamydia trachomatis* genital infection in 1995; ehrlichiosis in 1999; listeriosis in 2000; giardiasis and West Nile encephalitis in 2002; varicella in 2003), reflecting the changing epidemiological significance of various diseases.[6]

Communicable disease surveillance in Canada is coordinated by the Population and Public Health Branch of Health Canada, in cooperation with the Advisory Committee on Epidemiology consisting of provincial and territorial epidemiologists. Surveillance data and relevant articles are published in *Canada Communicable Diseases Report* as well as *Disease Surveillance On-Line*.

As most noninfectious diseases are not notifiable, their incidence and prevalence can only be determined by special studies, and usually are only available locally or regionally. One exception is cancer, as registries have been established in most Western countries, if not nationally, at least in major cities and various regions (see Case Study 2.1 in the previous chapter). All Canadian provinces have well-established population-based cancer registries. In the United States, the Surveillance, Epidemiology, and End Results (SEER) program organized by the National Cancer Institute (NCI) began case ascertainment modestly in 1973 in five states and two metropolitan areas. By 2003 it had collected and published cancer incidence and survival data on over 25% of the country's population, including substantial proportions of minority populations such as African

Americans, Hispanics, and American Indians. Through the CDC's National Program of Cancer Registries, established in the early 1990s to support, enhance, and standardize cancer surveillance at the state level, comprehensive and accurate incidence data are now available for some 80% of the U.S. population.[7]

The existence of universal health insurance plans in all Canadian provinces and territories, all of which maintain databases of all hospital and physician-care utilization, can potentially provide a source of data on morbidity. The Canadian Institute of Health Information (CIHI) maintains a Hospital Morbidity Database of key clinical and demographic data obtained from all acute care hospitals in Canada.[8]

In the United States, utilization databases exist for specific beneficiary populations such as Medicare (for the elderly) and Medicaid (for the poor), and for enrollees of prepaid health plans and health maintenance organizations such as the Kaiser-Permanente system. The Centers for Medicare and Medicaid Services (formerly the Health Care Financing Administration) maintain the data and statistical systems and provide datafiles to the public. At the national level, the United States has to rely on the National Health Care Survey, a family of annual surveys of samples of health care institutions and providers (such as hospitals, physician practices, nursing homes) and their patient records.[9]

It should be recognized that health service utilization does not entirely reflect the burden of illness in a population. Many factors, such as those relating to access to, and availability of, health care facilities and the practice styles of health professionals, may account for the observed pattern. For hospital morbidity, "case," "episode," and "discrete patient" may not be readily distinguishable when individuals have multiple admissions or multiple diagnoses.

To "capture" information on health conditions that do not result in any kind of formal contact with the health care system, the only way is to ask people directly about them. Health surveys solicit the participants' subjective judgment of their health and/or recall of past health events. They provide an opportunity to gather data on health behaviors, practices, attitudes, and beliefs—more "positive" measures of health beyond those of death, disease, and disability. From such surveys, a variety of scales and indices can be constructed.

Health surveys require the cooperation of the respondents. The accuracy of their answers to specific questions may be affected by a variety of factors. Perception of health may be influenced by temporary health problems present at the time of the survey. Recall of past events may not be accurate, or altered to conform with social desirability and to please (or to get rid of) the interviewer. Responses may vary according to the method of data collection—by telephone, face-to-face interview, the order of the questions, the precise phrasing, the use of a "proxy" such as a spouse or parent, and whether it is coupled with clinical and laboratory tests, which may be inconvenient and time-consuming at best and painful and even

BOX 3.2.   Never-Ending Health Surveys

In the industrialized countries, health surveys are conducted from time to time to assess the health of the population.[10] In the United States, the National Health Interview Surveys (NHIS) have been conducted annually since 1957. There are also periodic surveys involving clinical examinations and laboratory tests—the National Health and Examination Surveys (NHES), three of which were conducted during 1960–1962, 1963–1965, and 1966–1970. After NHES III, a nutrition component was added, and the 1971–1974 cycle was named National Health and Nutrition Examination Survey, or NHANES I. This was followed by NHANES II (1976–1980), a special Hispanic HANES (1982–1984) and NHANES III (1988–1994). Participants of NHANES I have also been resurveyed in the Epidemiologic Follow-Up Study (NHEFS) in 1982–1984, 1986, 1987, and 1992. A voluminous library of documents covering the design, methods, and results of these surveys has been published by the National Center for Health Statistics.

Beginning in 1999, NHANES became a continuous annual survey, which is linked to NHIS at the primary sampling unit level (the same counties, but not necessarily the same individuals, will be in both surveys). The 1999/2000 NHANES data include the following:

- Examination: body measures (height, weight, waist circumference, skinfolds); blood pressure; lower extremity (status of peripheral circulation); and muscular strength;
- Laboratory: heavy metals (lead, cadmium, mercury, etc.); iron deficiency; vitamins; cardiovascular risk factors (cholesterol, triglycerides, fibrinogen, homocysteine); diabetes; bone health; immune status (for various infections); and a variety of blood and urine tests for renal, hepatic, hematological, and endocrine function;
- Interview: sociodemographic (including language and ethnic origin); general health status; past health; family history, dietary intake; physical functioning, selected symptoms (pain, respiratory, cardiovascular, skin, etc.); health care utilization; preventive services; work environment; smoking; social support, etc.

In Canada, a series of health surveys has also been conducted, including: Canadian Sickness Survey (1950–1951); Nutrition Canada Survey (1970–1972); Canada Health Survey (1978–1979); Canada Fitness Survey (1981); Canadian Health and Disability Survey (1983–1984); General Social Survey (1985, 1991); Canada's Health Promotion Survey (1985, 1990); Health and Activity Limitation Survey (1986, 1991); and the series of provincial Heart Health Surveys (1986–1992). Beginning in 1994/1995, the National Population Health Survey (NPHS) was launched on a biannual basis, including a longitudinal component where a cohort of individuals is re-surveyed at each cycle. The corresponding survey for children is the

(continued)

National Longitudinal Survey of Children and Youths. In 2000/2001, the Canadian Community Health Survey was conducted with the specific objective of providing health information at the level of health regions.

Some of these consisted of telephone interviews only, others involved face-to-face interviews with or without physical measurements and laboratory tests. Many of these datasets are available to individuals for independent analyses.

During 2002 and 2003, the Joint Canada–United States Health Survey was conducted by Statistics Canada and NCHS, a one-time telephone survey of both countries using the same questionnaire and methodology. In 2002, WHO also initiated the first round of the World Health Surveys to collect standardized and comparable data at relatively low cost from countries around the world. The surveys consist of several modules (e.g., health status, risk factors, health care coverage and expenditure) from which participating countries can choose, based on their national priorities and available resources.

Table 3.2. Comparison of Different Methods of Questionnaire Administration in Health Surveys[11]

Issue	Face-to-face	Telephone	Mail
Certain of respondent identity	yes	no	no
Respondent likely to omit items	no	no	yes
Can assess understanding of question	yes	yes	no
Illiteracy may be a barrier	no	no	yes
Can rephrase question, prompt, or probe	yes	yes	no
Can use open-ended questions	yes	yes	no
Respondent may be confused by non-applicable/ skipped items	no	no	yes
Costly to administer	yes	no	no
Requires rigorous training of interviewers	yes	yes	no
Interviewer's personal attributes may affect response	yes	yes	no
Can use visual aids for complex questions	yes	no	yes
Can obtain basic demographic data from nonrespondents	no	yes	no
Wide geographical coverage	no	yes	yes

dangerous at worst. (Table 3.2 compares the advantages and disadvantages of various methods of questionnaire administration.) The respondents' understanding of health and disease is also dependent on their cultural and ethnic background, gender, and socioeconomic status. Many studies have been conducted to assess the accuracy of recall of past illnesses in a survey setting, often by comparison with medical records, with or without additional clinical and laboratory studies. But, medical records themselves are not without problems.[12]

Overall health status is often assessed by the respondents' self-rating (typically into categories of "excellent," "very good," "good," "fair," and "poor"), usually in absolute terms, but sometimes also in comparison to others of similar age or to themselves in the past. Remarkably, *self-rated health* has been shown by many studies in a variety of populations to be a valid indicator of health, with the ability to predict future health outcomes such as mortality, morbidity, and the use of health services. Several reasons have been put forward to explain this phenomenon. In providing an answer, respondents may take into account the full array of health problems and symptoms, some of which are not yet detectable medically; knowledge of family history; and an assessment of severity. Although surveys are cross-sectional, the respondents' summation may provide a dynamic rather than static perspective. Individuals who perceive their health as poor may engage in behaviors and pattern of health care use (or nonuse) that may adversely affect their health. Finally, self-rated health may also encompass the presence or absence of internal and external resources that affect their ability to cope with future illness.[13]

Self-rated health is an attractive health indicator because of its simplicity—it is based on a single question in a survey. Over the years, many questionnaires have been designed to measure specific dimensions of health, some of which consist of many questions and can be time-consuming (Box 3.3).

As the definition and concept of *health* becomes broadened from its original biomedical orientation, it tends to resemble, and sometimes becomes indistinguishable from, *quality of life*. Quality of life is a rather broad and elusive concept, and encompasses notions of happiness, satisfaction, wealth, and well-being. Clinical researchers (for example, oncologists and rheumatologists) are drawn to it as they need a tool to assess the effects of treatment beyond merely prolonging life and relieving symptoms. Quality of life is far more dependent on an individual's values and subjective judgment of what is desirable and undesirable than on an expert's objective assessment. In public health, rather than having to deal with the entire range of human experience, which is what "quality of life" implies, the more restrictive concept of *health-related quality of life*, or HRQOL, has gained popularity since the 1980s as an indicator of health disparities, service needs, and intervention outcomes. Donald Patrick and Pennifer Erickson defined HRQOL as the "value assigned to duration of life as modified by the impairment, functional states, perceptions, and social opportunities that are influenced by disease, injury, treatment, or policy."[14] There are many survey-based instruments to assess HRQOL. The CDC promotes the use of a relatively simple index called *healthy days*. It is based on one question to elicit self-rated health and three questions on the

---

BOX 3.3.   Assessing Health with Questionnaires

The comprehensive guide to health status measurement by Ian McDowell and Claire Newell described and evaluated some 88 rating scales and questionnaires.[15] Many of these are administered by clinicians for screening and staging specific diseases and evaluation of treatment. The following is a partial list of generic (rather than disease-specific) survey instruments intended for the general population which can be self-administered:

- Physical functioning and disability
  The OECD Long-Term Disability Questionnaire (1981): 16 items
  The Medical Outcomes Study Physical Functioning Measure (1992): 14 items
- Social health
  The Rand Social Health Battery (1978): 11 items
  The Medical Outcomes Study Social Support Survey (1991): 20 items
- Psychological well-being
  The Health Opinion Survey (1957): 20 items
  The Affect Balance Scale (1965): 10 items
  The General Health Questionnaire (1972): 60 items
- General health status and quality of life
  The Quality of Well Being Scale (1973): 18 items
  The McMaster Health Index (1976): 59 items
  The Sickness Impact Profile (1976): 136 items
  The Nottingham Health Profile (1981): 45 items
  The Short-Form-36 Health Survey (1990): 36 items
  The EuroQol Quality of Life Scale (1990): 5 items

---

number of days during the past month when physical health was not good, when mental health was not good, and when usual activities were limited because of poor physical and mental health.

The usefulness of different sources of health data, such as vital statistics, health insurance claims, and special surveys, can be enhanced when they are linked electronically, provided that they share some common identifiers such as a personal number, birthdate, etc. In the 1940s, Halbert Dunn, an early advocate of *record linkage*, used the analogy of assembling a "book of life" from birth till death with its pages consisting of all important life events. The tremendous advances in computer technology since then have made the process possible at relatively low cost and high speed. Not only does it provide comprehensive descriptive information on particular health conditions, data linkage can be used effectively to test specific etiological hypotheses through long-term

BOX 3.4.   The Capture-Recapture Method of Case Ascertainment

In order to determine if a data collection system or method is complete in its coverage or case ascertainment, the capture-recapture method can be used.[16] Originally developed for counting wildlife populations (whereby animals are captured, tagged, released, and recaptured) and by demographers working for the U.S. Census, this method requires obtaining the same data from two parallel systems; for example, disease registries vs. vital statistics; surveys vs. health services data.

	Source A		
Source B	No. reported	No. missed	Total
No. reported	R_{AB}	b	R_B
No. missed	a	X	
Total	R_A		N

The total number of cases identified by each source, R_A and R_B are known. By finding out those cases reported by both sources (R_{AB}), the total population (N), the number of cases missed by each source (a and b), and the unknown number of cases missed by both sources (X) can be determined as follows:

The probability of being captured by both sources (R_{AB}/N) is the product of the probability of being captured by source A (R_A/N) and the probability of being captured by source B (R_B/N):

$$\text{Thus, } R_{AB}/N = (R_A/N)(R_B/N) = R_A R_B/N^2$$

Solving the equation, $N = R_A R_B/R_{AB}$

From there, the rest of the table can be filled out.

$$\text{Since } R_A R_B = (R_{AB} + a)(R_{AB} + b) = R_{AB}^2 + aR_{AB} + bR_{AB} + ab$$
$$= R_{AB}(R_{AB} + a + b) + ab$$

$$N = R_A R_B/R_{AB} = [R_{AB}(R_{AB} + a + b) + ab]/R_{AB}$$
$$= (R_{AB} + a + b) + ab/R_{AB}$$

Since N is also equal to $(R_{AB} + a + b) + X$, therefore $X = ab/R_{AB}$

Note that some authors add a correction factor, such that

$$N = [(R_A + 1)(R_B + 1)/(R_{AB} + 1)] - 1$$

$$X = ab/(R_{AB} + 1)$$

(continued)

The completeness of ascertainment of source A is R_A/N, and for source B is R_B/N. An example can be found in Exercise 3.2.

Although the method is attractive, there are two important assumptions: (1) the two sources of capture should be independent of each other; and (2) all individuals have the same probability of being captured. These assumptions are not always met. Most data sources in the health system tend to function closely and cooperatively, and being captured by one source increases the likelihood of also being captured in the other. In any system, those who are clinically more severe tend to be captured more easily.

followup of large groups of individuals with specific exposures—for example, an occupational group or users of certain medications. Individuals who participated in a national survey can also be linked to the vital statistics database to study the mortality risks associated with specific lifestyles and behaviors.[17] To protect privacy and confidentiality, most databases in the public domain usually have the names of individuals deleted before they are made available to researchers. Depending on the number, type, and quality of unique identifiers, linkage can be made on the basis of an exact match (referred to as *deterministic* linkage) or based on a set of decision rules to assess the probability of two records' being from the same person (*probabilistic* linkage). Data linkage is technically complex and requires the services of experienced computer programmers.

Most sources of data on the health of populations are national in scope and they are usually funded and maintained by government agencies. Some individuals resent the intrusion and invasion of privacy that they involve. In the case of health surveys, there is provision for refusal to participate. Data linkage, on the other hand, can occur without the knowledge of individuals whose records from different databases are being linked. Some social scientists actually regard surveys and other tools of health surveillance as means of social control. In his *Political Anatomy of the Body*, a critique and "deconstruction" of medical knowledge, David Armstrong provided a history of the use of surveys in population health assessment in England. He observed that "the survey, a mechanism for 'measuring' reality, could be transformed into a technology for the 'creation' of reality; the tactics of the survey could make the operation of disciplinary power throughout a society more effective and more efficient." The extensive use of health surveys after World War II heralded in an era of "surveillance medicine," when everyone, healthy or ill, is targeted. Normality becomes "problematized" and illness becomes localized outside the space of the body.[18]

Summary Measures of Population Health

A type of health index that has gained increasing acceptance is one that combines both mortality and morbidity (or disability) in a single number. Unfortunately there is a multitude of such *summary measures of population health*, which have similar sounding names and confusing acronyms (DFLE, DALE, DALY, HALE, QALY, HLY, etc). They all comprise mortality, but differ in the way morbidity/disability is measured: whether activities of daily living, self-rated health, or activity limitation (both institutional and non-institutional) are used singly or in combination; and whether some sort of valuation or weighting is incorporated.

There are two basic types: *health expectancy* and *health gap* measures. Health expectancy is analogous to *life expectancy*. Instead of estimating the number of years just being alive, the number of years lived free of disability or in various shades of compromised health is computed. Health gap is analogous to premature mortality (one measure of which—*potential years of life lost*—is discussed in Chapter 2), and represents the difference between the current health of the population with an ideal situation where everyone lives to old age in full health. An example is *disability-adjusted life years* (DALY), which is the sum of the years of life lost due to premature mortality and the years lost due to disability.[19]

Figure 3.1 illustrates the conceptual difference between these two types. There are three survival curves, which show the proportion of the original members of a hypothetical cohort who die (line m) or become ill and disabled (line n) as time goes on. The two curves demarcate three areas, A, B, and C. Area C represents the years that are lost to death. Area A

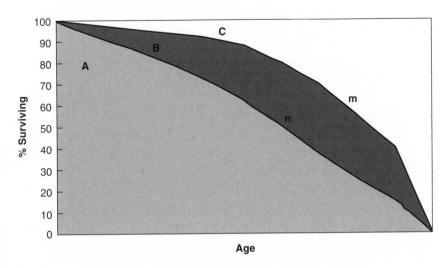

Figure 3.1. Survival curves of a hypothetical population.

encloses the years of perfect health (or at least free of disability, however defined). Area B includes different levels of health between death and perfect health. The population of Utopia would not follow either curve m or n, but go horizontally (along the top line of the rectangle) in perfect health until some ripe old age and then die (at the right-hand side of the rectangle). Health expectancy measures attempt to capture areas A or A and some portion of B. Health gap measures cover area C and some portion of B.

Summary measures of population health are now available for many countries. It is possible to construct time series of changes in *disability-free life expectancy* (DFLE) in several countries in Europe, North America, and Japan, with some dating back to the 1970s. In these countries the increase in life expectancy has not been accompanied by an increase in the time spent with severe disability. There is no clear trend, however, when the index is based on disability with all severity levels combined.

WHO began comparing summary measures of population health among member states in its *World Health Reports,* based on the massive amount of data collected by the Global Burden of Disease Project team of Christopher Murray, Alan Lopez, and others. It introduced *disability-adjusted life expectancy* (DALE) in the 2000 report, but changed its name to *health-adjusted life expectancy* (HALE) the following year. This differs from DFLE in that health or disability is not treated as dichotomous (yes/no, present/absent), but based on a set of health states and weights defined in terms of valuations. DALY, a health gap measure, was added to the 2002 WHO report, but had been used earlier in the 1993 *World Development Report* produced by the World Bank, which had health as its theme.

Again, it needs to be emphasized that numbers are not value-free. Summary measures such as DALY have been criticized for their explicit presupposition that disabled people's lives have less value than those of people without disabilities. Since such measures are used not just for describing the health of a population, but also advocated for use in resource allocation as a common "currency" across diseases, disabled people would become less entitled to scarce health resources for interventions that would extend their lives.[20]

Diagnosis and Classification of Diseases

In Chapter 1 various definitions of health are provided. In measuring health and disease in populations, a decision is often necessary to distinguish what is "normal" and what is "abnormal." Many biological variables, such as weight, blood pressure, and serum levels of various chemicals, are continuously distributed, and arbitrary cutoff points have to be used to categorize individuals into the normal (or healthy) and abnormal (or diseased). There are four approaches:

1. *Statistical*: Based on the distribution of the variable, an arbitrary level (e.g., 2 standard deviations from the mean, top 20%, etc.), is set beyond which a value is considered to be "abnormal." While convenient, this method is not suitable for comparing populations, since the level when abnormality begins is unique for each population. Yet, if the proportion of individuals with abnormal levels is to be compared, it will be exactly the same for all populations!

2. *Clinical*: For some physiological measures, extreme levels are often associated with clinical signs and symptoms (e.g., headaches for high blood pressure, fainting for low blood sugar). The levels at which such signs and symptoms are present can then be defined as "abnormal." These levels may not be consistent, however, and may cover too broad a range of values to be of practical use. Asymptomatic individuals may still be at risk for serious problems—hypertension and diabetes, for example, have been called the "silent killers."

3. *Prognostic*: If a long-term epidemiological study shows that a certain level is associated with an increased risk of developing or dying from a disease (e.g., diastolic blood pressure above 90 mmHg), then that level can be regarded as the boundary between "normal" and "abnormal." Data, however, are not always available for many conditions.

4. *Operational*: Individual practitioners in public health or clinical medicine may decide, based on whatever available evidence or criteria, that when certain levels are exceeded, some action will be instituted (e.g., drug therapy, dietary advice, mass hysteria!).

The task of assessing health status in a population is not a simple matter of dividing individuals into two groups, normal and abnormal. It is important to know what kinds of diseases there are and their relative frequency. In counting cases of disease, it is important to have a disease *classification system* and some means to ensure that different people doing the counting use the same *diagnostic criteria*. There must also be some means to assess the *diagnostic accuracy* attained, otherwise the whole counting exercise becomes meaningless. In these respects, the population health specialist has the same concern as the clinician in patient care.

Case definition is very important in epidemic investigations, particularly in situations where a new disease is discovered (such as AIDS or Lyme disease). Without an operational case definition, no estimate of the extent and severity of the problem can be relied on, and no rational means of control can be developed. As more knowledge accumulates, the case definition may be modified, which sometimes can create problems for comparison. A case may be temporarily assigned the status of "suspected" and upgraded to "probable" and "confirmed" as more information, especially laboratory tests, becomes available. Note that clear, unequivocal definitions and criteria are the exceptions rather than the rule in clinical medicine. For some diseases, there are international agreements on case

---

BOX 3.5.   Words and Origins

The classification, arrangement, and cataloguing of diseases is sometimes referred to as *nosology*, which may also be used to mean the study of disease classifications. Nosologists are usually to be found in medical records departments of health care institutions or vital statistics agencies. The word has nothing to do with *nose*, which comes from the Old English *nosu*, but is derived from the Greek *nosos*, meaning "disease." The branch of biology dealing with classifications is called *taxonomy*, from the Greek *taxis*, meaning "arrangement" (and not the four-wheeled variety).

An early work of nosology called *Nosologia Methodica* was published by François Bossier de Lacroix (1706–1777). William Cullen (1710–1790) published *Synopsis Nosologiae Methodicae* in 1785, a system that remained in use until the nineteenth century. While pioneers such as William Farr (1807–1883) made attempts at classification, it was Jacques Bertillon (1851–1922) who developed the first numerically based system arranged in chapters. It was adopted by the International Statistical Institute conference in 1893, the first of a series of international statistical congresses from which the modern disease classification system evolved.

Infections acquired in health care facilities are called *nosocomial* infections, whose control is an important task of hospital epidemiologists.

---

definition and diagnostic criteria; for example, the WHO criteria for diabetes mellitus, the Minnesota Code for resting electrocardiographs, and the Rose Questionnaire for symptoms of cardiovascular diseases. Increasingly new "diseases" are proposed that are characterized by chronic, vague somatic symptoms involving multiple body systems (chronic fatigue syndrome, Gulf War syndrome, multiple chemical sensitivities, sick building syndrome, etc.). They pose particular difficulty for developing and agreeing on case definitions and diagnostic criteria.[21]

The *International Classification of Diseases* (ICD) has been periodically revised under the auspices of the World Health Organization. The ninth revision was adopted in 1975. A modified version, called ICD-9-CM, was commonly used in North America for morbidity data derived from hospital and ambulatory care records. The long-overdue tenth revision was approved by the World Health Assembly in 1990 and the manual published in 1992. It was not until 2000 and beyond that countries such as the United States and Canada began to change over to ICD-10.[22]

The necessity of periodic revisions is evident from the fact that there was no Legionnaire disease, Lyme disease, or AIDS when ICD-9 was first adopted in the 1970s. Viral hepatitis has expanded from a single code to five separate ones in ICD-10. (The nosological saga of AIDS is described in Box 3.6.)

BOX 3.6.   The Changing Classification and Definition of AIDS

AIDS, the Acquired Immunodeficiency Syndrome, first came to the attention of the CDC in 1981, when an outbreak of the rare and deadly *Pneumocystis carinii* pneumonia was reported among homosexual men in San Francisco. It was soon followed by similar outbreaks in other cities. The clinical picture was characterized by severe and rare infections and also tumors (such as Kaposi sarcoma) that afflict immunosuppressed patients. Initially labeled "Gay-Related Immune Disease" (GRID), the etiology was finally elucidated in 1984 when almost simultaneously a French and an American team led by Luc Montagnier and Robert Gallo, respectively, identified the virus, which was eventually named Human Immunodeficiency Virus (HIV).[23]

The changes in the knowledge of the etiology of AIDS are reflected in how the disease was classified. In 1984–1985, AIDS was given the ICD-9 code of 279.19, after the existing 279.1 for "deficiency of cell-mediated immunity" in Chapter III (which groups immune disorders with endocrine, metabolic, and nutritional disorders). In 1986, code 795.8 was allocated, following the existing 795.7 for "other non-specific immunological findings" in Chapter XVI (Signs and Symptoms). After 1987, the NCHS created a new category of 042-044 for AIDS, firmly putting it among other infectious diseases in Chapter I. In ICD-10, AIDS occupies codes B20–B24. It has thus gone through both the clinical and pathogenetic stages of classification (as an immunodeficiency disease) to finally end up at an etiological one (a viral infection).

As the epidemic evolved, a working definition was established by CDC in 1982 to track the spread of the disease nationally. This was revised in 1985 and 1987. The complex definition, described in a 15-page booklet complete with flow diagrams and several appendices, took into account the results of the HIV test, with an expanded list of AIDS-associated diseases for persons who are HIV-positive.

In an investigation of the impact of the change in definition, it was found that 28% of AIDS cases diagnosed in the United States since the 1987 revision would not have been counted as cases under the previous definition. It also changed the distribution of risk groups. Thus, under the old system, heterosexual intravenous drug abusers (IVDA) accounted for only 18% of all cases; under the new system, they accounted for 35%. The proportion of cases who were homosexual non-IVDA men decreased from 63% to 43%.

In 1993 there was yet another revision of the case definition, although only involving relatively minor changes, with three additions to the 23 clinical conditions associated with AIDS. In 1999 a further revision consolidated both HIV infection and AIDS into a single case definition and incorporated findings from new DNA and RNA-based laboratory tests.

(continued)

American essayist and critic Susan Sontag published *AIDS and Its Metaphors* in 1988, as a follow-up to her earlier *Illness as Metaphor* where she explored the social stigmatization of people with cancer, when the "reputation of the illness added to the suffering of those who have it." Sontag considered that AIDS marked "a turning point in current attitudes toward disease in general and to medicine, as well as to sexuality and to catastrophe." The creation of the status of the HIV-positive person has radically expanded the notion of illness to include those who are "seemingly healthy but doomed," and a "new class of lifetime pariahs, the future ill."

There are many ways to classify diseases. At the most superficial and descriptive level is *clinical* classification. This is based on the signs and symptoms only; for example, the presence of fever. This may be superseded later with better understanding of the disease process by a *pathogenetic* classification. Ultimately we wish to be able to achieve an *etiological* classification; i.e., according to "causes." From a prevention perspective, diseases can also be classified according to their manner of control, which is often more useful in practice than a classification based on disease etiology or clinical characteristics (Box 3.7).

As Table 3.3 shows, the ICD is a mixture of different "axes" of classification, which may be based on anatomical site (diseases of musculoskeletal, nervous system), causal agent (infectious diseases, injuries), disease mechanism (neoplasms, metabolic diseases), or specific age-sex group (perinatal conditions, pregnancy and childbirth). Chapter I, for example, does not include all infectious diseases, as meningitis is grouped with the diseases of the nervous system, pneumonia with the respiratory system, pyelonephritis with the genitourinary system, etc. For injuries, Chapter XIX refers to the nature of the conditions such as burns, fractures, asphyxiation, etc., whereas Chapter XXI lists them by "external causes"; for example, motor vehicle collision, fires, falls, suicide, etc. Chapter XXI does not deal with diseases at all, but with the reasons for people making contact with the health care system; for example, well-child visits, insurance medical examination, screening tests, and so forth. Note that ICD-10 uses alphanumeric rather than numeric codes, a departure from previous editions.

Family doctors (and other primary-care practitioners) are often confronted with patients presenting with vague and ill-defined health problems rather than clear-cut, discrete diseases. The "reasons for encounter" include symptoms, complaints, concerns, fears, and psychosocial issues. The *International Classification of Primary Care* was developed by the World Organization of Family Doctors (WONCA) to capture more accurately the content of family practice. It strives to incorporate within one system the patients' reasons for visit, the doctors' diagnostic labels, and the interventions that ensued. The most recent version (ICPC-2-Electronic) was released in 2002. It is complementary and convertible to ICD-10.[24]

BOX 3.7.   A Prevention-Oriented Classification for Water and Sanitation-Related Diseases

In developing countries, many infectious diseases are associated with inadequate sanitation and water supply. While a common practice is to classify these diseases etiologically according to the organism into *viral, bacterial, protozoan,* and *helminthic,* from the standpoint of control measures, it is not very useful. A prevention-oriented system has been suggested:[25]

1. *Waterborne diseases:* Water as passive vehicle of transmission and contamination occurs through poor excreta disposal (e.g., cholera, typhoid, giardiasis, amebiasis, hepatitis A); control by improving water quality and sanitation.
2. *Water-washed diseases:* Insufficient water use and poor personal hygiene favor spread (e.g., scabies, skin infections, typhus, trachoma); includes also certain intestinal infections related to poor excreta disposal (e.g., dysentery, salmonellosis, enteroviruses, ascariasis, enterobiasis); control by increasing water quantity, improving personal hygiene and sanitation.
3. *Water-based diseases:* A necessary part of the life cycle of infectious agent is in an aquatic animal (e.g., schistosomiasis, dracunculosis); control by reducing contact with infested water, protecting water source, and improving excreta disposal.
4. *Water-related vector-borne diseases:* Spread by insects that breed in water or bite near it, unrelated to excreta disposal (e.g., yellow fever, filariasis, malaria, onchocerciasis, sleeping sickness); control by providing reliable water supply, avoiding contact with infested water sources; ecological management such as clearing bush, draining stagnant waters, etc.
5. *Excreta disposal diseases:* Not already included in above (e.g., fish tapeworms and liver flukes); control by improving sanitation and health education for eating well-cooked fish and seafood.

Health status encompasses more than mortality and morbidity. Measures of health should not be concerned just with the presence or absence of specific diseases and their diagnostic labels, but also their consequences in terms of disability and the functional status of the individual. The World Health Organization published in 1980 an *International Classification of Impairments, Disabilities and Handicaps.* It differentiates these three common, interchangeably used terms. *Impairments* refer to loss or abnormality of function or structure at the organ level (e.g., loss of eyesight). An impairment may result in a *disability* if it affects the functional activity of the individual (e.g., a blind person's inability to drive). A *handicap* results if

Table 3.3. Chapter Headings in ICD-10 and Corresponding ICD-9 Codes

Chapter	ICD-10 code	Rubric		ICD-9 code
I	A00–B99	Certain infectious/parasitic diseases	I	001–139
II	C00–D48	Neoplasms	II	140–239
III	D50–D89	Diseases of blood/blood-forming organs/	IV	280–289
		certain disorders involving the immune mechanism	III	279
IV	E00–E90	Endocrine/nutritional/metabolic diseases	III	240–278
V	F00–F99	Mental/behavioral disorders	V	290–319
VI	G00–G99	Diseases of nervous system	VI	320–359
VII	H00–H59	Diseases of eye/adnexa	VI	360–379
VIII	H60–H95	Diseases of ear/mastoid process	VI	380–389
IX	I00–I99	Diseases of circulatory system	VII	390–459
X	J00–J99	Diseases of respiratory system	VIII	460–519
XI	K00–K93	Diseases of digestive system	IX	520–579
XII	L00–L99	Diseases of skin/subcutaneous tissue	XII	680–709
XIII	M00–M99	Diseases of musculoskeletal system/connective tissue	XIII	710–739
XIV	N00–N99	Diseases of genitourinary system	X	580–629
XV	O00–O99	Pregnancy/childbirth/puerperium	XI	630–676
XVI	P00–P96	Certain conditions originating in perinatal period	XV	760–779
XVII	Q00–Q99	Congenital malformations/deformations/chromosomal abnormalities	XIV	740–759
XVIII	R00–R99	Symptoms/signs/abnormal clinical/laboratory findings	XVI	780–799
XIX	S00–T98	Injury/poisoning/certain other consequences of external causes	XVII	800–999
XX	V01–Y98	External causes of morbidity/mortality	Supplementary	E800–E999
XXI	Z00–Z99	Factors influencing health status/contact with health services	Supplementary	V01–V82

a disabled person cannot fulfill her or his usual role in his particular social and cultural milieu (e.g., a blind person's chronic unemployment due to discrimination). This was replaced in 2001 by the *International Classification of Functioning, Disability and Health* (ICF). ICF is not just a system of classification, but also a conceptual framework to describe and understand the components and domains of health and functioning in their social and physical environmental context.[26]

ICF consists of two parts, each with two components. Within the components are *domains*. Each component and domain can be expressed in positive and negative terms:

Part 1. *Functioning and Disability*:

    a. *Body Functions and Structures*: within this component are domains corresponding to the various body systems (e.g., the structure of the nervous system and mental function, the musculoskeletal system and movement). Each domain can be rated by an *impairment* scale from 0 (no impairment) to 4 (complete impairment).

    b. *Activities and Participations*: *Activities* refer to the execution of tasks or actions by individuals, while *participation* refers to involvement in life situation. Examples of domains include general tasks and demands, mobility, interpersonal interactions and relationships, and community, social, and civic life. Each domain is rated in terms of the extent of *participation restriction* and *activity limitation*, from 0 (no difficulty) to 4 (complete difficulty).

Part 2. *Contextual Factors*:

    c. *Environmental Factors*: refer to the physical and social environment in which people live and conduct their lives, and include access to products and technology, the extent of family support and social relationships, and societal attitudes and policies. Each domain can be rated in terms of *barriers* (from 0, no barrier, to 4, complete barriers) and *facilitators* (from 0, no facilitator, to +4, complete facilitator).

    d. *Personal Factors*: although recognized as part of the system, these are not formally classified or rated, but instead relevant factors to be recorded (e.g., social background, ethnicity, sexual orientation, past life events, etc.).

The ICF, although invaluable for clinicians, especially rehabilitation specialists, is also useful at the population level. Aggregation of individual assessments in institutions or communities can provide useful measures of health outcomes, quality of life, and health services needs, and serve as a tool for social policy design and public education.

Accuracy of Screening and Diagnostic Tests

The purpose of a test is to separate diseased from non-diseased individuals. *Screening* tests are usually simple affairs that can be done cheaply, quickly, and on a large scale (more about them in Chapter 7) but require further confirmation by more elaborate *diagnostic* tests. To assess how accurate a diagnostic or screening test is, it is necessary to compare its performance (in discriminating disease from non-disease) with some *gold standard*. Unfortunately, the gold standard is usually some other existing, established test. In clinical situations, autopsy or biopsy findings are usually considered closest to the truth as to whether pathology exists. In public health screening, the screening test is usually compared to a more cumbersome laboratory procedure (such as measuring height and weight and comparing them to various physiological measures of body fat). The relationship between the gold standard and results of the test can be shown in a 2×2 table.

Test results	"Truth/gold standard"		
	Disease	No disease	
Positive	a (TP)	b (FP)	(a + b)
Negative	c (FN)	d (TN)	(c + d)
Total	(a + c)	(b + d)	N

TP refers to *true positive*, FP to *false positive*, TN to *true negative*, and FN to *false negative*.

The ability of a test to identify correctly those who have the disease is referred to as its *sensitivity*, which is thus the proportion of those who test positive among those who truly (according to the gold standard) have the disease. The *specificity* is the ability of the test to identify correctly those who do not have the disease, and is the proportion of those who test negative among those who truly do not have the disease. Sensitivity is sometimes represented by α and specificity by β.

Expressed in terms of the 2×2 tables:

$$\text{Sensitivity} = a/(a + c) = TP/(TP + FN)$$
$$\text{Specificity} = d/(b + d) = TN/(FP + TN)$$

The proportion of individuals whose disease status a test correctly identifies (the sum of the true-positives and true-negatives) out of the total population is the *accuracy*.

$$\text{Accuracy} = (a + d)/(a + b + c + d) = (TP + TN)/(TP + TN + FN + FP)$$

It can be seen that terms that are in everyday use such as "accurate," "sensitive," and "specific" have been given very specific (!) meanings.

It is helpful also to express how many times a positive test is more likely to occur in someone who has the disease than in someone who does not—this is called the *likelihood ratio* for a positive test (LR+):

$$LR+ = \frac{a/(a+c)}{b/(b+d)} = \frac{\text{sensitivity}}{(1-\text{specificity})}$$

Alternatively, it is also the ratio of the proportion of true positives (TP) among disease cases to the proportion of false positives (FP) among non-cases.

Similarly,

$$LR- = \frac{c/(a+c)}{d/(b+d)} = \frac{(1-\text{sensitivity})}{\text{specificity}}$$

or the ratio of the proportion of FN among cases to the proportion of TN among non-cases. A test with a sensitivity of 90% and specificity of 80% will gives a LR+ of 0.9/0.2 or 4.5 and a LR− of 0.1/0.8 or 0.125.

From the perspective of the individual being tested, the most important question is: "If the test comes back positive (or negative), what does it mean to me? What are my chances of actually having (or not having) the disease?" Given a positive test, the probability that an individual will have the disease is called the *positive predictive value* (PPV). Given a negative test, the probability that an individual will not have the disease is the *negative predictive value* (NPV). From the table, it can be seen that:

Positive Predictive Value = a/(a + b) = TP/(TP + FP)

Negative Predictive Value = d/(c + d) = TN/(TN + FN)

Before a test, the only clue to how likely it is that a patient will have the disease comes from the prevalence of the disease in the patient's population; that is, (a + c)/N from our table. This is sometimes also called the *pre-test* (or *prior*) *probability* of disease. After the test, the *post-test* (or *posterior*) *probability* is none other than the positive predictive value. Tests that result in substantial changes between the two are useful to the clinician.

Terms such as *prior* and *posterior probability* are derived from *Bayesian* statistics, named after the Reverend Thomas Bayes (1701–1761), a major figure in that branch of mathematics known as *conditional probability*. Bayes' theorem (posthumously discovered) can be applied to the screening test situation (or indeed any clinical decision-making) as:

$$P(D_1|T) = P(T|D_1)P(D_1)/[P(T|D_1)P(D_1) + P(T|D_0)P(D_0)$$

The notation $P(x)$ refers to the probability of x, and $P(x|y)$ the probability of x occurring, given y, (i.e., conditional on y being present). $P(D_1)$ thus means the probability of disease, $P(D_0)$ the probability of non-disease, $P(D_1|T)$ the probability of disease given a positive test, $P(T|D_1)$ the probability of a positive test in the presence of disease, and $P(T|D_0)$ the probability of a positive test in the absence of disease.

$P(D_1|T)$ is the posterior probability of disease (positive predictive value)
$P(D_1)$ is the prior probability of disease (prevalence of disease)
$P(D_0)$ is the prior probability of non-disease (prevalence of non-disease)

The astute reader will notice that $P(T|D_1)$ is just another way of expressing the sensitivity (proportion of positive tests among the diseased) and $P(T|D_0)$ the proportion of false-positive among the non-diseased, or $(1 - \text{specificity})$.

Rephrasing Bayes' theorem, the positive predictive value is equal to:

$$\frac{\text{(sensitivity)(prevalence of disease)}}{[\text{(sensitivity)(prevalence of disease)} + (1 - \text{specificity})(\text{prevalence of non-disease})]}$$

It can be seen that the PPV of a test depends on its sensitivity and specificity as well as the prevalence of the disease. For a given sensitivity and specificity, PPV will fall as the prevalence decreases. This is shown numerically in Box 3.8. Screening tests are often used in different situations. In a population where the prevalence is high, such as among patients in a referral clinic, the PPV is higher than when the same test (with the same sensitivity and specificity) is performed in a predominantly healthy population. The negative predictive value, on the other hand, declines with increasing prevalence.

As the definition of abnormality in many diseases is based on often arbitrary cutoff points of physiological variables that are continuously distributed (e.g., plasma glucose for diabetes), moving the cutoff point up or down can have an effect on the specificity and sensitivity of a test (Box 3.9).

Where should one "draw the line"? This very much depends on the consequences of being wrong; i.e., whether it is preferable to be labeled FN or FP. If a disease is such that being labeled FN has grave consequences (e.g., an HIV-positive person incorrectly tested negative is given a false sense of security, and then carries on with unprotected sex, thus endangering others), one would want FN to be as low as possible, and the sensitivity as high as possible. If a disease is such that being FP is undesirable (e.g., a healthy woman incorrectly tested positive on Pap smear may be subjected to unnecessary surgery and/or radiation treatment), one would want FP to be as low as possible and the specificity as high as possible.

BOX 3.8.   Effect of Changing Prevalence on Predictive Values of a Test

Suppose a hypothetical screening test has a sensitivity of 90% and specificity of 80%. The same test is applied in three different populations where the prevalence of disease is 1%, 20%, and 50%. The notations a, b, c, d are as used in the previous 2 × 2 table.

	Prevalence		
	1%	20%	50%
Population (a + b + c + d)	1,000	1,000	1,000
No. of diseased (a + c)	10	200	500
No. of non-diseased (b + d)	990	800	500
No. of true positive (a) = 0.9 (a + c)	9	180	450
No. of true negative (d) = 0.8 (b + d)	792	640	400
No. of false negative (c)	1	20	50
No. of false positive (b)	198	160	100
Positive predictive value [a/(a + b)]	4.3	52.9	81.8
Negative predictive value [d/(c + d)]	99.9	97.0	88.9

It can be seen that, even with a good test with high sensitivity and specificity, applying it in a low-prevalence population will result in a disappointingly low PPV.

There is thus a trade-off between sensitivity and specificity—increasing one will be at the expense of the other. Altering the cutoff point for "normal" and "diseased" will affect the sensitivity and specificity of a test in identifying cases of disease. It is possible to plot a curve: called a receiver-operator characteristic (ROC) curve.[27] The ROC plots the sensitivity on the y axis and the false-positive proportion (the proportion of FP among the non-diseased, which equals 1−specificity). The diagonal straight line represents cutoff points where there is a 50:50 (random) chance that those with disease will show up positive or negative on the test. (Note that this is also where the LR is 1.0.) The point on the curve where it is the most convex—closest to the upper left corner—is the ideal cutoff point, offering the highest possible sensitivity with the lowest possible FP proportion (highest specificity). Note that the ROC can be replotted with sensitivity against specificity, which is a mirror image of the traditional ROC (see Exercise 3.3 for an example with "real" data).

The ROC can be used for finding the best cutoff point for a test, or it can be used to compare the performance of several tests for the same disease condition. (See Figure 3.2.)

BOX 3.9.   Effect of Changing Cutoff Points on Sensitivity and Specificity

Generally there is no problem in choosing a suitable cutoff point if the diseased (D_1) and non-diseased (D_0) populations are clearly separated according to the test measure:

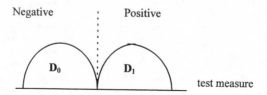

This does not happen very often, and some overlap between the two populations usually occurs:

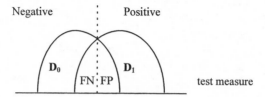

When the cutoff point is progressively moved up (the criteria becoming more stringent), FP is progressively reduced (and eventually eliminated), resulting in an increasing specificity:

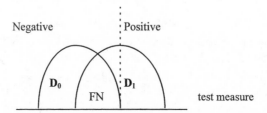

On the other hand, if the cutoff point is progressively moved down (the criteria becoming more lenient), FN is progressively reduced (and eventually eliminated), resulting in an increasing sensitivity:

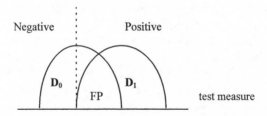

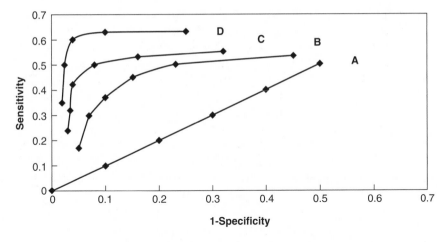

Figure 3.2. Receiver-operator characteristic (ROC) curves.

Curve A, a diagonal straight line, describes a situation where the test is of no use as sensitivity is equal to the FP at every cutoff point. Curves B and C are progressively better, and D is best. The value corresponding to the most convex part of each curve offers the best trade-off between sensitivity and specificity.

Other methods can be used to compare test results, which do not entail designating one test as the gold standard. There are occasions when comparisons need to be made between two different observers (e.g., pathologists and radiologists), or the results reported by the same observer at different times.

	Observer A		
Observer B	**Positive**	**Negative**	
Positive	a	b	(a + b)
Negative	c	d	(c + d)
Total	(a + c)	(b + d)	N

One way is to report the *percent agreement*, which is obtained from $(a + d)/(a + b + c + d)$. Note that this is essentially the same as *accuracy* as defined earlier. However, a high percentage agreement can occur because of the large number of negative tests (i.e., d is very large). This may obscure the considerable disagreement that may exist in reporting a positive test. One modification is to ignore the cases when both observers report negative results, eliminating d from both the numerator and the denominator:

$$\% \text{ agreement} = a/(a + b + c)$$

Another problem is that a certain degree of agreement will always occur simply by chance alone. (Students who are experts at multiple-choice
examinations will attest to the benefit of guesswork.) The kappa statistic
remedies this problem by providing a measure of agreement over and
above that which is due to chance. Its formula is as follows:

$$\text{kappa} = (P_o - P_e)/(1 - P_e)$$

where P_o is the proportion of subjects who are observed to be "concordant," to agree in terms of both "positive" and "negative"; and P_e is the
proportion of subjects expected to be concordant based on chance alone.

$$P_o = a + d$$

$$P_e = [(a + b)(a + c) + (c + d)(b + d)]/N^2$$

Kappa values can range from -1 (complete disagreement) to $+1$ (complete agreement), with 0 representing agreement due to chance. Most researchers tend to consider kappa values above 0.60 as good and above
0.80 as excellent.[28]

So far the 2×2 tables are applied when a screening or diagnostic test is
being evaluated. More often, the purpose of population screening is not to
evaluate a test, but to attempt to find out the prevalence of a disease or
characteristic. Suppose the screening reveals that the prevalence is x%.
Since the survey tool used is unlikely to be 100% sensitive and specific, the
true prevalence should exclude the false positives from among those who
have tested positive, but add on the false negatives from among those
who have tested negative. If the screening test one uses has known sensitivity (α) and specificity (β) established in other studies, one can adjust the
prevalence estimate as follows:

$$p = (p' + \beta - 1)/(\alpha + \beta - 1)$$

where p is the "true" (more accurately the "misclassification-adjusted")
prevalence and p' is the observed frequency of positive tests (consisting of
an unknown mix of TP and FP).[29] An example can be found in Exercise 3.4.

Surveillance and Epidemic Investigations

The ongoing systematic collection, analysis, and interpretation of outcome-
specific data for use in planning, implementing, and evaluating public
health practice is called surveillance.[30] Historically, *surveillance* refers to
the monitoring of cases of infectious diseases and their contacts. (The term
has a military and French origin, and was purportedly introduced into the
English language at the time of Napoleon.) Its use has been much broadened: for example, from infectious diseases to noninfectious diseases, to

the adverse effects of mass immunization programs (e.g., polio, swine flu), and new drugs on the market; and from diseases to risk factors such as nutrient intake, smoking, and alcohol use in the population. In its broadest sense, it encompasses the whole data-management function of population health practice and research.

By establishing baseline rates of disease and time trends through surveillance, it is possible to detect or anticipate disease outbreaks and to institute control measures. Continuing surveillance can also become an evaluation tool of the control program and policy. (Case Study 3.2 discusses the course of the diphtheria epidemic in the Russian Federation during the 1990s, and Exercise 3.5 is based on the investigation of the anthrax outbreak in the United States in 2001.)

Surveillance can be passive or active. *Passive* surveillance refers to the routine reporting of special health events (e.g., notifiable diseases) to health authorities by health care institutions and practitioners, usually mandated by law (but rarely enforced). The major drawback is a lack of compliance, resulting in gross underreporting of most conditions of interest. However, if the extent of underreporting is consistent, a passive system can still provide important trend data.

Active surveillance is more resource-intensive but tends to be more complete. It involves reaching out to various sources to solicit information on a regular basis.

Sentinel surveillance refers to the collection from a limited number of population sites and service providers of a limited number of health indicators. Even though the data may not be representative of the entire population, they can still provide important aids to policy, planning, and evaluation, whether to obtain a national picture of the burden of certain diseases, or more restrictively, in relation to specific health programs. It should be less expensive than full surveillance of the total population, and is particularly appropriate in jurisdictions where such a system is lacking. "Sentinel" conveys a sense of an "early warning"—like surveillance, "sentinel" also has a military origin. Hence one speaks of sentinel health events, sentinel sites, and sentinel providers.

In the course of surveillance, an *outbreak* of a particular disease may be detected. What should happen next? Note that the difference between "outbreak" and "epidemic" is subtle; the former is used more in the context of a local event, and the latter if it involves large numbers of people and covers a wider geographic area. The public tends to find "epidemic" more frightening than "outbreak." The key condition is that the number of cases must exceed the expected. Hundreds of cases of influenza in midwinter in a typical North American city by themselves are no cause for concern. A single case of smallpox, in a world where the disease has been eradicated, is a dire emergency. A *cluster* is used to refer to cases occurring together in time and space, which do not require any reference to the expected frequency.

Outbreak investigation usually applies to infectious diseases, but the same principles can be applied to hazardous exposures. Such investigations are characterized by the need for immediate action and decisive judgment. Sometimes it may also become necessary to compromise somewhat the usual standard of methodological rigor. The 1995 movie *Outbreak* (starring Dustin Hoffman) and best-sellers such as Richard Preston's *The Hot Zone* and Laurie Garrett's *The Coming Plague* have popularized the outbreak investigation and the threat of emergent infections. In the aftermath of the September 11, 2001, terrorist attacks in the United States, the threat of bioterrorism has refocused the public's (and governments') attention on the need to strengthen public health capacity and infrastructure.

An outbreak investigation follows several steps. These steps are not inflexible, and often several steps have to be taken simultaneously, or in circular loops, rather than in neat, linear sequence.

1. Prepare for fieldwork
2. Establish the existence of an epidemic
3. Verify the diagnosis
4. Establish a case definition
5. Characterize by time, place, and person
6. Develop a hypothesis
7. Test the hypothesis
8. Initiate control measures
9. Evaluate control measures
10. Communicate the findings

The time of occurrence of the cases can be plotted on an *epidemic curve* and the place (both workplace and residence) on a map. These often provide useful clues to the type of epidemic and possible routes of spread. John Snow (mentioned in Case Study 1.2 in Chapter 1) used such a map in investigating cholera deaths on Broad Street and its environs in London. Much progress has been made since Snow's "spot map," and today the medical geographer and spatial epidemiologist have at their disposal a sophisticated array of computer-based tools (both hardware and software) to capture, manage, analyze, and display health information, organized as a *geographic information system* or GIS.[31]

An epidemic can be characterized by its source, type of exposure, and the routes of spread. Many people may become exposed simultaneously to a *common source*—for example, drinking from the same contaminated well, eating spoiled food from the same wedding banquet. The epidemic curve is usually of short duration with a high peak and rapid decline. In a *propagated* epidemic, usually one person develops the disease first (the *index case*), who then passes it on to others, who in turn pass it on to still others; i.e., *person-to-person* spread. The epidemic curve may have a prolonged, "undulated" pattern. If the spread is rapid and explosive, however, the epidemic curve may resemble that of a common-source epidemic.

There are several common *routes of spread*—airborne, fecal-oral, skin contact, exchange of body fluids, parenteral, and vector-borne. A *vector* is usually an insect or other arthropod that carries the pathogen from an infected person to another person either directly (e.g., by biting) or by depositing it in his surroundings (e.g., food) from which he can then contract the disease. A *fomite* is an inanimate object that has been contaminated with the pathogen and can convey an infection to others (e.g., clothing, toys, and the public's greatest fear—toilet seats!).

The regularly updated *Control of Communicable Diseases Manual* published by the American Public Health Association provides useful advice on the appropriate control measures, such as isolation, disinfection, quarantine, treatment, prophylaxis, immunization, vector control, and so on.

The methods of the social sciences have an important contribution in *rapid field assessments* in the context of disease control programs. Intensive field research using such qualitative methods as key informant interviews, focus groups, and participant observations (see Chapter 6), covering a relatively small number of individuals or households in a limited time can often isolate the key behavioral and cultural variables, providing insight into and understanding of the cause of the epidemic and the likelihood of success in controlling it.[32]

Cultural Concepts of Health and Disease

It is a central theme of this book that social and cultural factors are critically important to the study and practice of population health. In this chapter the manner in which cultural knowledge and understanding of health and disease affect the assessment of population health status is discussed. Chapter 4 explores the role of culture as a determinant of health and disease, while Chapter 7 investigates sociocultural barriers to population health interventions.

It is important first to clarify certain basic concepts, and there are none as fundamental as the concepts of *culture* and *society*. A much-quoted definition of *culture* is that provided by Edward Tylor (1832–1917), one of the "fathers" of British social anthropology: "that complex whole which includes knowledge, belief, art, morals, law, custom, and any other capabilities and habits acquired by man as a member of society." There have probably been as many definitions since then as there are anthropologists, and any introductory textbook of anthropology will offer one. Much is also made of the distinction between "culture" and "society." Mervyn Susser, in his textbook of medical sociology, states that society is a:

> system of social relationships that characterizes some particular aggregate of individuals who are dependent upon one another for survival

and procreation, and who as a group enjoy some measure of political independence.

Culture, on the other hand, refers to a:

> system of values and meanings in terms of which social behavior takes place. It is pre-eminently symbolic in nature, a body of tradition borne, enacted and shared by members of a society and transmitted from one generation to the next. It includes norms, values, knowledge, and belief that serve as standards of behavior and that define a way of life peculiar to that society or a segment of it.[33]

It should be noted that most modern societies contain more than one culture. Societies are also stratified according to age, sex, education, ethnicity, income, language, etc. Former British prime minister Margaret Thatcher once claimed: "There is no such thing as society. There are individual men and women, and there are families." This is a rather extreme libertarian and individualistic view, and most population health researchers and practitioners would contend that "society" not only exists, it is more than just a collection of individuals and has its own characteristics and qualities. Indeed, increasingly, societal or community-level factors need to be considered alongside individual-level ones in models of disease causation.

It is also important to distinguish between *disease, illness*, and *sickness*, a distinction not often made in general usage or in the biomedical literature. Disease is the underlying structural and functional disturbance of the human body, which is observable by an individual or a health care provider as signs and symptoms and labeled as deviation from the norm. Illness is the personal and subjective experience of the disease, while sickness is the societal response to the individual's illness, affecting his or her relations with others. The psychiatrist Leon Eisenberg succinctly distinguished between the professional and popular ideas of sickness thus: "Patients suffer 'illnesses,' doctors diagnose and treat 'diseases.' " In a treatise on the doctor–patient relationship, Eric Cassell wrote:

> "Illness" stands for what the patient feels when he goes to the doctor and "disease" for what he has on the way home from the doctor's office. Disease, then, is something an organ has; illness is something a man has.[34]

In studying cultural phenomena, anthropologists often make the distinction between what is *emic* and what is *etic*. These terms have their origins in linguistics, having been extracted from "phon*emic*" and "phon*etic*." "Emic" refers to what is perceived and understood by members of a particular culture, while the "etic" represents the viewpoint of the external observer, who in the context of population health, is usually someone trained in the Western biomedical and scientific tradition. The Western biomedical model, while undoubtedly predominant and pervasive in the world today, is often automatically assumed to have universal validity. Yet it is but one of many conceptions of health and disease amidst the diversity of concepts and models developed by every human culture down the ages in every corner of the earth. The study of non-Western, indigenous medical systems is called *ethnomedicine.*

It is evident that ethnomedical approaches to disease diagnosis and classification need to be recognized in any exercise in health needs assessment, particularly in the cross-cultural setting. Traditional epidemiology, confident of its tools and techniques, has been criticized for forsaking the richness of a people's way of living for quantitative rigor.[35] The equivalence of disease concepts across cultures has to be painstakingly established through ethnographic field work, and is not simply a matter of translating names. Even the concept of life and death itself may be modified by culture. For example, infants who die shortly after birth before naming or baptism may not even be considered to have been born, let alone reported to a government agency. Ethnomedical knowledge would be essential in the detection of such "hidden" deaths and in establishing accurate causes of death.

In some cultures, the endemicity and prevalence of certain diseases may result in their signs and symptoms (e.g., hematuria in schistosomiasis, a parasitic disease) being considered as "normal" and not requiring medical attention. Thus culturally determined health-care-seeking behavior can affect a population's health status assessment, particularly in utilization-based morbidity indicators. Stigmas associated with certain diseases may also result in preventing their existence from being broadcast beyond the family or village, and thus have implications for disease surveys.

Implicit in the discussion so far is that Western biomedical knowledge is the "gold standard" against which ethnomedical concepts are gauged. There are social scientists who argue that Western biomedical knowledge is just as much a product of the Western culture. "Reality" and "objectivity" are "socially constructed" and do not have an independent existence. A disease exists because someone describes and defines it, reflecting prevalent social, cultural, and political values. For example, infant mortality is an important measure in population health. Yet it is not necessarily a universal, "natural" concept whose existence and importance is self-evident. Indeed it was not until the early 1900s that infant mortality came to be seen as "a problem about which something ought to be done." The medicalization of child care is considered by some to be a social construction, reflecting changing medical attitudes to infancy and associated with the ascendancy of the germ theory. On the other hand, the cultural anthropologist Alexander Alland, Jr., cautioned that an ethnomedical perspective can obscure the ecological relationships that constitute the real epidemiological patterns of a population (to which the relativist would retort that the patterns are "real" only in the mind of the Western scientist).[36] While it is important to recognize that there is a pool of infant deaths that are not being counted for cultural reasons, adopting the ethnomedical definition of infant death would in fact lead to an underestimation of a major public health problem. The factors that give rise to infant deaths would still persist, whether the deaths are counted or not.

The role of culture is even more important in the field of mental health. Of particular interest are the so-called *culture-bound syndromes*, usually first recognized by Western observers in "exotic" colonial lands and believed to be unique to the particular local culture without a parallel in Western biomedical nosology. A famous example is *amok*, a homicidal frenzy among the Malays, a term that has entered into everyday English vocabulary. Considerable debate has centered on whether these are different diseases or only different clinical manifestations, but culturally mediated versions, of diseases known to Western culture. There is a broader issue of whether there exists a universal, pan-human core group of psychiatric disorders that are "culture-free" and reducible to biological dysfunction. The psychiatrists' diagnostic bible, *Diagnostic and Statistical Manual of Mental Disorders*, now in its fourth edition, does address cultural issues in diagnosis but relegates culture-bound syndromes to a list of "exotica" in the appendix, reflecting the Western bias of the American Psychiatric Association. Some psychiatrists have argued that chronic fatigue syndrome and anorexia nervosa are just as culture-bound as various syndromes from non-Western cultures.[37]

Summary

This chapter continues the discussion on the methods of measuring health and disease in populations. It goes beyond the basic demographic indicators of birth and death to the use of health status indicators and indices. The sources of information include death certificates, morbidity data derived from health service utilization, special disease registries, and health surveys. The linkage of different health databases can enhance the ability to describe the health status of a population. Summary measures of population health include both health gap and health expectancy measures attempt to combine mortality with morbidity/disability in a single number. Any method to measure the magnitude and extent of a disease requires diagnostic criteria and a classification system, preferably ones that are internationally agreed upon. How a disease is defined and classified can affect the apparent frequency of its occurrence. The diagnostic accuracy of tests can be assessed using such measures as sensitivity and specificity, percent agreement, and the kappa statistic. The systematic collection, analysis, and interpretation of population health data is referred to as *surveillance*, which is essential to establishing baseline trends of disease occurrence. When the "usual" has been exceeded, an *outbreak* is said to occur, which should trigger a series of steps to investigate and control it. Finally, health status assessment does not occur in a social and cultural vacuum, but must take into consideration ethnomedical concepts of disease and approaches to diagnosis and classification.

Case Study 3.1.   Are Death Certificates Accurate?

Much of our knowledge of the changing pattern of mortality in populations is derived from death certificates. In a study comparing autopsy reports and death certificates in Connecticut, major disagreement was found in 29% of 272 cases, which would require reclassification of the cause of death in the death certificates.[38] For specific categories of diseases, the following 2×2 tables can be constructed:

		Cancer		Circulatory diseases		Respiratory diseases	
		Autopsy results		Autopsy results		Autopsy results	
		Yes	No	Yes	No	Yes	No
Death	Yes	41	7	59	20	5	11
certificate	No	6	218	13	180	10	246

Using autopsy results as the "gold standard," the "test" characteristics of death certificates with regard to the different diseases are:

	Cancer	Circulatory diseases	Respiratory diseases
Sensitivity	$41/(41+6) = 87\%$	$59/(59+13) = 82\%$	$5/(5+10) = 33\%$
Specificity	$218/(7+218) = 97\%$	$180/(20+180) = 90\%$	$246/(11+246) = 96\%$
Accuracy	$(41+218)/272 = 95\%$	$(59+180)/272 = 88\%$	$(5+246)/272 = 92\%$
PPV	$41/(41+7) = 85\%$	$59/(59+20) = 75\%$	$5/(5+11) = 31\%$
NPV	$218/(6+218) = 97\%$	$180/(13+180) = 93\%$	$246/(10+246) = 96\%$

Put in other words:

- "Of those who truly died of cancer, the death certificate was able to identify 87% of cases";
- "Of those who truly did not die of circulatory diseases, the death certificate was able to identify 90% of cases";
- "With regard to death from respiratory diseases, the death certificate was able to identify correctly their presence or absence in 92% of cases";
- "If a death certificate indicates a death from cancer, there is a 85% chance that the deceased did indeed die from cancer; for respiratory diseases, there is only a 31% chance";
- "If a death certificate indicates that someone did not die from circulatory diseases, there is a 93% chance that that person truly did not die from them."

Beyond the problem of diagnostic accuracy, there is also the issue of single vs. multiple causes of death. Mortality statistics have traditionally been based on a single cause for each death. This is adequate for infectious diseases but not so appropriate for the chronic diseases, many of which may coexist in the same individual. Multiple cause-of-death data are particularly useful in providing more accurate trend data, explaining mortality differentials between populations, investigating associations between diseases, and examining the impact of removing competing risks.

For some years the proportion of deaths, even hospital deaths, that are followed by an autopsy has been declining in most jurisdictions in North America. In remote regions and most developing countries, the lack of adequate resources results in even lower autopsy rates. Furthermore, a high proportion of deaths occurs among individuals with little or no medical care prior to death, making an "intelligent guess" about the cause of death difficult. One approach to improve the quality of mortality data is the *verbal autopsy*, which involves questioning the next-of-kin or other informants using symptom lists and diagnostic algorithms for classification.

Case Study 3.2.   Diphtheria in Russia—Return of a Vanquished Foe?

Diphtheria is an acute infectious disease caused by the bacteria *Corynebacterium diphtheriae*. It is characterized by the formation of a false membrane in the throat, other mucous membranes, or skin. There the bacteria produce a toxin, which causes damage in other parts of the body, including the heart and nerves, and can be fatal. Although antibiotics kill the bacteria, antitoxin is needed to counteract the effects of the bacterial toxin already in the body. Infection can be prevented by vaccination with a toxoid, a substance that acts like the toxin in provoking an immune response from the body. (Use of the toxoid vaccine is called *active immunization*, whereas the use of antitoxin, which contains ready-made antibodies, is called *passive immunization*).

At the beginning of the twentieth century, diphtheria was a leading cause of childhood mortality in the industrialized countries in the temperate zone. With the introduction and widespread use of an effective vaccine since the 1930s and 1940s, there has been a rapid decline in the incidence and mortality of the disease. In North America, the annual incidence rate is at the level of 0.05/100,000.

During the 1990s, following the dissolution of the Soviet Union, an explosive epidemic of diphtheria occurred in many of the newly independent states, especially in the Russian Federation, Central Asia, the Caucasus, and the Baltics. The causes, course, and control of this epidemic provide many valuable lessons for public health. It

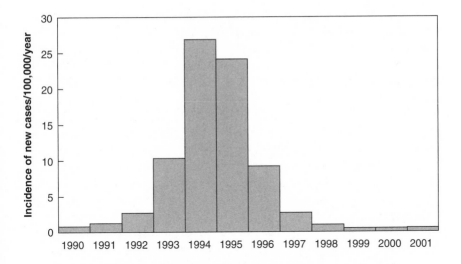

demonstrates that an old, and long thought to be vanquished, disease can reemerge in modern society and cause extensive illness and death.[39]

Universal childhood immunization was implemented in the USSR in the late 1950s. By the mid-1970s, the incidence rate of diphtheria was comparable to that of the United States, at $<0.1/100,000$. It gradually crept up in the early 1980s, reaching a peak of $0.9/100,000$ in 1984. Vigorous control measures brought the rate down to $0.3/100,000$ in 1989. Then, in the 1990s, as the above epidemic curve shows, it went through the roof, reaching a peak of $27/100,000$ in 1994.

Of the 115,000 new cases reported in the Russian Federation during 1990–1997, there were 3,000 deaths (a case–fatality ratio of about 3%). Most of the cases and deaths occurred among adults. The tide was turned towards the end of the decade, and by 2001, the incidence was finally brought down to the level of the 1980s.

Many factors, some biological, others sociopolitical, are believed to be responsible for the upsurge of a disease that had been under control. A high proportion of adults were susceptible to the disease, with the waning of vaccine-induced immunity during childhood in the absence of routine adult revaccination, setting the stage for the epidemic. There may have been introduction of new strains of the bacteria. Most urban dwellers live in crowded apartments, which promoted the transmission of the bacterial agent. The economic crisis of the post-Soviet era exacerbated the poor living conditions. With a large standing army of conscripts, huge numbers of susceptible young adults were brought together from across the land into crowded barracks and then redistributed afterwards, facilitating the spread. The breakup of the Soviet Union also resulted in large-scale population movements, especially of ethnic Russians back to the Russian heartland from the Far East, Central Asia, and the

Caucasus. The deterioration of the health care infrastructure, which had begun even before the breakup, hampered the production and distribution of vaccines and delayed the implementation of controls.

Aggressive measures were undertaken, with massive, nationwide immunization campaigns directed at both children and adults, at work sites, and in house-to-house visits. School entry booster dosing, which had been dropped in the mid-1980s, was reinstituted. By the end of 1995, childhood coverage with the primary series at one year of age had exceeded 90%, compared to less than 70% in 1990. Adult coverage with one or more doses in the previous 10 years was estimated at 75%. The worst of the epidemic was finally over.

Case Study 3.3.   Is Schizophrenia Universal?

Schizophrenia, one of the psychoses, is characterized by such signs and symptoms as delusions, hallucinations, disorganized speech, catatonic behavior, and flattening of the affect. It is associated with considerable social dysfunction and is a major cause of long-term institutionalization in mental hospitals. While the disease has probably existed since antiquity, the modern clinical concept originated with the seminal work of psychiatrists Emil Kraepelin (1855–1926) and Eugen Bleuler (1857–1939). The psychiatric profession has long been curious whether schizophrenia exists across cultures. Indeed, the "universality" of schizophrenia has important implications for our understanding of its etiology and treatment.

In the late 1970s, the World Health Organization sponsored a collaborative study on the frequency and clinical features of schizophrenia in 12 catchment areas in 10 countries. Cases of individuals with suggestive psychotic symptoms were searched from a variety of "helping agencies," including health and social services, religious centers, and traditional healers, who then underwent standardized diagnostic procedures. It was found that in eight sites with good coverage, the first-contact incidence varied from 1.5 to 4.2 cases/10,000 age 15–54/years, using a "broad" definition; whereas the range was much narrower, from 0.7 to 1.4, if a "restrictive" definition was used. The researchers concluded that there was a core syndrome that appeared to vary little across cultures.

The WHO study has been criticized by various scholars for its bias in favor of "universality" and for ignoring the cultural context in which the illness occurs.[40] Arthur Kleinman, a psychiatrist and anthropologist, called the imposing of nosological categories developed in one particular culture on another culture for which it lacks coherence and validity, *category fallacy*.

Even neighboring European countries such as England and France differ significantly in the first admission rate of schizophrenia, its

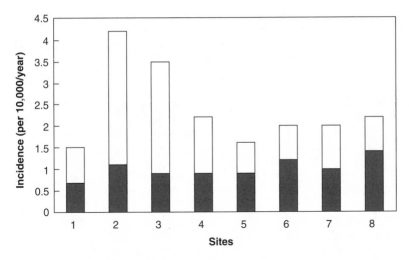

Note that the total height of the bar represents the incidence according to the *broad* definition; the dark-shaded area represents the *restrictive* definition.

age-specific incidence, and time trend. This is attributed to the different diagnostic practices of the psychiatric professions in the two countries, which have very different medical and intellectual traditions, between "Anglo-Saxon empiricism and continental rationalism— between trying to reach the truth through experiment and trying to reach it through ideas."

Notes

1. See the reviews by Donovan et al. (1993) and McHorney (1999).
2. The definition of a health indicator appears in Last (2001:83), and the distinction between data, information, and intelligence is made by Spasoff (1999:59). The ranking of countries according to the human development index appears annually in the UNDP's *Human Development Report* (www.undp.org). Up until 2000, Canada had ranked number one, when it was edged out by Norway and Sweden, much to the consternation of politicians who had been claiming credit. The United States ranked sixth.
3. See WHO (1981), Zucconi and Carson (1994), and the *Healthy People 2010* web site (www.health.gov/healthypeople/).
4. See the report by the IOM Committee on Summary Measures of Population Health (Field and Gold, 1998).
5. Teutsch and Churchill (2000:33).
6. Description of the National Notifiable Disease Surveillance System and the current list of diseases can be found in the Epidemiology Program Office's web site (www.cdc.gov/epo/). Health Canada's Disease Surveillance On-Line, which also includes cancer, cardiovascular diseases, and injuries, can be accessed at www.hc-sc.gc.ca/pphb-dgspsp/dsol-smed/.

7. Connecticut has the oldest population-based cancer registry in the United States. In 2002, *United States Cancer Statistics: 1999 Incidence* was released, based on data collected from cancer registries from 37 states, six metropolitan areas, and the District of Columbia, which have met stringent criteria for accuracy, completeness, and timeliness. It is available from the CDC web site (www.cdc.gov/cancer/ npcr/uscs/).

8. The health insurance database in the Canadian province of Manitoba has been the source of many health services research projects, examining surgical procedures, screening and preventive services, physician practice patterns, and the incidence and prevalence of chronic diseases. Considerable effort has been devoted to determining the quality and accuracy of such an administrative database (Roos et al., 1993). Two supplements to *Medical Care* (vol. 33, no. 12, Dec. 1995; and vol. 37, no. 6, June 1999) focused on research using this unique database. CIHI, an independent, not-for-profit organization, was established in 1994 by amalgamating the private Hospital Medical Records Institute and various health information programs of Health Canada and Statistics Canada. Its mandate was established jointly by federal, provincial, and territorial health ministers. It publishes *Health Care in Canada* annually. It maintains a variety of health services databases and registries. For more information, see www.cihi.ca.

9. A list of Medicare and Medicaid databases is available from www.cms. hhs/gov/. More information on the surveys included under the National Health Care Survey umbrella (e.g., National Ambulatory Medical Care Survey, National Hospital Discharge Survey, etc.) can be found in the NCHS web site (www.cdc/ gov/nchs/nhcs.htm). For a review of the use of Medicaid and Medicare data in descriptive and analytical epidemiological studies, see Bright et al. (1989) and Lauderdale et al. (1993), respectively. Caution must be exercised in using automated systems of patient discharge abstracts as sources of morbidity data. A study of the U.S. Veterans Administration system (Lloyd and Rissing, 1985) found 82% discordance, with physicians contributing to over 60% of the errors. Many diseases that were treated affected length of stay, or used hospital resources were not coded and captured by the database.

10. Further information on national health surveys can be found in the web sites of NCHS (www.cdc.gov/nchs/) and Statistics Canada (www.statcan.ca). The World Health Surveys are described in the WHO web site (www3.who.int/whs). For a review of the Canadian national health surveys, see Kendall et al. (1997). For an international perspective on the contributions of national health surveys to health policy, see Kars-Marshall et al. (1988). The NCHS publishes the *International Health Data Reference Guide*, a compendium of major national health surveys from many countries.

11. For further details, see Chapter 13 of Streiner and Norman (1995).

12. Harlow and Linet (1989) reviewed the concordance of survey data with medical records. Table 3.2 is based on Chapter 13 of Streiner and Norman (1995). Studies have been done to compare various data collection methods in terms of costs and quality of data; e.g., by O'Toole et al. (1986) among Australian veterans and by Siemiatycki (1979) in an urban Canadian population, with different results.

13. See the comprehensive review by Idler and Benyamini (1997). A classic study was that of Mossey and Shapiro (1982), who showed that elderly Canadians' self-rated health was a better predictor of seven-year survival than medical records. Segovia et al. (1989) showed that self-rated health correlated also with utilization-based morbidity measures such as physician visits and hospital days.

14. See Patrick and Erickson (1993:22) for the definition of HRQOL and chapters 3 and 4 for the theoretical foundations of the concept. The CDC's Health Days

instrument has been used in both the Behavioral Risk Factor Surveillance System (BRFSS) and National Health and Nutrition Examination Survey (NHANES). There is also a longer, 14-question version (HRQOL-14). See www.cdc.gov/ncchphp/hrqol/pdfs/mhd.pdf.

15. See McDowell and Newell (1996), who provide references to the original publications, studies using and evaluating them, and contact addresses.

16. For a more detailed methodological discussion, see Hook and Regal (1995). Tilling (2001) suggested improving incomplete registers by identifying patient characteristics related to the probability of capture through multivariate modeling.

17. See Dunn (1946), now a classic, and the handbook by Newcombe (1988). Spitzer et al. (1992) linked the Saskatchewan Prescription Drug Plan with mortality and hospital data to determine if the use of certain asthma drugs is associated with an increased risk of death and near-death. Yassi et al. (1994) linked a cohort of workers in an electrical transformer manufacturing plant with the Canadian Mortality Database to determine if exposure to polychlorinated biphenyls (PCBs) is associated with an increased risk of cancer.

18. See Armstrong (1983:43) and Armstrong (1995).

19. The concept was advanced by Sanders (1964) and a method of computation proposed by Sullivan (1971). For further discussion of methodological issues, see the critical review by Murray et al. (2000) and Gold et al. (2002). Robine et al. (1999) analyzed international trends in DFLE. The *active life expectancy* (Katz 1983) uses an index of activities of daily living (ADL) as the morbidity measure. At the NCHS, Erickson et al. (1995) computed *years of healthy life* using both self-rated health and activity limitation from the National Health Interview Survey, whereas Molla et al. (2001) used only self-rated health from the NHIS. In Canada, Wilkins and Adams (1983) developed a *quality-adjusted life expectancy* based on both survey data on activity limitation and institutional data on long-term care, while Wolfson (1996) computed a version of *health-adjusted life expectancy* using the Health Utilities Index, which is a survey-based preference measure of functional status.

20. The methodology used by WHO in creating DALE/HALE and DALY is detailed in a series of working papers of its Global Programme on Evidence for Health Policy (www3.who.int/whosis/discussionpapers/). See also Murray (1994) and Mathers et al. (2001), and the ethical critique by Arnesen and Nord (1999). The Global Burden of Disease project is described in a series of four papers in the *Lancet* by Murray and Lopez (1997).

21. The diabetes criteria can be found in WHO (1985). The Minnesota Code and the Rose Questionnaire can be found in the manual for cardiovascular survey methods (Rose et al., 1982). Hyams (1998) discusses the poor specificity of diagnostic criteria for the new syndromes.

22. A brief history of the evolution of ICD can be found in the Introduction to volume 2 of ICD-10 (WHO, 1992). The dates of the various revisions are: 1st (1900), 2nd (1910), 3rd (1920), 4th (1929), 5th (1938), 6th (1946), 7th (1955), 8th (1965), 9th (1975), 10th (1990). Until the sixth revision, it was called *International List of Causes of Death*. With the sixth revision, the word *Diseases* was added before *Causes of Death*. The ninth revision is called *International Statistical Classification of Diseases, Injuries, and Causes of Death*, while the tenth simplified the title to *Diseases and Related Health Problems*.

In the United States, the NCHS began using ICD-10 for mortality statistics only in 2000. No date has been set for the implementation of ICD-10-CM. In Canada, ICD-10 is used by Statistics Canada for mortality applications. CIHI is preparing an enhanced version (ICD-10-CA) for morbidity classification to replace ICD-9-CM.

23. For revisions of the CDC case definition of AIDS, see *MMWR* 1985; 34:373–75; 1987; 36 (Suppl 1); 1993; 41(RR–17); and 1999; 48(RR–13). The study on the effects of change in definition was conducted by Selik et al. (1990). The quotations are from Sontag (1988:12, 72, 33–34).

24. The scheme originated in the work in East Africa by White, Bradley, and White described in *Drawers of Water*. It has been adapted and reproduced in Saunders and Warford (1976) and Cairncross et al. (1980).

25. The ICPC was first published in 1987 and displaced other systems then in use, including ICHPPC (*International Classification of Health Problems in Primary Care*), which first appeared in the 1970s, and last revised in 1983 as ICHPPC-2-Defined. ICPC-2 was first published in book form in 1998. See Lamberts and Wood (2002). The WONCA web site is www.globalfamilydoctor.com.

26. The ICF can be ordered from WHO through its web site. The introductory chapter and a clinician checklist (which shows all the components, domains, and categories) can be downloaded (www.who.int/classification/icf/).

27. ROC can also be used to compare different screening guidelines (e.g., plasma cholesterol) in identifying individuals at risk for coronary heart disease (Grover et al. 1995).

28. Kappa can be readily computed by most statistical analysis software packages. "Kappa," more specifically "Cohen's kappa," was first used in the educational and psychological testing fields. See Feinstein and Cicchetti (1990) for further discussion. Maclure and Willett (1987) cautioned about its use, especially in studies comparing ordinal variables.

29. More advanced readers may want to find out the derivation of this formula from Rogan and Gladen (1978).

30. Comprehensive monographs on public health surveillance (Teutsch and Churchill, 2000) and field epidemiology (Gregg, 2002) are available. Goodman et al. (1990) provided a review of epidemiological field investigations.

31. See the text on medical geography by Meade and Earickson (2000) and spatial epidemiology by Elliott et al. (2001). Cliff and Haggett (1988) provide a comprehensive and richly illustrated review of different approaches to mapping disease distributions.

32. Manderson and Aaby (1992) discuss the use of anthropological methods in rapid assessments in disease-control programs.

33. Tylor's definition of *culture* appeared in his *Primitive Culture*, first published in 1871, and was cited in Helman (1994:2). The other definitions are quoted from Susser et al. (1985:132–33). Thatcher's 1987 remark can be found in the *Oxford Dictionary of Modern Quotations*.

34. The differences between *impairment, disability*, and *handicap* discussed earlier in this chapter can be seen as one example of this broader distinction between *disease, illness*, and *sickness*. The two quotations are from Eisenberg (1977) and Cassell (1976:48).

35. This rigor may be so extreme that it becomes rigor mortis! (Nations 1986:97). Nations's review provides copious examples of how cultural practices and beliefs influence the recognition of disease, concepts of causation, and approaches to treatment.

36. *The Social Construction of Reality* is the title of an influential book by Berger and Luckmann (1966). For a full discussion of the infant health example, see Wright (1983). Alland's (1970) small but influential book is a classic in medical anthropology.

37. *DSM-IV* text revision was published in 2000, which updated the text but made no changes to the criteria from the 1994 version. For a survey and classification

of culture-bound syndromes, see Simons and Hughes (1985). Hahn (1995:40–56) provides a critique of the concept.

38. The data are from Kirchner et al. (1985). Riboli and Delendi (1991) provided a comprehensive monograph on the contributions of autopsy studies to epidemiology and medical research. See Israel et al. (1986) on the use of multiple cause-of-death data and Chandramohan et al. (1994) on the use of verbal autopsies among adults.

39. The data are from Vitek and Wharton (1998), Dittman et al. (2000), and Markina et al. (2000). Time series of global diphtheria incidence data can be obtained from the WHO web site (www-nt.who.int/vaccines/globalsummary/timeseries/TSincidenceDip.htm).

40. The WHO study (Sartorius et al. 1986) has been criticized by Kleinman (1987) and Corin (1994). The Anglo-French study of schizophrenia was reported by Van Os et al. (1993).

EXERCISE 3.1.   Validity of Self-Reports of Chronic Diseases

In a linkage study, individuals participating in a population health survey (the Manitoba Heart Health Survey of 1990–1991) were linked with the provincial database of health care utilization, consisting of claims submitted by physicians and hospitals for reimbursement under the universal health insurance system. Each claim contained personal data as well as the diagnoses of the conditions treated. It was found that of 2,719 survey participants, 193 had a self-report of diabetes, 174 had a physician/hospital claim for diabetes, and 133 had both. If we take the physician and hospital claims data as the "gold standard,"

(a) What is the sensitivity of survey self-report as a means of detecting diabetes?

(b) How would you define "specificity" in this situation?

(c) If someone in the survey reports having diabetes, what is the likelihood that he or she actually has a physician or hospital claim for diabetes?

(d) What do you call what you have just calculated in (c)?

(e) What is a "linkage study," and what can one use to link two databases?

Source: Robinson et al. (1997)

EXERCISE 3.2.   Surveillance of Fetal Alcohol Syndrome

In a study estimating the birth prevalence of fetal alcohol syndrome (FAS) among Alaska Natives, two sources of cases were used: the Indian Health Service and private physicians. During 1982–1989, the former generated 45 cases and the latter 13 cases. Common to both sources were 8 cases.

(a) Using the capture-recapture method of case ascertainment, what is the total number of FAS cases among Alaska Natives?

(b) How complete are the two sources of data in ascertaining cases of FAS?

(c) Given that the total number of live births was 19,914, what is the birth prevalence of FAS based on each of the two sources?

(d) What is the ascertainment-adjusted prevalence of FAS: that is, the prevalence that takes into account the number of cases missed by both sources?

Source: Egeland et al. (1995)

EXERCISE 3.3.   Prostate Cancer Screening in the Community

A population-based study from Olmstead County, Minnesota, evaluated the prostate-specific antigen (PSA) test as a screening tool for prostate cancer. For each cutoff point of PSA separating cancer and non-cancer cases, the corresponding sensitivity and specificity are shown in the table below:

PSA level	Sensitivity	Specificity
1.0	0.99	0.43
1.5	0.97	0.62
2.0	0.94	0.75
2.5	0.92	0.81
3.0	0.90	0.84
3.5	0.87	0.89
4.0	0.85	0.91
4.5	0.82	0.93
5.0	0.80	0.95
6.0	0.73	0.97
7.0	0.66	0.98

(a) Plot the ROC curve; i.e., sensitivity against (1−specificity).

(b) Plot also the sensitivity against specificity.

(c) From the table or the graph, which cutoff point in PSA level offers the best trade-off between sensitivity and specificity?

Source: Jacobsen et al. (1996)

EXERCISE 3.4.   Verbal Autopsy in Establishing Causes of Death

In a study of the causes of mortality in the Morogoro District of Tanzania in East Africa using verbal autopsy (VA), it was found that the combined number of deaths from tuberculosis (TB) and/or AIDS accounted for 20.8% of all deaths among adults during the study period. This is the *cause-specific mortality proportion*, sometimes incorrectly referred to as the proportionate mortality "rate" or PMR.

In a validation study conducted in another district of the country, comparing VA with hospital diagnosis as the gold standard, the sensitivity (α) of VA was determined to be 76% and the specificity (β) 93%.

Using the formula for "adjusting" prevalence estimates with known values of α and β (p. 96), what is the adjusted mortality proportion from TB/AIDS in Morogoro District?

(Note: In this exercise, the denominator of the proportion is the total number of deaths from all causes, and not the population. The calculation, however, is the same).

Source: Chandramohan et al. (2001)

EXERCISE 3.5.   An Outbreak of Bioterrorism

In October 2001, shortly after the September 11 terrorist attacks in the United States, the first inhalational anthrax case in the country since 1976 was identified in a media company worker in Florida. Anthrax is caused by the bacterium *Bacillus anthracis,* and is usually acquired through exposure to infected animals or contaminated animal products such as wool. Because the bacteria can persist in the environment for long periods of time as a spore, it can be used, especially in a powdered form, as a military or terrorist weapon.

The relevant demographic and epidemiological data of the known cases are summarized in the table below:

No.	Date (onset)	Date (Dx)	State	Age	Sex	Occupation	Type	Outcome
1	Sept. 22	Oct. 19	NY	31	F	B	Skin*	Alive
2	Sept. 25	Oct. 12	NY	38	F	B	Skin	Alive
3	Sept. 26	Oct. 18	NJ	39	M	A	Skin*	Alive
4	Sept. 28	Oct. 15	FL	73	M	A,B	Inh	Alive
5	Sept. 28	Oct. 18	NJ	45	F	A	Skin	Alive
6	Sept. 28	Oct. 12	NY	23	F	B	Skin*	Alive
7	Sept. 29	Oct. 15	NY	0.6	M	C (child of B)	Skin	Alive
8	Sept. 30	Oct. 4	FL	63	M	B	Inh	Dead
9	Oct. 1	Oct. 18	NY	27	F	B	Skin	Alive
10	Oct. 14	Oct. 19	PA	35	M	A	Skin	Alive
11	Oct. 14	Oct. 28	NJ	56	F	A	Inh	Alive
12	Oct. 15	Oct. 29	NJ	43	F	A	Inh	Alive
13	Oct. 16	Oct. 21	VA	56	M	A	Inh	Alive

(continued)

EXERCISE 3.5 (*Continued*)

No.	Date (onset)	Date (Dx)	State	Age	Sex	Occupation	Type	Outcome
14	Oct. 16	Oct. 23	MD	55	M	A	Inh	Dead
15	Oct. 16	Oct. 26	MD	47	M	A	Inh	Dead
16	Oct. 16	Oct. 22	MD	56	M	A	Inh	Alive
17	Oct. 17	Oct. 29	NJ	51	F	C	Skin	Alive
18	Oct. 19	Oct. 22	NY	34	M	A,B	Skin*	Alive
19	Oct. 22	Oct. 25	VA	59	M	A	Inh	Alive
20	Oct. 23	Oct. 28	NY	38	M	B	Skin	Alive
21	Oct. 25	Oct. 30	NY	61	F	C	Inh	Dead
22	Nov. 14	Nov. 21	CT	94	F	C (retired)	Inh	Dead

Notes: Occupation: (A) mail handlers—including U.S. Postal Service staff, mailroom staff in offices; (B) media company employees—newspapers and television stations; (C) other.
Inh—inhalational; * suspected only, not confirmed.
Date (Dx)—Date of diagnosis.

Based on the information provided,

(a)   Plot the epidemic curve, using the date of onset (which differs from the date of discovery or diagnosis). Can you detect any spatial and temporal clustering of cases?

(b)   What is the median age of the victims. Explain why median is preferable to mean in this situation.

(c)   What is the case–fatality ratio during this anthrax outbreak?

(d)   Can you speculate on the mode of transmission of the pathogen?

Source: Jernigan et al. (2002)

4
Modeling Determinants of Population Health

Models and Pathways of Health

In the previous chapter, methods and concepts in assessing the health status of populations were discussed. While it is important as a first step to describe the extent and magnitude of various conditions along the health–disease continuum, the study of population health also requires seeking explanations of why the health status is what it is: in other words, what the *determinants* of health are. While health determinants are associated with the development of health problems, they themselves are not considered to be health problems. The title of a collection of essays, *Why Are Some People Healthy and Others Not?*, succinctly sums up the concept and explanatory power of health determinants.[1]

A simple, long-hallowed model used in epidemiology to explain why infectious diseases occur is the *host-agent-environment* triad:

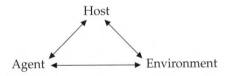

Thus, tuberculosis requires an agent—the micro-organism *Mycobacterium tuberculosis*; a susceptible host—the patient, who may be a malnourished alcoholic; and an environment—perhaps the sharing of an overcrowded shelter for the homeless with others who may have been infected.

In *Uses of Epidemiology*, Jerry Morris expanded this concept. *Host factors* can refer to both inborn characteristics and those acquired through experience and life situations. The *environment* may refer to the natural world or to society—living conditions, technology, human groups and institutions, social networks, values, and culture. For the chronic, non-communicable diseases, *agent* can be substituted with *personal behaviors*.[2] Ischemic heart disease then can occur in a host who is obese, whose work environment is such that he is sedentary much of the time, and for whom there is no compensatory increase in leisure-time physical activity. Into such a scenario one then adds an agent in the form of tobacco smoke—the result is first myocardial infarction at age 45!

In 1974, the Canadian government released a working document called *A New Perspective on the Health of Canadians*. It introduced a framework for the analysis of health determinants, called the *health field concept*, which categorizes the determinants of health status into the four fields of *human biology, environment, lifestyles,* and *health care organization*.[3] This scheme is still useful in broadening the focus of health care planners, practitioners, and administrators, traditionally solely concerned with issues relating to the delivery of health care services. In fact, the use of health services is more appropriately thought of as a consequence of health status rather than a determinant.

There have been more recent attempts to refine and expand the concept of the determinants of health and the relationship between health status and health care. One such model is that proposed by economists Robert Evans and Gregory Stoddart, reproduced in Figure 4.1. Of note is the direct impact of *health care* on *disease* but not on *health and function*, or on *well-being*, although there is a negative impact on *prosperity*, through a net drain on the wealth of the community, which is not offset by short-term economic spin-offs of health care.[4]

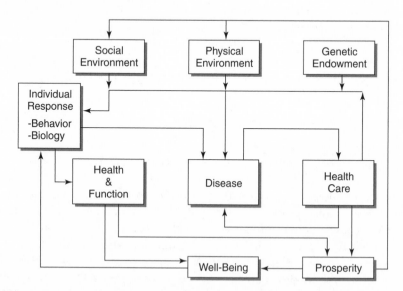

Figure 4.1. A model of health determinants, health status, and health care. Reproduced from Evans RG, Stoddart GL. Producing health, consuming health care. *Social Science and Medicine* 1990; 31:1347–63, with kind permission from Elsevier Science Ltd, The Boulevard, Langford Lane, Kidlington, OX5 1GB, United Kingdom.

In the rest of this chapter, the various major determinants of health are discussed in turn. It should be emphasized that the division is artificial—these determinants should be considered as working together in producing health and disease in individuals and in populations, best characterized by the notion of a *web of causation* (more in Chapter 5). The naïve analytical approach of throwing every potential determinant together in a multivariate "soup" to see which ones emerge as "independent predictors" of the disease or health outcome being investigated fails to reflect the complexity of most causal relationships. It is unfortunately endemic in the research literature, having been greatly aided by the existence of push-button, user-friendly statistical software packages. As an empirical science, population health is often seen to be "data-driven" and the need for any *conceptual framework* is not often recognized. The development of *multilevel, hierarchical modeling* is a response to the need to explain the interrelationships between different determinants operating at different levels (from the molecular to the societal) and at different times.

Some researchers regard the existing, predominantly *linear*, research paradigm as inadequate to understand the complex nature of disease causation, and that further gains need to incorporate *nonlinear dynamics* (of which the highly popularized *chaos theory* is a special case). Nonlinearity does not assume that the probability of an outcome is the sum of its component forces or that the outcome is predictable. Given the same set of determinants, the multiple pathways and feedback loops can produce unexpected outcomes in different individuals. Nonlinear dynamics can also lead to the persistence of the disease process even when the initial, remote exposure has been discontinued. Nonlinear approaches have been used in the basic biomedical sciences, but their applications in population health are few and far between, for example, in modeling the transmission of infectious diseases.[5]

Genetic Susceptibility

It has been recognized for a long time that heredity plays an important role in the causation of diseases and their variation in populations. *Genes* are the basic units of heredity that are passed from parents to offspring. In the era of molecular biology, genes have a physical existence—a segment of DNA (*deoxyribonucleic acid*) endowed with a specific function, usually the production of a specific protein. All the DNA contained in an organism (found in the chromosomes of the cell's nucleus and also in the mitochondria) constitutes its *genome*. The DNA molecule has the shape of a double helix (like a twisted ladder) with the rungs made up of *base pairs*; that is, pairs of the chemicals adenine (A), thymine (T), guanine (G), and cytosine (C), the four letters of the *genetic code*. All genes are made up of stretches of these four bases in different ways and in different lengths. It is estimated that there are between 30,000 and 40,000 human genes. A major milestone in the modern history of science was the completion of sequencing the entire human genome's three billion base pairs in 2003 by the Human Genome Project, 50 years after the landmark publication on the structure of DNA by James Watson and Francis Crick.[6]

The observable traits or characteristics of an organism (e.g., height, eye color) are referred to as *phenotypes*. In the context of disease, the clinical features can be considered the *phenotypic expression* of the underlying genes for that disease in the individual's *genotype*.

Note that a disease may be *congenital*, referring to the fact that it is present at birth, without necessarily having a genetic etiology. Similarly, *familial* only means that the disease occurs in several close relatives ("runs in families") who share not only genes but also environments. A trait may be transmitted from generation to generation by cultural rather than genetic means, such as language, surnames, aristocratic titles, and certain behaviors and practices.

Diseases differ in the degree of genetic involvement. *Single-gene* diseases are caused by a *mutation*, a transmission error in the reproduction of DNA, which leads to some disturbance in protein structure or function and disruption in the functioning of particular cells, tissues, and organs and manifested as clinical signs and symptoms. Some of the earliest diseases in this category to be recognized are the various *inborn errors of metabolism*, a term coined by Archibald Garrod (1857–1936) and used in the title of his 1909 book. An example is phenylketonuria, a disorder of the metabolism of the amino acid phenylalanine, which may result in mental retardation.

The relatively simple mode of inheritance (autosomal dominant, autosomal recessive, and X-linked) is often referred to as *Mendelian*, after the father of modern genetics, Gregor Mendel (1822–1884).[7] The sex chromosomes are designated X and Y (women are XX and men XY). All other chromosomes are called autosomes, of which there are 22 pairs. If an autosomal gene must be present on both chromosomes to express itself as clinical disease, it is called *recessive*. If the gene needs only be present in one chromosome, it is *dominant*. A person with only one copy of a recessive gene is referred to as a *carrier*, who does not actually become sick but in whom the gene can be detected by special tests. (An example is sickle-cell anemia, discussed in Case Study 4.1). A gene located on the X chromosome is called *X-linked* (e.g., color blindness). One copy will be enough to cause disease in men since they have only one X chromosome. In women, for the disease to occur the gene must be present in both X chromosomes if it is recessive and in only one X chromosome if it is dominant.

Chromosomal disorders occur as a result of changes in the number or structure of chromosomes. A prime example is Down's syndrome, formerly called "mongolism," a form of which is due to trisomy 21 having an extra (three instead of two) chromosome number 21.

Most diseases are *polygenic*, involving many genes, and indeed *multifactorial*, with both genetic and non-genetic causes. Several genes may act

BOX 4.1. The Burden of Genetic Diseases in a Population

Patricia Baird and her colleagues estimated the prevalence of different types of genetic disorders from one million consecutive births in British Columbia during 1952–1983.[8] Among children and adults under 25 years of age, genetic disorders occurred with a frequency of 53/1,000 live births, divisible into:

Single gene disorders

Autosomal dominant	1.4/1,000 (e.g., neurofibromatosis	0.08/1,000)
Autosomal recessive	1.7/1,000 (e.g., cystic fibrosis	0.23/1,000)
X-linked	0.5/1,000 (e.g., hemophilia A	0.06/1,000)
Chromosomal disorders	1.8/1,000 (e.g., Down's syndrome	1.22/1,000)
Multifactorial disorders	46.4/1,000 (e.g., spina bifida	0.34/1,000)
Uncertain mode of inheritance	1.2/1,000	

This was one of the few attempts to provide a comprehensive estimate of genetic diseases in a defined population. The genetic contribution to a population's disease burden is not easily determined, since genetic diseases are not labeled as such in mortality databases nor constitute a distinct category in the International Classification of Diseases. Baird's data were obtained from the British Columbia Health Status Registry. First established in 1952 as the Crippled Children's Registry, the registry receives information on handicapping conditions, congenital anomalies, and familial disorders from multiple sources, including vital statistics and health care utilization databases.

Thousands of genetic diseases have been identified. Victor McKusick has been engaged for some years in the task of cataloging them, an ever-expanding and rapidly outdated enterprise. The twelfth edition (1998) of his catalogue *Mendelian Inheritance in Man* contains 8,587 entries (93% of which are autosomal), compared to 1,487 in the 1966 edition.

---

together to determine the susceptibility of the individual to disease, while environmental factors determine the likelihood of disease among the genetically susceptible.[9]

Finally, there are diseases and health conditions in which genetics probably play no or little role, such as most infections, injuries, and insults from chemical and physical agents.

It should be recognized that even diseases in the last category are not entirely without genetic influence. The association between the sickle-cell gene and reduced susceptibility to malaria (Case Study 4.1) is a classic example that has been known for decades. While such single-gene examples are rare, human genetic variation (*polymorphism,* see below) is an important determinant of susceptibility to such infectious diseases as tuberculosis, leprosy, and HIV.[10]

While a motor vehicle collision cannot be said to be genetically determined, genetic factors do contribute to the susceptibility to, initiation of, and recovery from injuries. Rare genetic syndromes of bleeding disorders and brittle bones cause afflicted individuals to be more susceptible to serious injuries from relatively mild energy transfers. There is also an increasing body of literature on the genetics of substance abuse, violent behaviors, and suicide.[11] As can be expected, many of the conclusions and interpretations are controversial. It should be emphasized that the existence of genetic susceptibility and biological pathways does not undermine the importance of psychosocial factors in causation and interventions.

On the other hand, single-gene and chromosomal diseases may also have environmental influence in clinical expressions of disease or environmental "trigger." Individuals who carry the gene for phenylketonuria need not suffer from mental retardation if they are not exposed to phenylalanine in the diet—which is the rationale for neonatal screening and dietary restriction therapy. Radiation, an environmental (and in the case of nuclear fallout from the atom bomb, manmade) agent causes genetic damage that may be transmitted.

Therefore, almost *all* diseases/health problems involve *some* degree of genetic–environmental interaction.

In assessing the health status of populations, the demonstration of geographic or ethnic variation in disease risk often suggests a possible role for genetic factors, although alternative explanations that favor a stronger environmental influence may sometimes be more plausible. Where the degree of racial or ethnic admixture of individuals or populations is known, it is possible to compare disease rates across groups categorized on such a basis. The correlation of diabetes prevalence with degree of Native American ancestry ("blood quantum") has been reported among the Pima in the Southwest. Mexican-Americans are a hybrid population with both European (mainly Spanish) and Native American ancestry. Diabetes prevalence among Mexican-Americans tends to be intermediate between that of Native Americans and non-Hispanic Whites. Within the Mexican-American population, diabetes prevalence also increases with increasing Native American admixture, as measured by various genetic markers and skin color reflectometry.[12]

Because twins are genetically alike [indeed identical in the case of monozygotic (MZ) twins], studying them with regards to the differential risk of disease among twins reared together and apart is akin to a natural experiment where the influences of genetics and the environment can be separated. The concordance of a disease (i.e., the likelihood that one twin will also have the disease if the other one has it) among MZ twins should

BOX 4.2.   Tracking the Health of Migrant Populations

Studies of migrants, by comparing them with the population that stays behind and the population of the new country, are intended to investigate environmental factors (such as diet) of various diseases while "holding constant" the genetic makeup of the population. Further information can also be obtained by comparing first-generation immigrants with their descendants in the new country, and also the risk of disease by duration of residence in the new country.

Migrant studies have often been used in cancer epidemiology.[13] One of the most studied migrant populations is the Japanese in the United States. Other groups that have been studied include Europeans in Australia, Indians in England, and the various dialect groups of Chinese in Singapore. The results from the many studies are quite consistent in showing that, for virtually all cancers, the migrants' incidence and mortality rates tend to approach those of the native-born in the new country with increased duration of residence or in succeeding generations. For example, for breast cancer among women and colon cancer among men, the Japanese in Japan, Japanese migrants in the United States, and migrant descendants in the United States all have rates lower than U.S.-born whites; among the three Japanese groups, the migrant descendants have the highest rate. In the case of colon cancer, it approaches the rate for U.S.-born whites.

Migrant studies have also been conducted in cardiovascular diseases. In the 1960s and 1970s the Ni-Hon-San Study followed a cohort of 11,900 men of Japanese ancestry aged 45–64 in Hiroshima and Nagasaki, Honolulu, and San Francisco. [Note that the study's acronym— "Ni" for Nippon or Nihon (Japan), "Hon" for Honolulu, and "San" for San Francisco—happens to mean also "Japanese" in Japanese, with the "san" suffix being a form of polite address.] Japanese men in Hawaii

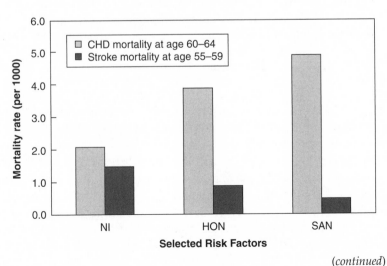

(continued)

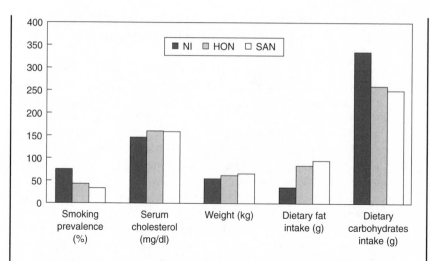

tend to occupy an intermediate position between Japan and California in terms of coronary heart disease and stroke. For coronary heart disease, all three Japanese groups were markedly lower than U.S. whites, whereas for stroke, Japan has the highest rates, with Japanese-American rates comparable to those of U.S. whites.

In terms of cardiovascular risk factors, gradients are observed in a variety of physiological (blood pressure, plasma glucose, cholesterol, body weight), behavioral (smoking), and dietary (total calories, total fat, total carbohydrates) variables:

Migrant studies are not quite natural experiments, as genetic background may change because of intermarriage with the host population (gene flow), while environmental factors may not change as much as anticipated because of the retention of some "old-country" customs and habits even for several generations, while some habits of the host population are readily adopted (acculturation). Migrants also tend to be a highly self-selected group. They are generally not representative of the country of origin, as they may originate predominantly from a specific geographic region or socioeconomic stratum.

be higher than for dizygotic (DZ) twins, who are no closer than mere siblings, and may approach 90%–100% in strongly genetic diseases.

To quantify the degree to which a trait is genetically determined, a *heritability index* (H) can be constructed, based on regression analyses of studies involving twins and close relatives. It is the proportion of the observed variance of a character in a population that can be attributed to genetic causes: $H = V_G/V_T = V_G/(V_E + V_G)$, where V_G is the genetic component to the variance and V_E the environmental component. V_T is the total measured variability.[14] It should be remembered that this is a statistical measure—a ratio of variances and not of actual phenotypic values. The same trait in different populations may have different indices. The value of the index also does not convey any information about the genetic mechanism involved.

At a particular site on a chromosome (locus), different forms of a gene (alleles) may be found. Heterozygous individuals have two different alleles at a particular locus, whereas homozygous individuals have two copies of the same allele. Genes that have multiple alleles occurring at relatively high frequencies (1% or more) in populations are called *polymorphic*. The DNA sequence of any two individuals is 99.9% identical—it is the variations that contribute to our differences, including differences in disease risks. Many polymorphic genes (variant alleles) serve as genetic markers, and their association with the occurrence of disease in populations has been extensively studied. Such markers as blood groups, various enzymes, serum proteins, and the human leukocyte antigens (HLA) have been much studied in the pre-molecular era. These are called *gene products* since it is not the genes themselves that are measured biochemically. Note that what the geneticists call *association studies* are what epidemiologists would call *case-control studies* (see Chapter 6), in that the phenotype (or disease) is the outcome of interest, with the genetic markers serving as the exposure variable. Polymorphism at the level of the DNA molecule can also be used to study disease associations. The degree to which a gene's action is fully expressed phenotypically is called *penetrance*. Much of the genetic contribution to chronic diseases such as cancer and coronary heart disease results from a large number of low-penetrant genes. High-penetrant genes are infrequent in the general population, and they tend to be concentrated in particular groups or families. Table 4.1 provides a classification of the various types of disease-associated variant alleles, showing the range in gene–gene and gene–environment interactions.[15]

Geneticists also devote considerable attention to the aggregation of disease in families. One approach, called *segregation analysis*, investigates the distribution of phenotypic traits in families or pedigrees and assesses its fit with a known model of Mendelian inheritance. The other approach is *linkage analysis*, which attempts to locate the position of the gene in the human genome. Until the advent of molecular techniques of *gene mapping*, this is primarily a statistical exercise. Genes that are located close together on a chromosome are "linked," i.e., more likely to be inherited together. By studying the pattern of inheritance of specific traits in families, it is possible to infer the relative positions of different genes.

When populations are large, gene frequencies do not vary much from generation to generation—they are said to be in *equilibrium*. The famous *Hardy-Weinberg Law* in population genetics explains mathematically how relative gene frequencies are maintained and how recessive genes do not readily disappear from a population.[16]

Table 4.1. Types of Disease-Associated Alleles

1. High-risk variant alleles, high-penetrant with little environmental influence: e.g., the *RB* gene associated with retinoblastoma, a malignant tumor of the eye occurring in childhood.
2. High-risk variant alleles, with variable penetrance as a result of the modifying action of alleles at other loci: e.g., the *BRCA1* gene for breast cancer.
3. Modifier alleles that alter the penetrance of other genes: e.g., the *Mom1* gene, which modifies the penetrance of the *Apc* gene for familial adenomatous polyposis (or adenomatosis polyposis coli).
4. High-risk variant alleles, with different effects across generations as a result of changes in environmental exposures: e.g., the *MSH2* alleles in hereditary non-polyposis colorectal cancer (HNPCC) families—the impaired capacity to repair DNA damage is inherited, but the site where the failure occurs and ultimately leads to cancer varies.
5. Low-penetrant, high-prevalent alleles that have an effect only in the presence of relevant environmental exposures: e.g., the *MTHFR* C677T variant, which increases the risk of colorectal cancer only when serum folate levels are low (due to dietary deficiency).
6. Alleles that confer protection from, rather than susceptibility to, disease: e.g., *APOE* in coronary heart disease, and PPARγ in type-2 diabetes.

At equilibrium, the relative frequencies of three genotypes AA, Aa and aa (for a gene with two alleles, A and a) is p^2, $2pq$, and q^2, where p is the frequency of A and q the frequency of a, and $(p + q = 1)$. Under conditions of random mating, the following matings and their respective genotypes are possible:

Frequency:		p^2	$2pg$	q^2
	Genotype:	AA	Aa	aa
p^2	AA	p^4	$2p^3q$	p^2q^2
$2pq$	Aa	$2p^3q$	$4p^2q^2$	$2pq^3$
q^2	Aa	p^2q^2	$2pq^3$	q^4

The prevalences of the AA, Aa, and aa among the offspring are then:

AA: $p^4 + 2p^3q + p^2q^2 = p^2 (p^2 + 2pq + q^2)$
Aa: $2p^3q + 4p^2q^2 + 2pq^3 = 2pq (p^2 + 2pq + q^2)$
aa: $p^2q^2 + 2pq^3 + q^4 = q^2 (p^2 + 2pq + q^2)$

The ratio AA : Aa : aa reduces to $p^2 : 2pq : q^2$, since the quantity $(p^2 + 2pq + q^2)$ cancels out. This ratio is identical to that of the first generation.

Over time, the frequency of particular genes (including disease genes) in a population does change. This can be brought about by a variety of means.

New genes appear in a population primarily through mutation. Mutations are generally rare events. While they occur spontaneously, their rate of occurrence can be affected by environmental factors. Only mutations affecting germ cells (i.e., sperm and eggs) can be transmitted to the next generation (the germline). Mutations affecting somatic cells (all other cells in the body) cannot be transmitted but they do cause important diseases such as cancer.

Whether mutant genes become established in the population depends on the ability of an individual to contribute his or her genes to subsequent generations through natural selection. Mutant genes which kill the individual, reduce her or his resistance to disease, or interfere with his or her ability to reproduce, will be "selected against" and reduced or eliminated from the population over time. On the other hand, "advantageous" genes are more likely to persist and spread (see Case Study 4.1).

In small populations, the gene pool (i.e., the sum total of genes and their variants) is small and the sampling variation is much greater. Since the next generation must be sampled from the current generation, the sampling error will compound and gene frequencies may change substantially. This is known as *genetic drift*. Another effect of random variation is the founder effect. When a small group of people breaks off from a larger population, the sample of genes in that population may not be typical of the home population. Over many generations, the descendants may show unique patterns of gene frequencies, sometimes manifested in the prevalence of disease. Rare genetic diseases have been found in high frequency in populations such as the Amish in Lancaster County, Pennsylvania, and French Canadians in the Saguenay region of Québec, which can be traced to the arrival of specific individuals in North America generations ago.

The "randomness" of sampling from the gene pool does not always hold true. Non-random mating occurs when there is inbreeding (marrying close relatives) or assortative mating—choosing one's mate based on certain visible characteristics (hair color, height, beauty, size of wallet), some of which are themselves inherited.

The study of genetic factors in diseases is an important task of population health. It involves assessing the burden of illness, determining the relative roles of genes and environment in disease causation, predicting disease risks in individuals and families, and controlling the problem through genetic screening, genetic counseling, and other preventive strategies. It is an enterprise that is fraught with ethical dilemmas and often politically sensitive.

Physical Environment

As a health determinant, "environment" is usually discussed as separate from "genetics" or "biology" and encompasses all that is external to the human body.[17] It is usually further divided into "physical" and "social" and conceived of as expanding concentric circles representing the home, the worksite, the community, and ultimately the entire planet Earth. The physical environment is what Hippocrates referred to as *airs, waters,* and *places,* and its influence on health has long been recognized. In our time, the World Health Organization's Commission on Health and Environment released its report *Our Planet, Our Health* in 1992. Its main theme is the close interrelationships between human activities and the integrity of the natural environment and how they interact to influence the health of populations.

The many environmental factors that have an adverse impact on health can be organized according to the nature of the hazard (biological, chemical, and physical); their source (natural, industrial, and agricultural); where they occur (air, water, soil, and food); the site of exposure (home, school, work, community); and the route of exposure (by inhalation, ingestion, contact, and bites).

The health effects of environmental hazards are many. Exposure to a sufficient quantity may result in symptoms of acute toxicity, which may even lead to instant death. However, long-term, chronic health effects from low-dose exposure are of greater concern since they are often difficult to assess, affect large numbers of people, and are associated with complex social, economic, and political factors that make them more than just the responsibilities of the health sector. Many effects are mild signs and symptoms of irritation (skin, eyes, lungs), allergic reactions, and psychological distress. Others are more serious and may lead to various types of cancer (carcinogens), birth defects (teratogens), and genetic change (mutagens). In children, growth and development, both physical and neurobehavioral, may be delayed.

Microorganisms pose the most serious biological hazards in the environment. Molds, viruses, and bacteria are capable of causing many human diseases when inhaled, ingested, or introduced to the body through contact and bites. They can be found in the air (expelled from an infected person through coughing); in the water (contaminated by sewage); in food (handled by unhygienic food vendors); and in the soil (growing among decaying organic materials). Where they are maintained and multiply is referred to as the *reservoir,* which can be animate or inanimate. Often they are carried by *vectors,* such as insects and rodents, and brought into closer contact with humans. While infectious diseases are the major health effects, biological agents such as dander from furry pets and pollens can also cause allergic reactions and trigger acute attacks of asthma.

Toxic chemical substances exist as fumes, dusts, suspended particles, and liquids that have been released into air, water, soil, and the food chain

BOX 4.3.   Of Pests and Chemicals

Pesticide can be broken down into its Latin roots *pesti*, from which the word *pestilence* is also derived, and *cida*, meaning "killer." A pest is any living being whose presence near us is considered undesirable, because it causes disease, damages our economy, or simply offends our sense of esthetics. Human beings have developed a whole array of chemicals that can kill anything and names to indicate the victims. *Herbicides* kill weeds, i.e., undesirable plants. There are *-cides* to go along with *insecti-, fungi-, bacteri-, rodenti-, avi-, nemati-, mollusca-, pisci-,* and *ovi-*, referring respectively to insects, fungi, bacteria, rodents, birds, nematodes, snails, fish, and eggs.

Mao Tse-tung (1893–1976), founder of the People's Republic of China, composed a poem in 1963:[18]

On this tiny globe
A few flies dash themselves against the wall,
Humming without cease,
Sometimes shrilling, sometimes moaning. . . .
    Away with all pests!
    Our force is irresistible.

He was referring to human pests, better known as "enemies of the people," who must be crushed, whether figuratively or literally.

Abbreviations may be a bane of normal everyday conversation and correspondence, but they are absolutely essential for the myriad chemical substances that are potential environmental pollutants.

DDT stands for dichlorodiphenyltrichloroethane, an insecticide once used worldwide in the control of malaria but now banned. The organophosphates (parathion, malathion) break down more easily than the organochlorines and have generally replaced them as insecticides. PCB (for polychlorinated biphenyls) is a collective name for some 200 chemicals formerly widely used as fire retardants and insulators. The manufacture of PCBs has been banned in North America since the late 1970s. In the late 1960s an outbreak of poisoning occurred in Yusho, Japan, when cooking oil was contaminated with PCB. *Dioxin* refers to polychlorinated dibenzodioxins, a group of 75 chemicals structurally linked to the 135 or so furans, or polychlorinated dibenzofurans, formed as industrial byproducts. The most notorious of the dioxins is 2,3,7,8-tetrachlorodibenzoparadioxin (TCDD), used in Agent Orange, a defoliant used during the Vietnam war by U.S. forces. An industrial accident in Seveso, Italy, in July 1976 resulted in a TCDD cloud covering some 80 hectares and exposing the population, many of whom developed an intractable, severe form of skin disease called *chloracne*.

inadvertently, deliberately, or unavoidably by human actions. Chemicals have become indispensable to modern society, whether as products or intermediaries in industrial processes and the manufacture of consumer goods. Chemical hazards may be classified according to their functions (e.g., pesticides, solvents), the target tissues (neuro-, nephro-toxic) or chemical structure. Beyond simple division into organic and inorganic, there are many different ways of grouping chemicals. Familiar classes include the heavy metals (e.g., mercury, lead, cadmium); the organochlorines, which include synthetic materials such as polyvinyl chloride, and insecticides such as DDT, lindane, and chlordane; the polychlorinated hydrocarbons, which include PCBs, dioxins, and furans; organophosphates, found in many pesticides; chlorofluorocarbons (CFCs), used in solvents, aerosol propellants, and refrigerants; and polycyclic aromatic hydrocarbons (PAHs) released by fossil fuels.

Toxicity is a relative rather than absolute characteristic. It is determined by the frequency, duration, and intensity of exposure, and host factors such as genetic susceptibility, nutritional status, immunocompetence, and rate of metabolism. Solvents used daily in household chores, pesticides used by farmers to ensure a healthy crop, and particulates released by the burning of fossil fuels become "pollutants" when they appear in excessive quantities in unintended places and have overcome nature's capacity to break down or dilute them. Not all toxic chemicals are man-made—heavy metals such as mercury can also be found in nature and be incorporated into the food chain.

Examples of physical hazards include radiation, temperature extremes, and excessive noise. Radiation may be ionizing or non-ionizing; natural or manmade (see Box 4.4). Fatalities from cold exposure and heat waves remind us that our rather limited range of physiological adaptation cannot protect us from the elements without technical innovations (clothing, shelter, central heating). Noise (from machinery, sonic booms, rock concerts) may only be a nuisance, but it can induce stress and hearing loss.

Determining the role of the physical environment on human health requires measurements of environmental quality, extent of human exposure, and health effects. *Dose* refers to the amount of a contaminant deposited in the body; it needs to be absorbed, and once in the body, it interacts with a target site and alters its function, producing a biological effect.

Environmental quality is often determined by sampling and analysis of air, water, and soil. The concentration or level is often expressed as parts per million (ppm) or units of weight of the contaminant per unit volume of air (cubic meter) or water (liter). With the increasing sensitivity and sophistication of laboratory instruments, ever smaller concentrations are being detected. Some contaminants are measured in parts per billion, trillion, and even quadrillion! In the case of highly toxic minerals such as asbestos, the actual number of fibers or particles per unit volume is measured.

BOX 4.4.   A Small Dose of Radiation Physics

Radiation in physics refers to the emission and transport of energy in the form of waves or particles. Some radiation is *ionizing* because it causes the formation of ions in substances through which it passes, including DNA in living cells. It comprises cosmic rays, gamma rays, and X-rays that occupy the short-wavelength, high-frequency end of the electromagnetic spectrum, as well as protons, neutrons, and various other particles designated as α (helium nuclei) and β (electrons).[19] *Non-ionizing* radiation refers to several forms of electromagnetic radiation of wavelengths longer than those of ionizing radiation that do not have the same damaging effect on tissues and cells. These include ultraviolet, visible light, infrared, microwave, radiofrequency, and extremely low frequency radiation from power lines, electrical appliances, and video display terminals.

Ionizing radiations are produced when charged particles are accelerated and interact with matter, and from the natural decay of radionuclides. *Decay*, or disintegration, is the emission of particles from the nuclei of a chemical element resulting in a new element with a different atomic weight. It occurs as a series until a stable, non-radioactive element is formed; e.g., the transformation from ^{235}U to ^{207}Pb. *Radioactivity* is the property of certain unstable chemical elements that emit radiation as the result of spontaneous nuclear decay. The time it takes for 50% of the original nuclei to disintegrate is referred to as the *physical half-life* (τ_P). The time required for 50% of the absorbed radiation to be eliminated from the body is the *biological half-life* (τ_B). These two can be combined to produce an *effective half-life* τ_{eff}, where $1/\tau_{eff} = 1/\tau_B + 1/\tau_P$.

The major sources of ionizing radiation humans are exposed to are natural: cosmic rays from outer space, radiation from radioactive elements in the earth's crust, and most important of all, radon gas, formed naturally from the decay of radium and uranium. Man-made sources include medical X-rays and agents used in nuclear medicine, the production of nuclear energy, and nuclear weapons testing.

One measures radioactivity by the amount produced at the *source* emitting it, the amount reaching an object (the *exposure*), and the amount absorbed (the *dose*). How radioactive a substance is can be measured by the number of disintegrations per second, or *becquerel* (Bq). It replaces the older unit *curie*, Ci ($1\,Ci = 3.7 \times 10^{10}\,Bq$).

Measures of exposure and dose are derived from measures of energy (basic unit the *joule*, J) and of electrical charge (basic unit the *coulomb*, C). The unit for exposure is C/kg of air. It replaces the *roentgen*, R ($1\,R = 2.58 \times 10^{-4}\,C/kg$). These units measure how much ionization is induced and electrical charge liberated in a fixed quantity of air. The energy imparted per kilogram of irradiated material is the *absorbed dose*, and is measured in *grays*, Gy ($1\,Gy = 1\,J/kg$). It replaces the rad, which stands for radiation absorbed dose ($1\,Gy = 100\,rad$).

(continued)

The various types of radiation have different biological effectiveness, according to their *linear energy transfer* (LET). Alpha particles have high LET; i.e., they are capable of producing a high density of ions and depositing a large amount of energy along their path. Gamma rays, x-rays, and β particles, on the other hand, have low LET. By assigning different weighting factors to the different types of radiation, an *equivalent dose* can be converted from the absorbed dose. It is measured in *sieverts* (Sv), which replace the older unit *rem* (1 Sv = 100 rem), abbreviation for roentgen-equivalent-man. By summing individual equivalent doses for all members of a population, one can obtain a collective dose equivalent, measured in man-Sv. The equivalent dose is measured for an organ or tissue. Since body organs and tissues differ in their sensitivity to radiation and risk of carcinogenesis in the long term, it is possible to assign weighting factors to different radiosensitive organs and tissues and produce an effective dose equivalent for the whole body by summing the weighted individual contributions.

The figure below summarizes the pathways of transfer of radionuclides to humans, a model used by the United Nations Scientific Committee on the Effects of Atomic Radiation (UNSCEAR).

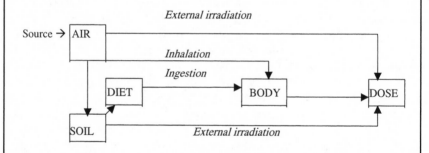

Exposure can be measured using a spectrometer which can be installed in a car and driven around the countryside. Assumptions need to be made in terms of the shielding provided by buildings and the average time people spend indoors and outdoors. Internal radiation can be directly measured using whole-body scanning. Indirect estimation of dose can be made using complex computer modeling, taking into account meteorological factors, amount of ground deposition, uptake by plants and animals, and patterns of food consumption, etc.

Certain indicator substances are used to measure overall environmental quality. The levels of sulfur dioxide and total suspended particulates are common indicators of air quality. General indicators of water quality include BOD (biological oxygen demand) and total suspended solids. As a measure of fecal contamination, the coliform count is often used. Note that the *E. coli* bacteria being counted are not the actual cause of diarrheal disease but form part of the normal intestinal flora.

In measuring specific physical, chemical, and biological agents in the environment, it should also be recognized that a certain amount of a substance may "normally" or "naturally" occur (the *background level*) even in the absence of contamination from man-made sources.

Human exposure, while dependent on environmental quality, is also affected by human activities (intensity, duration) that allow the pollutant to be ingested, inhaled, or absorbed into the body. It can be measured by the use of personal monitors (dosimetry badge for radiation workers); questionnaires, diaries, job and residence histories, and biological monitoring; and the testing of specific markers in blood, urine, saliva, breath, breast milk, and other body specimens. Some markers are the exogenous substances themselves, whose presence indicates exposure. Others reflect biochemical changes in the body as a result of exposure. (A *biomarker* is defined as any substance, structure, or process, or its products, that can be measured in the human body that may influence or predict the occurrence or outcome of disease.[20]) There is a hierarchy among the different types of measurements in terms of how close they truly represent exposure. The strongest are personal measurements, followed by ambient measurements of the immediate vicinity. Least accurate are surrogate measures (e.g., water consumption), and duration of residence and employment in an area or distance from it.

Most developed countries have regulatory agencies that set standards of environmental quality and limits for human exposure, based on available evidence. Often, the only data are toxicological, derived from animal studies. A *NOAEL* (for "no-observed-adverse-effects-level") can be determined from dose-response curves. To determine acceptable or maximum levels of human exposure, regulators tend to set them far below (100th or 1,000 times) the levels at which adverse health effects have been observed. This is the "margin of safety" approach. It does not actually assess the probability or size of the health risk, which is assumed to be so miniscule as to be nonexistent.

The tasks of a population health system, having recognized the existence of the different types of environmental hazards, measured their occurrence, and assessed their risk to health, also include designing and evaluating effective interventions to ensure and maintain the basic requirements for a healthy environment: clean air; safe and sufficient water; adequate and safe food; safe and peaceful shelter; and a stable global ecosystem.

Air

We all need air, more precisely oxygen, to survive. With every breath we inhale not just oxygen and nitrogen, but a host of air pollutants as well. Air pollution first became a problem in the cities of Europe where the Industrial Revolution started in the early nineteenth century and soon went into full swing. The first serious health emergency involving air pollution occurred in December 1930, when a dense fog descended on the Meuse Valley in Belgium. In December 1952, a similar fog enveloped London and caused some 4,000 excess deaths, mainly from respiratory problems among the elderly and infirm. Such fogs, whose consistency has been compared to pea soup, are the result of temperature inversion, when warm air lies on top of cool air, trapping air pollutants at ground level. By the end of the twentieth century, air pollution had become a global problem, with the worst occurrences in the megalopolises of the Third World and the industrial wastelands of Eastern Europe formerly under Communism.

The main sources of air pollution are the burning of fossil fuels such as oil and coal, releasing sulfur dioxide and suspended particulate matter (SPM); and motor-vehicle emissions of carbon monoxide, oxides of nitrogen, and hydrocarbons. These substances have acute and chronic effects on the respiratory, cardiovascular, and central nervous systems. Air pollution has declined in regions where there has been a switch to hydroelectricity and natural gas as energy sources, and where emission controls have been instituted in industries and motor vehicles. It has grown worse in areas faced with rapid urbanization and unfettered industrialization, where antiquated industries cannot afford expensive pollution-control technologies, and where laws regulating emissions are lacking, lax, or unenforced.

Of increasing concern in recent years is indoor air pollution. It is far more serious than outdoor pollution because of the increased concentration of pollutants in enclosed space, its occurrence among rural populations far from cities and industries, and the heavy exposure of women and young children who stay at home. The main sources of pollutants include tobacco smoking; cooking and heating, especially the use of wood-burning stoves, kerosene heaters, and gas-fired stoves (which emit combustion products such as NO_x, SO_x, CO, CO_2, and polycyclic aromatic hydrocarbons); furnishing and construction materials (which may release formaldehyde gas and asbestos fibers); household chemicals; and radon gas, which may infiltrate the house from underlying rocks and soil. Indoor air quality is compromised also by biological agents such as bacterial spores, molds, dust mites, and dander.

The building of energy-efficient and virtually airtight homes and offices has exacerbated the indoor air pollution problem. Large number of workers appear to be affected by the "sick building syndrome," a collection of mostly mild but often incapacitating symptoms. Improved ventilation and reduction or elimination of the sources of contaminants will improve indoor air quality.

Water

Like air, water is essential to life. In the environment, water exists as surface water (rivers, lakes, seas), groundwater, and precipitation, all of which can potentially be subjected to pollution. Despite the fact that 75% of the earth's surface is covered by water, less than 3% is fresh water.

A substantial proportion of the world's population has no access to a safe and sufficient source of water. It is often not recognized that the quantity of water has a stronger impact on health outcomes than its quality, especially in developing countries. High standards for water quality are unrealistic and unattainable in many locations, and scarce resources should be directed as a priority towards increasing water supply and improving excreta disposal. Standards of quality are not absolute but depend on the intended uses—drinking, recreation, irrigation, aquatic life, or industrial processes.

Water quality varies as a result of natural (geological, climatic, and biological) processes, even in the absence of contamination from human activities. Health hazards found in water include the full array of pathogenic microorganisms and chemicals resulting from sewage, industrial effluent, and agricultural land use (pesticides, trihalomethanes, heavy metals, nitrates and nitrites, etc.).

Many diseases can results from unsafe and inadequate water.[21] In Chapter 3, a scheme for the classification of infectious diseases related to water and sanitation is presented in Box 3.7.

Food

Food and health are intimately related. Some populations suffer from undernutrition, which stunts the physical growth and intellectual development of children and increases their susceptibility to, and mortality from, infections. Other populations direct much of their health promotion effort at "overnutrition" and its health effects (e.g., heart disease, diabetes). Everywhere there lurks a variety of contaminants to threaten the safety and wholesomeness of our foods.

Contaminants come in the form of food-borne infections, toxic chemicals, and radionuclides. Pathogenic microorganisms originate and proliferate in human or animal excreta and infect humans via the fecal–oral route. Biological agents such as plants, fungi, fish, and shellfish (actually algae ingested by shellfish) can also produce toxins that can cause acute poisoning, including fatal paralysis. Contaminants in the soil and water can bioaccumulate; that is, their concentration increases as they advance up the food chain, ultimately reaching the dinner table of humans. Human activities in agriculture and cattle-raising provide ample opportunities for contamination from pesticides, fertilizers, antibiotics, and growth hormones. Additional contamination can occur during food processing, packaging, and storage. Food additives and irradiation reduce the threat from biological hazards, yet may introduce new and uncertain health risks from physical and chemical agents.

Shelter

While the basic purpose of housing is to provide shelter from the elements, housing offers a focus for family and communal life. Unfortunately, the dwellings in which most of the world's population lives fail to satisfy such basic needs, and instead expose them to serious health risks.

The health effects of poor housing have been recognized for a long time. Major advances in public health in the developed countries occurred in the nineteenth century when the dismal living conditions of the urban poor were ameliorated. In recent decades, the attention has shifted from gross dilapidation and unsanitary conditions to problems associated with indoor air quality and other chemical and physical hazards in the home. In terms of health effects, psychological well-being and injuries have become as important as severe morbidity and mortality from infectious diseases.[22]

The quality of shelter is compromised by overcrowding, inadequate sanitation facilities, presence of fire and other safety hazards, poor ventilation, thermoregulation, and illumination. Most jurisdictions have building codes that regulate the construction of buildings to safely sustain the loads expected from the type of occupancy and to be reasonably safe from fire and similar hazards. Housing standards, on the other hand, define the health requirements of "decent" housing and ensure that the dwelling is safe, sanitary, and fit for human habitation. The American Public Health Association (APHA) has been in the forefront of promoting the establishment of standards on housing and guidelines to evaluate its quality and impact on health. As early as 1938, its Committee on the Hygiene of Housing, chaired by Charles-Edward Winslow, published *Basic Principles of Healthful Housing*.[23]

Housing is more than a physical structure designed to keep its occupants dry, warm, safe, and free from disease. People's homes are meaningful places, intimately connected to their sense of security, confidence, self-esteem, and overall social and emotional well-being.

People's perception of housing quality varies tremendously from one culture to another. The perception of overcrowding differs substantially between that of North American suburbanites and residents of a public housing estate in an Asian city. Architectural and aesthetic qualities of housing reflect prevalent cultural values—for example, the spatial orientation of the building, the allocation of space for family activities, the social roles of children and the elderly, and attitudes towards privacy. Within a community, the physical location of houses can have a major impact on social interactions, a fact often overlooked in refugee resettlement schemes. Thus, failure to respect the territoriality of clans or other subgroups, to accommodate the needs of extended families, and to provide equitable access to open spaces and water resources can lead to social conflicts.

Global ecosystem

Risks to human population health from global environmental changes are a new departure from the conventional concerns with specific hazards in the environment. The United Nations convened in 1983 a World Commission on Environment and Development, chaired by Gro Harlem Brundtland, then prime minister of Norway. The Commission's 1987 report, *Our Common Future*, took stock of the situation and urged action to ensure a viable future for the human species. This was followed by the WHO's Commission on Health and the Environment, which reported in 1992. At the beginning of the twenty-first century, several problems of global significance have emerged: the greenhouse effect, resulting in global warming and other climatic changes; stratospheric ozone depletion, resulting in increased exposure to ultraviolet radiation; the release of acid rain from the combustion of sulfurous fossil fuels and its long-range transport; land degradation from over-intensive agriculture and excessive grazing, contributing to soil erosion, salinization, desertification, and the depletion of underground acquifers; loss of biodiversity from the destruction of habitats such as the rainforest and extinction of many species of plants and animals; and overpopulation leading to increased competition for limited resources, rural–urban migration, and the creation of large urban slums.[24]

The effects of such changes tend to be general, affecting the well-being and indeed the survival of the species, rather than specific diseases. Predicting such effects is fraught with problems since there are usually no precedents, and existing data are greatly limited. Often computer simulation models have to be relied upon. On the other hand, inaction while waiting for definitive answers is not a prudent alternative.

Personal Lifestyles and Behaviors

It is increasingly recognized that many personal behaviors or lifestyles are associated with the development of a variety of diseases and health problems. Of particular importance are such individual behaviors as smoking, diet, alcohol and drug use, physical activity, sexual behavior, and safety practices. The modification of such behaviors has become the mainstay of current efforts in health promotion.

Smoking

The most important lifestyle determinant of health is smoking. Because tobacco use is a form of addiction, some would consider it a disease in its own right, and not just a risk factor for other diseases. Indeed, in ICD-9, tobacco dependence is given a code (305.1). In ICD-10, there is a category (F17) labelled "mental and behavioral disorders due to the use of tobacco."

Nicotine is the addictive substance in tobacco. There are, however, myriad chemical substances in tobacco that are responsible for an ever-increasing list of diseases and adverse health effects (Box 4.6). See also Case Study 6.3 in Chapter 6, which traces the evolution of our understanding of the causal link between cigarette smoking and lung cancer. Box 5.3 in Chapter 5 demonstrates how mortality attributable to smoking is calculated.

BOX 4.5.   Words and Origins

Lifestyle has been defined as "the culturally, socially, economically and environmentally conditioned complex of actions characteristic of an individual or group . . . as a pattern of habituated behaviors over time that is health related but not necessarily health directed."[25]

The term *lifestyle* comes from the German *Lebenstil*, which was used in the sociological writings of Karl Marx (1818–1883) and Max Weber (1864–1920). The term represented the characteristics of social groups, a forerunner of the modern concept of socioeconomic position. In the 1920s the concept was incorporated into the personality theories of psychiatrist Alfred Adler (1870–1937). The application of the term *lifestyle* to individual behavior was confined to the field of clinical psychology until the 1960s. *Index Medicus* did not index articles under "lifestyle" until the early 1970s, when it was differentiated from "personality development" as a separate subject heading. Since then the use of the term *lifestyle* in the health literature has burgeoned, although the majority of articles used it to refer to specific personal behaviors identified as disease risk factors. The *Adlerian* definition is still provided in standard dictionaries. The *New Shorter Oxford Dictionary* (1993), for example, defines it as "a person's basic character as established early in childhood which governs his or her reactions and behavior."

The prevalence of smoking has declined in North America since the 1960s, when about half of all adults were smokers. By 2000 only about one in three were smokers. The decline has been more rapid and substantial among men than women, so that the prevalence of smoking among women, while still lower, now approaches that of men. Figure 4.2 shows that U.S. men born during 1911–1930 achieved the highest prevalence of 66%. Birth cohorts after 1931 experienced successively lower peak prevalences. Women began to smoke in substantial numbers much later in the century than did men. The highest peak prevalence among women occurred for the 1931–1940 cohort, reaching 44% in 1965.[26] (This is an example of *age-period-cohort analysis*. A further example is given in Case Study 6.1 in Chapter 6.)

Another estimate of a population's exposure to tobacco is the per capita consumption, derived from sales data and applied to the entire adult population, smokers and nonsmokers included. In the United States, an adult smoked on the average 50 cigarettes a year at the beginning of the twentieth century, increasing to over 4,000/year in the 1960s, and declining since then to under 3,000 in the 1990s.

The prevalence of smoking only conveys one aspect of the pattern of smoking in a population. Based on responses to questions in surveys about smoking initiation and cessation, respondents can be divided into

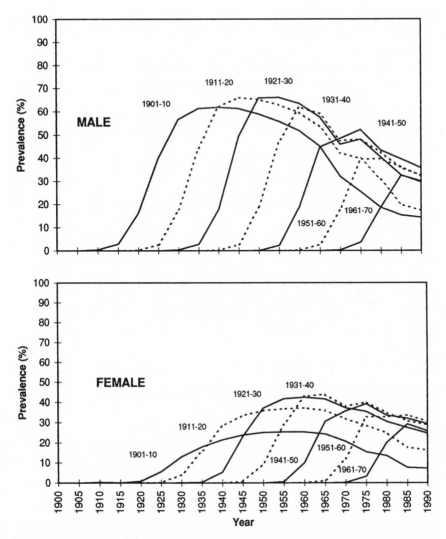

Figure 4.2. Prevalence of cigarette smoking among successive birth cohorts of Americans.

never and *ever* smokers, the latter into *former* and *current* smokers, who can be further divided into *regular* and *occasional* smokers. Current smokers differ in terms of the number of cigarettes they smoke per day, and can be designated *heavy, moderate,* and *light* smokers. In many epidemiological studies, the duration of smoking is often incorporated into an index with *pack-years* as the unit.

In addition to indicators from surveys that must rely on recall, there are also biochemical methods that can be used to validate the questionnaire response. These involve measuring nicotine, its metabolite cotinine, or thiocyanate (a metabolite of cyanide) in various body fluids such as blood, saliva, and urine. Carbon monoxide can also be measured in the breath.[27]

Smoking patterns vary between countries—the prevalence and consumption is much higher in the developing countries. Within countries, they differ according to geographic regions, ethnic groups, age, sex, and socioeconomic status. In general, the prevalence of smoking tends to be higher among people with less education and lower income.

The reasons why people smoke are varied and complex, including the pharmacological action of nicotine, individual personality, social

---

BOX 4.6.   Tobacco Smoke: Chemical Hazards and Health Risks

The burning of tobacco releases *mainstream* smoke (MS), which travels through the tobacco column and is inhaled; and *sidestream* smoke (SS), which is emitted into ambient air from the smouldering cigarette.[28] Over 4,000 chemicals have been identified in tobacco smoke in the vapor phase and as particulates. The concentration of many of these substances is higher in SS than MS. Many are also present in smokeless tobacco.

At least 40 chemicals in tobacco smoke are known carcinogens or mutagens, including: carbon monoxide, hydrogen cyanide, arsenic, nickel, cadmium, lead, benzene, vinyl chloride, polycyclic aromatic hydrocarbons, N-nitrosamines, aldehydes, aromatic amines, aza-arenes, and others.

According the Cancer Prevention Study (CPS-II), the risks of mortality from various causes among current smokers aged 35+, relative to nonsmokers, are:

	M	F		M	F
Cancers:			**Respiratory Diseases:**		
Lip, oral cavity, pharynx	27.5	5.6	*Bronchitis, emphysema*	9.7	10.5
Trachea, bronchus, lung	22.4	11.9	*Other respiratory diseases*	2.0	2.2
Larynx	10.5	17.8			
Esophagus	7.6	10.3	**Cardiovascular Diseases:**		
Kidneys and urinary tract	3.0	1.4	*Cerebrovascular disease (ages 35–64)*	3.7	4.8
Bladder	2.9	2.6	*Ischemic heart*	2.8	3.0
Pancreas	2.1	2.3	*disease (ages 35–64)*		
Cervix	–	2.1	*Other heart disease*	1.9	1.7

In addition, smoking is associated with complications of pregnancy, perinatal and neonatal mortality, sudden infant death syndrome, and child growth retardation.

interactions, market forces, and the legislative and regulatory environment. Knowledge of the health consequences of smoking plays only a minor role in deterring people from smoking.[29]

Smoking can be described as a "career," with different stages: from initiation, to habitual use, to cessation. Cessation is characterized by contemplation, quitting, maintenance, and relapse. Different influences and actions are in play at different stages.

Nicotine is rapidly absorbed into the bloodstream and delivered to the brain, where nicotine-specific receptors have been demonstrated. Nicotine exerts an euphoric and anxiolytic effect, and is capable of reinforcing behavior even in laboratory animals. It is associated with physical and psychological withdrawal symptoms. The desire to smoke, however, is more dependent on conditioning to cues associated with smoking than on blood nicotine levels.

Psychological studies have linked smoking to rebelliousness, impulsiveness, and identity assertion in adolescents. Depending on ethnic and socioeconomic status, a poor self-image and low achievement may also be predictors. Peer and parental (or spousal) models influence smoking initiation and inhibit attempts at quitting.

The availability of cigarettes, a function of price and the compliance of retailers with age limits, has a major influence on smoking behavior, especially among adolescents. The tobacco industry devotes massive resources towards sales promotion, including advertising and sponsorship of public events. It is highly targeted at specific socio-demographic groups. Brands cater to those who like to conceive of themselves as "macho" men, "liberated" women, or "cool" teenagers. Endorsement by the medical profession, incredible as it seems now, was once common.[30]

Societal measures such as enacting and enforcing laws to regulate sales and promotion, prohibit smoking in public places and the workplace, and increase taxation of tobacco products, have a strong impact on smoking behavior. Such measures reflect the growing social unacceptability of smoking, and they in turn reinforce and promote not smoking as a social norm.

Alcohol use

There are many parallels between smoking and alcohol use. At one point, both were considered vices, and North America actually experienced the official prohibition of alcohol. One can view tobacco and alcohol as examples of an array of pharmacological agents that human societies have discovered through the ages that are capable of producing pleasurable effects.

The assessment of the extent and impact of alcohol use is hampered by the limited sources of epidemiological data. In the ICD-10, a variety of codes make direct reference to alcohol. Mental and behavioral disorders due to the use of alcohol are designated F10, with subcategories for harmful use, dependence, withdrawal, delirium, psychotic disorders, amnesia, and other residual effects. (F11–F19 are similarly organized for the other

---

BOX 4.7.   Terms of Use and Abuse

There is considerable confusion in the terminology denoting the use and abuse of alcohol and other psychoactive substances.[31]

The ICD-10 distinguishes between *harmful use* and *dependence syndrome*. The former refers to use that causes damage to health, and is synonymous with *substance abuse*. *Dependence* is defined as "a cluster of behavioral, cognitive, and physiological phenomena that develop after repeated substance use" and is associated with "a strong desire to take the drug, difficulty in controlling its use, persisting in its use despite harmful consequences, a higher priority given to drug use than to other activities and obligations, increased tolerance, and sometimes a withdrawal state." It is synonymous with *drug addiction*, and if alcohol is the substance used, *chronic alcoholism*.

The American Psychiatric Association's *Diagnostic and Statistical Manual*, the 1994 edition of which is referred to as *DSM-IV*, is generally compatible with ICD-10. It recognizes both *substance abuse* and *substance dependence*. Both refer to a maladaptive pattern of use leading to clinically significant impairment or distress—although for a patient to be designated as dependent, the criteria of tolerance, withdrawal, and compulsive use need to be present, whereas abuse refers only to the consequences of repeated use. *Abuse* and *dependence* can be applied to alcohol and a host of other substances. The terms *alcoholism* and *addiction*, however, do not appear in *DSM-IV*.

The term *alcoholism* continues to be favored by some specialists in the field. The National Council on Alcoholism and Drug Dependence and the American Society of Addiction Medicine proposed a definition of alcoholism: "a primary, chronic disease with genetic, psychosocial, and environmental factors influencing its development and manifestations . . . often progressive and fatal . . . characterized by impaired control over drinking, preoccupation with the drug alcohol, use of alcohol despite adverse consequences, and distortions in thinking, most notably denial."

---

psychoactive substances.) Alcoholic liver diseases (K70) comprise alcoholic hepatitis and cirrhosis. Poisoning and exposure to alcohol are given codes of X45 for accidental, X65 for intentional, and Y15 for undetermined intent. Some diseases have an "alcoholic" epithet attached; for example, alcoholic cardiomyopathy (I42.6), alcoholic gastritis (K29.2), and alcoholic pancreatitis (K86.0). Alcohol also plays a contributory role in many injuries, various gastrointestinal cancers, infectious diseases, and nutritional deficiencies. The impact of alcohol extends into the second generation in the form of fetal alcohol syndrome (Q86.0).

Beyond disease and injury, alcohol disrupts the social and economic well-being of families and communities. Data collected by the law enforcement and justice systems can provide additional information on the impact of alcohol on the community.

Alcohol, however, is not without health benefits. Many studies in diverse populations have demonstrated an inverse association between "moderate" alcohol intake and coronary heart disease. Individuals who consume one to three drinks a day have a 10%–40% lower risk than abstainers. The beneficial action of alcohol is probably mediated through changes in serum lipids and hemostatic factors. The risk decreases linearly with alcohol intake up to about three drinks a day. At higher consumptions, disease risk increases: thus the relationship can be described as U-shaped. It should be noted that for the other health outcomes, there are different "risk curves": for cancers, it is linear; for cirrhosis, it is curvilinear, with disproportionately higher risk at high consumption levels; with hypertension, there is probably a threshold effect, i.e., there is no dose–response relationship below a certain level of consumption.[32]

To assess the extent of alcohol use in the population that is not dependent on contact with any health and social service, a survey needs to be conducted. Questions can be designed to determine the frequency, quantity, and type of alcohol use. Biomarkers such as serum levels of the liver enzymes glutamyl transferase (GGT) and aspartate aminotrasferase (AST) can also be used to complement and validate responses to questionnaires.

Illicit drugs

Other drugs (prescribed and nonprescribed, legal and illegal) that have an impact on health include opioids, cannabinoids, sedatives and hypnotics, cocaine, stimulants, hallucinogens, and volatile solvents. Different populations "favor" certain drugs over others, depending on availability, social preferences, law enforcement practices, and cultural beliefs.

One approach to illicit drug use as a public health problem goes under the label of *harm reduction*. Harm reduction focuses on reducing the health and social consequences of drug use rather than eliminating drug use itself (thus the "harm" refers to the harm of HIV and hepatitis infections as consequences of intravenous drug use, rather than to the harm of heroin addiction itself). It originated in the Netherlands in the 1980s and has spawned programs of needle exchange, safe houses, state-supplied drugs, medically supervised use, and calls for decriminalization. It is at the opposite end of the spectrum of drug policies from the "war on drugs," which emphasizes military or police operations against producers, seizures of assets, tough sentences for offenders, and surveillance and drug-testing programs. Critics of the harm reduction strategy charge that it condones and even encourages drug use, while supporters point to successes in curbing the spread of HIV. Proponents of the harm reduction approach highlight four basic assumptions: (1) it is a public health alternative to the moral/criminal and disease models of drug use and addiction; (2) it recognizes abstinence as an ideal outcome but accepts alternatives that reduce harm; (3) it is a grassroots approach based on addict advocacy rather than top-down policy established by addiction professionals; and (4) it promotes low-threshold access to services through outreach, eliminating preconditions, and reducing stigma.[33]

The harm reduction approach is also diametrically opposite to the current health promotion approach to the other major addiction, tobacco use. Both pose serious health risks to human populations and are difficult to control. For tobacco, currently a legal product, the dominant approach is regulatory, restrictive, and punitive, affecting sales, advertising, and consumption in public places. The goal is cessation, rather than "social" smoking, switching to low-tar cigarettes, or providing enhanced cancer screening services for smokers.

Why do people use substances such as tobacco, alcohol, and illicit drugs? There is no lack of theoretical perspectives in the social sciences literature—one review counted 14 theories! These could be grouped into four categories:

1. Cognitive-affective theories, which posit that substance use involves a decision-making process whereby the consequences of the behavior are weighed against the values placed on it. An example is the *theory of reasoned action* of Icek Ajzen and Martin Fishbein (more about this in Chapter 7);
2. Social learning theories, which emphasize the effects of substance-using role models, an example being the *social cognitive theory* of Albert Bandura;
3. Conventional commitment and social attachment theories, which identify factors that promote withdrawal from conventional society, detachment from families, and attachment to substance-using peers;
4. Theories that attribute behaviors to intrapersonal processes such as personality traits, affective state, and biological predispositions.

These diverse theories can be organized into a framework consisting of three types of influences: social/interpersonal; cultural/attitudinal; and intrapersonal, which operate at the proximal, distal, and ultimate levels along the causal pathway.[34]

Nutrition and diet

The importance of nutrition and diet as a determinant of health status is well established.[35] The human diet consists of macronutrients (proteins, carbohydrates, and fats), vitamins, fiber, minerals (e.g., calcium, magnesium, iron, iodine, trace elements), electrolytes (e.g., sodium, potassium, chloride), and water. The macronutrients are the main sources of energy needed by the body to perform its functions. Various metabolic and neurobehavioral processes are involved in the maintenance of energy balance. An excess of intake (as in overnutrition) or a reduction in energy

BOX 4.8.   Criteria for Obesity and Overweight

Obesity is the excess of body fat or of adipose tissue.[36] The human body can be conceptualized as having several compartments. If viewed chemically, these compartments are total body fat (TBF) and fat-free body mass (FFM), the latter being composed of water, proteins, minerals, and glycogen. If viewed anatomically, the body can be regarded as being composed of adipose tissue (AT) and lean body mass (LBM), which consists of bones, skeletal muscles, and other soft tissues. The two schemes do not coincide exactly, due to the presence of non-fat in adipose tissue, or fat-free adipose tissue (FFAT). Thus FFM = LBM + FFAT and AT = TBF + FFAT.

Strictly speaking, the only true direct measure of human obesity would involve dissection of the body and chemical analysis of its components, an approach advisable only for cadavers. For live human beings, three basic approaches are commonly used:

1. Anthropometry—height and weight, skinfold thicknesses, and waist and hip circumferences;
2. Measures of percent body fat by estimating the various compartments, using techniques such as hydrodensitometry, isotope dilution, neutron activation, bioelectrical impedance, and infrared interactance;
3. Direct visualization of body compartments using clinical imaging techniques such as x-radiography, computer tomography, ultrasonography, and magnetic resonance, at different cross-sections of the body.

Most of these methods, with the exception of anthropometry, are cumbersome and unsuitable for large population surveys. Indices based on height and weight are attractive because of their ease of measurement and reproducibility. The body mass index (BMI), also called Quetelet's index, named after the Belgian statistician Adolphe Quetelet (1796–1874), is widely used. It is computed from the formula (weight in kg)/(height in meters)^2. Both WHO and NIH recommend using BMI and have almost identical cutoff points.

Underweight: <18.5
Normal: 18.5–24.9
Overweight: 25.0–29.9
Obese: ≥30.0

The "obese" category can be further divided into three classes of increasing severity: I (30.0–34.9), II (35.0–39.9), and III (≥ 40.0). In addition, there is substantial evidence showing that the regional distribution of body fat is an important and independent risk factor for many chronic diseases such as diabetes and coronary heart disease.

(continued)

There are two types of fat patterning:

1. Central, also called abdominal, android, truncal, upper-body, or "apple"
2. Peripheral, gluteo-femoral, gynecoid, centripetal, lower-body, or "pear"

It is (1) that is associated with adverse health outcomes. The ratio of waist-to-hip circumference (WHR) is a common measure of regional fat patterning. It has now been replaced by simply the waist circumference. Adult men with waist circumference >102 cm and women with >88 cm are considered at increased risk of adverse health effects.

Because children and adolescents are rapidly growing with changing body dimensions, the "one-size-fits-all" criteria for adults are not appropriate. For this group, the criteria need to be age- and sex-specific, and require comparison with a "standard" population distribution. The CDC published a new set of revised growth charts in 2000 for boys and girls aged 2–20 years, and overweight is defined as BMI at or above the 95th percentile. These charts are derived from nationally representative data from the National Health and Nutrition Surveys. (The older 1977 version was also adopted for international use by WHO.)

Obesity is the new epidemic of the twenty-first century. The U.S. Surgeon General has issued a "call to action" to prevent and decrease its prevalence. It is no longer a problem exclusively of the developed countries, but has become a global one.

expenditure through physical inactivity can lead to obesity, itself a risk factor for some diseases.

It should be remembered that human beings eat foods, not nutrients, and that foods are very complex chemically. Some nutrients are distributed over many foods. Evidence for disease causation or prevention would be strengthened if an effect could be demonstrated for a nutrient as well as foods rich in that nutrient.

In much of the world, the priority still remains the attainment of an adequate food supply for the whole population and the elimination of nutritional deficiency diseases, such as protein-calorie malnutrition, blindness resulting from vitamin A deficiency, rickets from vitamin D deficiency, endemic goiter from iodine deficiency, and iron deficiency anemia. (In Chapter 1, Case Study 1.4 introduces pellagra, a vitamin-deficiency disease that is now only of historical interest.) Nutritional deficiency diseases have not entirely disappeared from the developed countries, and may still affect specific, usually economically disadvantaged, segments of the population. Increasingly, the diet–health relationship is now focused on the chronic diseases, especially cardiovascular diseases (ischemic heart disease, stroke, hypertension), certain cancers (gastrointestinal tract, liver, lung, prostate), diabetes, gallbladder disease, osteoporosis, and dental caries. The epidemiological evidence linking these diseases with specific nutrients is extensive but inconsistent.

The emergence of chronic diseases is closely related to the changes in dietary pattern of the human species. Modern humans have been called "stone-agers in the fast lane." While still possessing the genetic makeup of the late Pleistocene hunter-gatherers, which has hardly changed in 10,000 years, modern humans live in a nutritional environment very unlike that to which our ancestors have adapted. For many populations, the transition to the "Western" or "affluent" diet occurred relatively recently and rapidly.[37]

Based on the current state of knowledge, various government health agencies, national cancer societies, and heart associations have issued nutritional advice, guidelines, or recommendations. These aim to encourage the public to adopt a dietary pattern that will provide the amounts of nutrients required by the body while reducing the risk of diseases. While aimed at individuals, these can also be regarded as population health goals to be achieved by a combination of education and public policy. The U.S. Department of Agriculture and the Department of Health and Human Services have since 1980 jointly published the *Dietary Guidelines for Americans* every five years.[38] The 2000 version offers these advice:

1. Aim for fitness:
   - Aim for a healthy weight
   - Be physically active each day
2. Build a healthy base:
   - Make food choices from the "food guide pyramid" (consisting of five food groups with recommended servings)
   - Choose a variety of grains daily, especially whole grains
   - Choose a variety of fruits and vegetables daily
   - Keep food safe to eat
3. Choose sensibly:
   - Choose a diet low in saturated fat and cholesterol and moderate in total fat
   - Choose beverages and foods to moderate intake of sugars
   - Choose and prepare foods with less salt
   - If one drinks alcoholic beverages, do so in moderation

Other guidelines are more specific, indicating the proportion of energy to be obtained from fat and carbohydrates. Government agencies also issue recommended nutrient intakes (RNI) or recommended dietary allowances (RDA), expressed in quantitative units such as μg, mg, or g of nutrients per day. These are intended to meet the needs of almost all individuals and so exceed the actual requirements of almost all. They are neither the average nor usual intake of members of the population. RNI and RDA are originally established in the days when the concerns were primarily with inadequate intakes. With many nutrients, the concern has now shifted to excessive intake. Some guidelines now also include a "safe range" to minimize the risk of both excess and inadequacy.

There are many methods in the quantitative assessment of nutrient intake. There are direct methods, which involve food diaries, direct observations, weighing, and chemical analyses of food. Others are based on responses to surveys, such as 24-hour dietary recall and food frequency questionnaires (FFQ). The FFQ reflects long-term, usual intake and is essentially a list of preselected foods with a choice of frequency responses. Some FFQs are semi-quantitative, including questions on the number of servings and serving sizes, aided by actual models of plates, glasses, heaps, spoons, etc. Food consumption data obtained from surveys are then translated into nutrients using food composition tables. The adequacy of some nutrient intake can be measured using biochemical markers in various body fluids or tissues, although the relationship between dietary intake and body burden is often not straightforward.[39]

Physical activity

Participation in physical activity, whether at work or during leisure time, has been shown to prevent some cardiovascular, metabolic, and musculoskeletal problems and promote an overall sense of well-being. Physical activity need not be strenuous to achieve health benefits. Men and women of all ages benefit from a moderate amount of physical activity, which is a function of frequency, intensity, and duration.[40]

Terms such as *physical activity, exercise,* and *fitness* are often used interchangeably but in fact represent very different concepts. *Physical activity* is defined as any bodily movement produced by skeletal muscles that results in energy expenditure above the basal level. Energy is measured in *kilojoules* (kJ) under SI (*le Système international*), which replace the old familiar unit of *kilocalories* (kcal) [1 kcal = 4.184 kJ]. Exercise is a type of physical activity that is planned, structured, and repetitive, with a final or intermediate objective of improving or maintaining physical fitness. While the intensity of physical activity can be categorized in descriptive terms as *mild, moderate,* or *vigorous,* a quantitative measure is *metabolic equivalents* (METs), which is the amount of oxygen consumed by the activity. One MET equals the resting metabolic rate, about 3.5 milliliter of oxygen per kilogram of body weight per minute. Intensity is also commonly expressed relative to the individual's *maximal oxygen uptake* (% VO_2 max).

Physical fitness is a set of attributes that are either health- or skill-related. The former includes cardiorespiratory endurance, muscular endurance, muscular strength, body composition, and flexibility. These are far more important to population health than attributes of athletic ability; namely agility, balance, coordination, speed, power, and reaction time.

There is an armamentarium of tests and procedures. Some of these are complex, time-consuming, and require the expertise of specialists in exercise physiology, or *kinesiologists* (*kinesis* is Greek for movement). Other measures are simple and can be used in population surveys, either based on self-reports (responses to questionnaires, activity diaries/logs; quantitative histories) or direct monitoring (behavioral observation; mechanical/electronic devices; physiological measurements).

Sexual and reproductive behaviors

The use of contraceptive devices, the age at onset and frequency of sexual intercourse, and the number of sexual partners, are important risk factors for such problems as sexually transmitted diseases (STDs) and unplanned pregnancies. Such practices are increasingly of interest in view of the rise of the AIDS epidemic. STDs are in turn risk factors for other health problems, including genital cancers, pelvic inflammatory diseases, ectopic pregnancies, infertility, and adverse pregnancy outcomes such as prematurity and low birth weight.

The spread of STDs in populations is determined by three sets of conditions:

(1) The probability of exposure: The likelihood of an uninfected person's being exposed to an infected individual varies according to the number of sexual partners, the extent of a high-risk sexual network, and the presence of an indiscriminate pattern of partner recruitment. The engagement in high-risk behavior, especially by adolescents, needs to be understood from a multisystem perspective that goes beyond the individual to the family, peer group, and the broader social environment.

(2) The probability of transmission: When an encounter occurs, transmission of the pathogen from the infected to the uninfected depends on the virulence of the microorganism, the infective dose, and the host's susceptibility, which are affected by vaginal ecology, male circumcision, and the use of barriers.

(3) The duration of infectiousness: An infected person remains infectious until such time he or she is diagnosed and receives appropriate treatment. This is dependent on health-care-seeking behavior by the individual, and health care system issues such as accessibility of services and providers' attitudes and behaviors, which may discourage use.[41]

Much of the current emphasis in sexual health promotion can be summed up under the slogan "safe sex," centered around the use of the condom. Education programs promoting safer sex are directed at high-risk groups such as adolescents and college students, as well as the general public at large through the mass media.

The prevalence of safe sex practices can be determined only by surveys, which must rely on the accuracy of the recall and truthfulness of the response. Condom use as a behavior is influenced by demographic characteristics such as age, education, marital status, and sexual orientation, as well as many other cultural, religious, and socioeconomic factors. Availability (cost and ease of purchase) affects use. Incorrect beliefs about the inhibition of pleasure, insufficient knowledge of the risk of disease transmissibility, and alcohol and drug use at the time hinder its use by men. Furthermore, a woman's desire to protect herself is not simply a matter of individual choice but involves negotiation with her partner, whose outcome often reflects the different power relationships based on gender roles and economic status.[42]

Safety practices

Injuries are major causes of mortality and morbidity, especially among children and young adults.[43] Among the causes and determinants of injuries are individual behaviors related to the safety practices in the home and during the operation of a vehicle. The extent of practices related to fire safety (presence of a functional smoke detector near sleeping area); scald prevention (control of hot water temperature); poison control (telephone access to poison control centers and having ipecac on hand to induce vomiting); car safety (use of seatbelts and appropriate child restraint devices); boat safety (use of flotation devices), etc., can be determined in health interview surveys.

As with most individual behaviors, knowledge, belief, and intent do not always translate into practice. Safety practices are also sensitive to socioeconomic factors such as household income, education, employment, ethnicity, and family structure and size. Surveys have shown that the adoption of preventive measures relating to car safety and fire prevention tend to be high. Parents tend to be less concerned about safety issues and injuries among children than they are about child abduction and drug abuse, both of which receive considerably more media publicity. Many parents believe that "being careful" is an effective and adequate preventive measure.

Social, Cultural, and Economic Factors

The association between the social environment and health has been observed for a long time. In Victorian England, the landmark study by Edwin Chadwick (1800–1890), *Report on the Sanitary Condition of the Labouring Population of Great Britain* (1842), used maps and statistics to establish the link between unsanitary living conditions and the poor health of workers. His report sparked a series of reforms that led to the creation of the modern public health system. At about the same time, Friedrich Engels (1820–1895) published *The Condition of the Working Classes in England* (1844) and described vividly the urban squalor and its impact on health.[44] Case Study 4.4 at the end of this chapter highlights research in "social medicine" in Germany at the beginning of the twentieth century.

The term *social epidemiology* first appeared in the 1950s and had its origin in medical sociology. In the 1970s it gained prominence through the work of John Cassel (1921–1976), who studied the rural poor in the Appalachians. In the 1990s, there was renewed interest in health disparities between social groups, and the investigation of the social determinants of health has become the dominant focus of population health.[45]

A remarkable and consistent finding in the social epidemiology literature is the gradient across different socioeconomic groups, no matter how they are defined, and regardless of the measures used for health outcome, whether mortality or morbidity, and applicable both to individual diseases and when all causes are combined. This gradient has persisted despite major improvements in the health and wealth of many populations. For some diseases, the association with socioeconomic status has actually reversed over time. Thus ischemic heart disease, long identified as a "disease of affluence," has become a disease affecting mainly the lower socioeconomic status groups, at least within developed countries.[46]

Globally, the health of nations is also very much correlated with their wealth. In international comparisons, health indicators like life expectancy vary according to the gross domestic product (GDP) of countries, although the relationship is not linear (Figure 4.3). Higher per-capita incomes, through steady and stable economic growth, increase a nation's capacity to purchase the necessary economic goods and services that promote health. The relationship between health and the economy in fact goes in both directions. Development economists are increasingly coming to the realization that health is a form of human capital and improving health is a necessary condition for the achievement of economic prosperity.[47]

In examining the relationship between the health and the wealth of nations, researchers such as Richard Wilkinson proposed that it was not just overall poverty that determined the health of nations, but also income inequality within nations. In a landmark study of nine OECD countries, Wilkinson found a strong correlation between life expectancy and income inequality, the latter measured by the share of the total income earned by the bottom 70% of the population. Combined with the gross national product per capita, income inequality accounted for three-quarters of the variance in life expectancy, whereas GNP per capita by itself could explain less than 10%. This study generated considerable debate and has been criticized on methodological grounds. The relationship was replicated by studies of mortality in American states and metropolitan areas but was inconsistent when different selections of countries and different measures of health status and income inequality were used. For example, the inclusion of Canadian provinces and metropolitan areas resulted in a strong North America–wide correlation between mortality and income

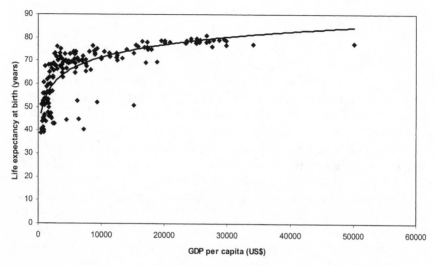

Figure 4.3. Correlation of infant mortality rate and gross national product.

inequality, but within Canada itself there was no corelation, suggesting that national policies directed at income distribution may have reduced the effects of inequality on health. In an editorial in the *British Medical Journal*, where much of this research was published, Johan Mackenbach concluded that the weight of the evidence was against an association, but considered it useful to have focused research on contextual factors for population income and reinforced the importance of individual income.[48]

The terms *socioeconomic status* (SES) and *social class* are often used loosely and interchangeably by health researchers. While they are both used to denote some kind of ranking and grouping of individuals within society, there are distinct concepts embedded in these terms that require clarification. *Class* refers to a social group formed by interdependent economic relationships among people, based on their position within the economy, with regard to property ownership, and the production, distribution, and consumption of goods and services. Classes "co-define" each other (e.g., employer/employee) and they tend to be in competition or conflict with one another; in a sense, one class gains at the expense of the other. The sociologist Erik Wright defined social classes on the basis of (1) ownership of capital assets; (2) control of organization assets; and (3) possession of skill or credential assets. He developed a three-question survey that captures hierarchy within the organization (manager, supervisor, and worker), participation in decision-making, and the opportunity to supervise others.[49]

The Registrar-General in England (with a long history dating back to the pioneer days of William Farr—whose acquaintance we have made in Chapter 2) has since 1913 used a "social class" scale based on the occupation of the "head of household": I, professional; II, intermediate; III, skilled labor (subdivided into non-manual and manual); IV, partly skilled; and V, unskilled. These categories are ranked according to the degree of "skill" involved and they broadly reflect social prestige, education level, and household income. (Queen Victoria may have been head of state, but being a woman, was not counted as the head of household—so the story goes!) Revisions are made periodically to account for new occupations and changes in skills and status attached to existing ones. Over time, the composition and size of these classes change. As can be expected, this system has been much criticized for its class and gender bias in the political sense. A major deficiency is its exclusion of individuals or groups outside the formal paid labor force: for example, the unemployed, retirees, students, homemakers, and those engaged in the "underground economy." This can be partly remedied by using proxy measures such as spouse's and parents' occupation, and "last occupation prior to retirement/unemployment." The scheme persists because it is a convenient measure and relatively simple to use, and it still has utility in demonstrating gradients in health indicators within populations.

SES, or *socioeconomic position*, which is preferred by some researchers, encompasses possession of material and social resources (such as income and education) and rank or status within a social hierarchy in relation to access to and consumption of goods, services, and knowledge. SES can be measured at the level of the individual, household, and neighborhood, as well as within different points in the life course (infancy, childhood, etc.). In many research studies, different components of SES (e.g., education, income, employment) may be measured separately. As these variables tend to be interrelated, many studies simply use one measure to represent the total construct of SES. Alternatively, multiple regression techniques can be used to determine which of several SES variables are independently predictive of health outcome. However, one can refine the analytical process by taking into account the temporal ordering of the SES variables in the causal pathway. Thus one can conceive of education as the most "distal"; it in turn affects occupation, and ultimately income, which is the most "proximal" to the outcome variable (see figure below).

Yet another approach is to combine the different components into a single index of SES, based on a mathematical formula.[50]

Some types of data are more conveniently available at the neighborhood (or census-tract) level, and they are often applied at the individual

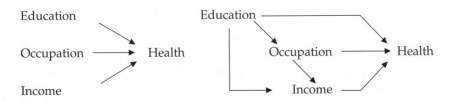

level. For example, an individual living in an area with a high average income is presumed to be rich. Aggregate level data such as neighborhood safety, pollution level, social disorganization, etc., however, are important in their own right, and they need to be taken into consideration alongside individual SES to provide a multilevel understanding of the social production of health.

The preoccupation with individual-level variables is detrimental to a full understanding of the social determinants of health. The concept of *social capital*, well known to sociologists, has been applied to explain why some communities or populations are healthier than others (as well as possessing attributes such as less crime and more democracy). Social capital is the "features of social organization such as the extent of interpersonal trust between citizens, norms of reciprocity, and density of civic associations, that facilitate cooperation for mutual benefit."[51] A substantial body of evidence has now been accumulated that shows the association between the lack of social capital and higher mortality and poorer self-rated health, even after other SES factors have been adjusted for.

Social factors are often measured to be "controlled for," as confounders (see Chapter 6), and their role as explanatory variables in their own right is sometimes neglected. When SES is touted as the "cause" of a disease, it is often treated very much like a "black box," with little concern for or interest in the precise mechanisms of how social factors influence health. While health interventions that ignore the social and economic forces predisposing and contributing to ill health are unlikely to be successful, to aver that all one needs to do is to "change society" (usually according to the dictates of one's preferred political ideology) and good health will ensue, is overly simplistic.

There does not appear to be a threshold effect for SES. The health gradient does not just occur between the highest and lowest status groups, but throughout the entire spectrum. Poverty is not the entire explanation. In the era of infectious diseases, high SES promotes health, most likely through better housing and nutrition, which reduce the opportunity for infection and improve the outcome of disease. How SES improves health in the era of chronic diseases is by no means agreed. Some believe that better access to medical care by the higher SES groups is the key. Subscribers to the McKeown-McKinlay thesis on the limited role of medical care measures on health (see Chapter 2) would disagree. Certainly in countries such as Canada and the United Kingdom, where there is universal access to essentially free medical care, SES gradients in health status persist. In the United Kingdom, the 1980 *Black Report* on the inequalities of health, which sparked considerable debate, pointed out that the gaps between social classes had in fact widened, despite the existence of the National Health Service since 1948.[52]

While an association between SES and health is undisputed, there are two perspectives on their temporal sequence. The *social causation* school

BOX 4.9.   Race or Ethnicity

Like age and sex, race and ethnicity are often included as demographic variables in studies on population health. Race is a particularly contentious issue, and there is an ongoing debate about whether it has any validity at all, whether it is appropriate to collect information about it, and whether anything useful can be obtained from studies that distinguish participants on the basis of race.[53] Although race and ethnicity are often used interchangeably, in general, *race* implies biological inheritance and genetic differences, whereas *ethnicity* is socially and culturally defined. Both are often also confounded by socioeconomic position or social class.

The attempt to classify human beings has a long history. Karl von Linné (1707–1778), the great Swedish taxonomist, better known by his Latin name, Linnaeus, proposed the system of naming animals and plants by their genus and species. He named humans *Homo sapiens* (sapiens means "wise," a quality that is not always evident). The species could be further divided into subspecies called *americanus, europaeus, asiaticus,* and *afer,* corresponding to Native Americans, Europeans, Asians, and Africans; as well as fanciful creatures called *ferus* (hairy, four-footed) and *monstrosus* (which is self-explanatory)! The German anthropologist Johann Blumenbach (1752–1840) introduced the terms "Caucasian" and "Mongolian" in 1781, which are still widely used today (sometimes in the form of "Caucasoid" and "Mongoloid"). Since that time there have been many efforts to define and name races, and the number of races has ranged from three to over 60!

Many biologists and anthropologists today agree that there is no biological basis for the designation of races, as races are based on externally visible characteristics such as skin color, hair color and texture, facial features, and shape of the skull. The geneticist Luca Cavalli-Sforza catalogued and mapped the genetic variation of all the peoples of the world. Rather than "races," there are "clusters" of populations defined on statistical, geographical and historical grounds. Genetic variation is greater within than between these clusters. All clusters overlap when single genes are considered, and in almost all populations, all alleles are present but in different frequencies. From an evolutionary perspective, these clusters of populations could be ordered "in a hierarchy that represents the history of fissions in the expansion to the whole world of anatomically modern humans," which most anthropologists today regard as originating from East Africa some 150,000 years ago. Using complex statistical analyses of gene frequencies, phylogenetic trees can be constructed that show the genetic distances (or relatedness) between populations. In the era of genomics, the debate now centers on whether human variation at the molecular level facilitates the categorization of human populations at the "continental" level.

(continued)

In the United States, the 2000 Census first asked if someone is "Spanish/Hispanic/Latino" (and then asked the person to specify whether Mexican, Puerto Rican, Cuban, or other). A second question asked about "race," with several categories: White, Black/African American/Negro, American Indian/Alaska Native, and several categories of Asians based on country of origin (e.g., Chinese, Filipino) and Pacific Islanders (e.g., Hawaiian, Samoan). Race, called "population group," was reintroduced in the 1996 Canadian census, and includes a mixed group based on "colors" (Black, White), countries of origin (Japanese, Korean), and broad geographic regions (Arab, South Asian, Latin American). This is in addition to questions on aboriginal origin and ethnic origin (defined as where one's ancestors came from).

Despite charges of racism (directed variously at inclusion or exclusion of racial categories), studies comparing disease burden in racial and ethnic groups are still being done. Their advocates point to several uses: providing clues to etiology, targeting underserved or vulnerable population subgroups for interventions, and understanding potential differences in disease mechanisms.

attributes ill health to the adversity, deprivation, and stress associated with low SES, whereas the *health selection* school asserts that unhealthy persons (e.g., the mentally ill) drift down to, or fail to escape from, low SES. It is believed that selection probably occurs between childhood and early adulthood, as individuals move from their parents' SES category to their own achieved SES. A cohort study (see Chapter 6) of 17,000 British babies born during a week in 1958 and surveyed at ages 16, 23, and 33 years found that those who reported poor health at age 23 were more likely to have moved down than stayed in the same social class. The contribution of social mobility to health inequalities, however, is minor compared to the cumulative lifetime social circumstances, determined by social class at birth, childhood, and young adulthood.[54]

SES may mediate through behavioral and environmental factors, such as the use of preventive health services (e.g., screening for breast and cervical cancer), engagement in healthy lifestyles (low-fat diet and smoking), and exposure to environmental hazards (unsafe work sites and residence near waste disposal sites). SES may also operate through stressful life events (death in the family, retirement, job loss, etc.). Psychosocial distress is unlikely to be directly pathogenic in the unidimensional manner of microorganisms, but acts in producing a nonspecific general susceptibility to disease. Research among British civil servants—the Whitehall Study—shows that a gradient exists across different administrative grades even in a relatively homogeneous "industry" and suggests the lack of personal control over the work environment is the key process linking SES and disease.[55]

Research into risk factors of cardiovascular disease, especially from the Human Population Laboratory in Alameda County, California, has identified social networks and social support as predictive of disease outcome independent of traditional individual attributes such as smoking and hypertension. A *social network* is the web of social relationships that surround an individual; members of a network provide emotional, financial, and other support to one another. How do networks enhance health and prevent disease? Beyond material mutual assistance, networks offer social intimacy and integration, a sense of belonging in a large and impersonal world. Within a network, an individual learns about nurturing behavior (e.g., toward the young, the elderly), and is reassured of his or her individual worth and contributions. Through networks, individuals can also gain access to valuable contacts and information, which may have both direct and indirect health benefits. Various survey instruments have been developed to measure and characterize networks in terms of their type, density, size, reciprocity, proximity, homogeneity, and accessibility.[56]

Other lines of research into how SES operates as a health determinant have delineated the processes of social discordance (or status discrepancy) and social mobility or *change*. *Social discordance* can be further divided into status inconsistency within individuals and status incongruities between individuals. The discrepancy refers to the different dimensions of SES, such as income and education. An individual with a Ph.D. earning less than "what he deserves" is an example of status inconsistency; a married couple is incongruent if the wife has a Ph.D. and the husband is a high school dropout. It is hypothesized that within- and between-individual discrepancy leads to role conflicts, psychosocial stress, and ultimately disease.[57]

Another process whereby SES induces health effects is change in one or more dimensions over time. This can occur at the level of the individual or the population. An individual may undergo change in social status over his lifetime—he can be upwardly or downwardly mobile. Social mobility can also occur between generations, as in children of blue-collar parents graduating from university and joining a profession.

Entire populations can undergo social and cultural and economic change, examples being urbanization, industrialization, and modernization. There may be actual mobility in the physical sense; i.e., migration. When groups of people belonging to different cultures come into contact, one or both groups may undergo cultural change, a process referred to as *acculturation*. This is particularly acute in the case of "traditional" cultures coming into contact with "modern" cosmopolitan culture.

The degree to which cultural identity has been retained by an individual or group in a new environment can be measured in terms of variables such as proficiency in the original language, participation in traditional cultural activities, consumption of specific foods, and so forth.

Culture affects health in different ways. Among traditional cultures, there are many examples of how cultural beliefs and practices expose people to, or protect them from, diseases and injuries, including dietary customs, child care practices, religious rituals, migration patterns, agricultural techniques, kinship relations, medical therapies, and funerary rites.[58]

In populations undergoing culture change, health becomes affected when there is discrepancy between modern and traditional values, analogous to the inconsistency and incongruity in social and economic status mentioned earlier. Conflicts at the cultural level can reinforce individual vulnerability and provoke disease among those already susceptible.

In response to the stresses of cultural change, individuals and groups may develop coping strategies, building on their cultural repertoire. But these stresses may be so strong and novel that the protection of traditional culture can be overcome.[59]

A Life Course Approach to Health

Since the 1990s, the term *life course* began to appear in the population health literature. A life course approach to health has been defined as "studying the long-term effects of exposures during gestation, childhood, adolescence, and adulthood on disease risk."[60] Although a developmental perspective is hardly new, especially in fields such as pediatrics, research by David Barker and colleagues into the association between low birth weight and adult cardiovascular diseases in the 1980s stimulated new research into the links between exposures during early life, and indeed fetal life, and health outcomes several decades later in adult life. Besides cardiovascular diseases, the early-life origins of diabetes, cancer, mental illness, and neurocognitive development have also been studied.

Two models of how early exposures affect later life have been proposed. One model postulates a critical period during which time a perinatal or early infancy exposure has lasting, lifelong effects on the individual's biological systems ("programming"), which may or may not be modified by later experience. An alternative, and not necessarily incompatible, model envisions the increasing frequency and duration of exposures over time as having a cumulative effect on the body.

Initially the operative factor was attributed to maternal nutrition, which resulted in low birth weight. This has now been replaced by a more refined nutritional hypothesis that focuses on fetal nutrition. This is conceived of as the net supply of metabolic substrates along a "supply line" that starts with maternal dietary intake, through the mother's metabolic and endocrine status, uterine and umbilical blood flows, placental transport and metabolism, and ultimately is delivered to the fetus. Although birth weight is a convenient summary indicator of fetal growth, it is the endpoint of several possible and different intrauterine growth trajectories (e.g., normal, early growth restriction, late restriction with fetal wasting, and late restriction with catch-up growth). Thus different newborns with the same birth weights may have different body composition and different adult disease risks.[61]

Childhood experiences occupy an important place in the causal pathway between early life and adult disease. The existence of long-term followup studies such as the British birth cohort study (already cited earlier in this chapter) provides a wealth of data to indicate that early childhood, adolescence, and adult factors all contribute to the prediction of adult health. A multilevel analysis of the determinants of self-rated health at age 33 identified social class at birth, height at age 7, social and emotional adjustment and social class at various ages during childhood and adolescence, and educational attainments by the end of schooling, as well as measures of occupational and socioeconomic well-being in contemporary adulthood as independent predictors. In a Dutch longitudinal study, low childhood SES (measured as father's occupational class) was found to be associated with poor adult health outcomes (self-rated health, health complaints, and mortality). Childhood SES is also associated with adult health-related behaviors (alcohol use, smoking, physical activity, and obesity), which are independent of adult SES. Moreover, childhood SES has an independent and direct effect on adult health, which is only partially mediated through its influence on behaviors.[62]

The several major categories of health determinants discussed in this chapter can operate at any point in the life course. The life course approach can link two hitherto disparate disciplines of child health and aging. Indeed, increasingly the determinants of population health are understood in an inter-generational context.

A Biopsychosocial Model of Health

How do the various health determinants discussed in this chapter work together to influence health? Clearly, broad environmental influences must ultimately act on the human body to produce pathophysiological changes. What pathways and mechanisms are involved?

The health determinants discussed in this chapter operate at different levels. The outermost layer is the "macro" level of social structures, which includes the political and economic system of the state and the extent of social inequalities in society. The next-lower level, the "meso," comprises social institutions such as the workplace, family, and social clubs. Such health determinants as social networks and supports, work control, autonomy, and family conflicts represent interpersonal relationships within the meso-level. Macro- and meso-level social processes lead to perceptions and psychological processes at the individual or "micro" level. This in turn interacts with biology and behavior in influencing health.[63]

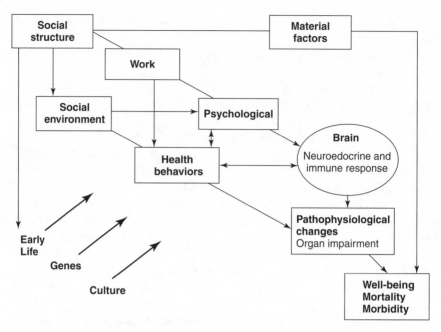

Figure 4.4. A biosocial model of health determinants. Reproduced from Brunner E, Marmot M. Social organization, stress and health. In: Marmot M, Wilkinson RG (eds.), *Social Determinants of Health.* Oxford: Oxford University Press, 1999:20.

A considerable body of research has now been accumulated that suggests that the brain plays a pivotal role in mediating external influences through the neuroendocrine and neuroimmune systems. One such model is shown in Figure 4.4.

That social gradients have been found in many different diseases supports the model that disease vulnerability is mediated through common psychoneuroendocrine (PNE) and psychoneuroimmune (PNI) pathways. It should be possible to identify biochemical substances or biomarkers along these pathways, which can serve as population-level indicators of susceptibility to poor health outcomes.[64]

Contributions to Global Disease Burden

In this chapter the major groups of health determinants are identified. How important are they in contributing to the observed pattern of health and disease in the world today? The importance of a health determinant depends on its prevalence, the size of its effect, and the strength of the evidence for causality. The Global Burden of Disease project of WHO has developed a methodology to compare diverse disease risk factors as a tool of public health planning. It estimates the reduction in mortality (or a summary measure of population health such as DALY—discussed in Chapter 3) that would result if the population distribution of exposure to that risk factor were reduced to a theoretical minimum. Whether this is currently achievable in practice is another matter. The minimum exposure would be zero in most cases (e.g., smoking) or the lowest observed level in some population (blood pressure, cholesterol). The results were published in the *World Health Report 2002*, which for the first time presented data not just on the burden of disease but also the proportion that can be attributed to specific risk factors (Chapter 5 explains the concept of population attributable risk).

A total of 26 risk factors or health determinants were selected on the basis of their health impact, data availability, evidence for causality, and potential modifiability. These determinants all fall under the rubric of "physical environment" and "personal lifestyles and behaviors" as used in this chapter. Figure 4.5 ranks the top 20 determinants in terms of their contribution to the total global burden of disease expressed in DALYs.[65]

It should be recognized that health determinants are not equally important across regions or countries of the world. On the basis of the level of child and adult mortality, the countries of the world can be divided into three groups:

A. Low-mortality countries—these are the highly developed countries of Western Europe, North America, Australasia, Japan, and Singapore;
B. Medium-mortality countries—these are the countries of Eastern Europe, the Middle East, and many Latin American and Asian countries;
C. High-mortality countries—these are the least developed countries in Sub-Saharan Africa, and some of the poorest Asian and Latin American countries.

Table 4.2 lists the top 10 determinants in the three groups of countries and shows how they overlap.

Certain factors are shared by all three groups of countries—tobacco, blood pressure, cholesterol, and iron deficiency. This highlights the growing importance of chronic diseases even in the developing countries, where they once were rare. The use of illicit drugs is the only top-ranking determinant in the developed world not shared by other countries; poor water and sanitation and nutritional deficiencies are important risk factors in the developing, but not in the developed, world.

This risk assessment project demonstrates that there is only a relatively small number of determinants that can account for a large proportion of the total disease burden in the world. None of the top 20 are particularly novel—their role as disease risk factors has long been established, and strategies to reduce the population's exposure to them are available. The corollary is that global health would be much improved if sufficient resources were targeted at these determinants.

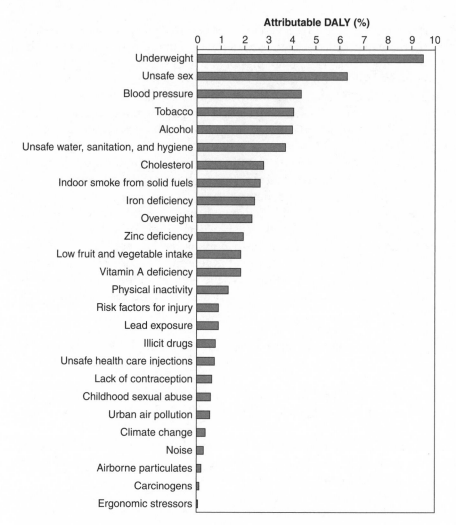

Figure 4.5. Contribution of selected health determinants to the global burden of disease.

Table 4.2. Top 10 Health Determinants in High-, Medium-, and Low-Mortality Countrie

C	B	C	B	A	B	A
	Undernutrition		Tobacco		Alcohol	
	Indoor smoke from solid fuels		Blood pressure		Overweight	
			Cholesterol		Physical inactivity	
			Iron deficiency		Low fruit/vegetable intake	
	Unsafe water/sanitation/hygiene		Unsafe sex		Illicit drugs	
	Zinc deficiency					
	Vitamin A deficiency					
C		C		A		A

The epidemiologists Robert Beaglehole and Paul Magnus pointed out that four risk factors (high blood pressure, high cholesterol, smoking, and physical inactivity) account for some 75% of the new cases of coronary heart disease. Continuing the search for new risk factors is therefore not an efficient use of scarce research resources. What is needed is narrowing the gap between knowledge and action.[66]

Summary

This chapter proceeds from the earlier chapters concerned with describing the health of populations, to understanding why some populations are healthier than others. Discussing various determinants individually (albeit grouped under genetic susceptibility; physical environment; personal behaviors; and social, cultural, and economic factors) does not imply that they act alone. The pathway to health and disease involves complex interactions of all these factors in varying degrees.

The genetic contributions to the disease burden in a population is substantial, including single-gene, chromosomal, and polygenic diseases. Indeed there are few instances where gene–environment interactions cannot be demonstrated.

The environment encompasses all that is external to the human body and is usually divided into the physical and the social. *Physical environment* refers to the physical, chemical, and biological hazards that exist in the air, water, soil, and food. Increasingly, concerns are directed at global environmental change. The risks to population health are general and difficult to define but may well affect the very survival of the human species.

Human beings constitute the social environment. Individual behaviors, the so-called healthy lifestyles such as not smoking, moderate alcohol use, physical activity, diet, sexual practices, and safety precautions, have been shown to promote health or prevent the development of diseases. Such behaviors themselves also have biological and social determinants, and they are not all under the control of the individual.

The differentiation of individuals into social and economic classes on the basis of education, income, and occupation occurs in most human populations. That such divisions have an impact on health status has been demonstrated repeatedly for different diseases in different countries at different times. Social factors can be understood at the macro level in terms of the structure of society and the unequal distribution of resources, or at the meso level in terms of social processes such as status discrepancy and social mobility, social network and support, which ultimately interact with the individual at the micro level. Within the organism, it is now believed that external influences are mediated by the brain and psychoneuroimmune and psychoneuroendocrine pathways, resulting in health and disease.

Health determinants operate throughout the life course, and many adult diseases have their origin in early and fetal life. Increasingly, health is viewed in a multigenerational context. Globally, a relatively small number of risk factors accounts for a large proportion of the disease burden. Some of these are universal (such as tobacco and blood pressure), while others affect only the highly developed countries (illicit drugs) or least developed countries (unsafe water and nutritional deficiency). Identification of these factors and their contribution to the global burden of disease provide the evidence needed for the planning of public health programs and services.

Case Study 4.1.   The Sickle-Cell Trait and Protection from Malaria

Sickle-cell anemia is an example of a single-gene, autosomal recessive disease.[67] The sickle-cell gene causes the substitution of one amino acid in the β-chain of the hemoglobin (Hb) molecule, resulting in an abnormal hemoglobin Hb^S. The red blood cells (RBC) of individuals homozygous for the gene (SS) are deformed, and the patients suffer from painful crises and may die from the severe anemia that results. Heterozygous individuals (AS)—i.e., individuals with Hb^S in one chromosome and the normal hemoglobin gene Hb^A on the other—appear healthy. Their RBCs, however, tend to "sickle" when exposed to certain chemicals, which is the basis of a clinical laboratory test using sodium metabisulphite. SS individuals are said to have the disease, while AS individuals carry the sickle-cell *trait*. The blood of both can be distinguished from unaffected individuals (AA) using electrophoretic techniques.

The disease was first recognized in 1910. In the early 1950s, its molecular basis was elucidated by chemists such as Linus Pauling (1901–1994) and its mode of inheritance clarified by geneticists such as James Neel (1915–2002). The disease and trait affect primarily, though not exclusively, Africans (and descendants of Africans in America and elsewhere), in a geographic belt that includes much of tropical Africa, the Mediterranean, and the Indian subcontinent. For example, in the Musoma district of Tanganyika (now Tanzania in East Africa), a survey in the 1950s showed that, of 287 infants tested, 65.9% were AA, 31.0% AS, and 3.1% SS. Genetically speaking, these are *genotype* frequencies. They can be converted into *gene* or *allele* frequencies:

The frequency of the Hb^A gene $= 0.659 + (0.31/2) = 0.814$

The frequency of the Hb^S gene $= 0.031 + (0.31/2) = 0.186$

That is, the Hb^S gene was present in 18.6% of individuals. One can also estimate gene frequency from genotype frequency using the

Hardy-Weinberg Law. Since the prevalence of SS individuals was 0.031, indicated as q^2, then q, the frequency of $Hb^s = \sqrt{0.031} = 0.176$. Similarly the frequency of Hb^A is $p = (1-q) = 0.824$.

How can the sickle-cell gene, if the disease it causes is so lethal, be maintained in so many populations at such high frequencies? Fresh, recurrent mutations cannot keep up with the constant elimination of the gene through death. Perhaps the gene offers some sort of *selective advantage*. Since homozygous individuals tend to die in infancy in areas lacking modern medical care and do not live long enough to reproduce, the advantage must be conferred on heterozygotes.

In 1954, A. C. Allison conducted a survey of Ugandan children aged five months to five years around Kampala and tested for malarial parasites in the blood. The prevalence of malarial parasitemia among those with the sickle-cell trait ("sicklers") was 28%, of whom 67% had a low density of parasites. Among non-sicklers, the prevalence was 46%, of whom only 34% had a low density. Allison further conducted an experiment among adult volunteers by injecting malarial blood into 15 sicklers and 15 non-sicklers. By the fortieth day, 14 of the 15 non-sicklers developed malaria and had to be treated, while only two of the sicklers developed mild disease.

The age-specific prevalence of the sickle-cell trait provides further evidence that AS individuals are protected. In a study in the former Belgian Congo (which became Zaire, and has now reverted to the name of Congo), the trait frequency was 10.3% among children under the age of three, but increased to 22.6% among those aged 3–15 years, suggestive of a higher mortality among non-sicklers under the age of three, the age when acquired immunity to malaria generally develops.

Laboratory scientists confirmed the protective effect of the sickle-cell trait in *in vitro* studies. The rate of invasion and growth of malarial parasites was retarded in cell cultures of RBCs from AS individuals compared to AA individuals under conditions of low oxygen tension.

By studying the geographic distribution of the sickle-cell trait, its variation among linguistic groups, the history of migration, and the diffusion of agriculture, anthropologists were able to study the adaptation of malaria to human settlement and ecological change, demonstrating that humans and microbes co-evolve and coexist.

Case Study 4.2.   Chernobyl: Aftermath of an Environmental Catastrophe

In the early morning of April 26, 1986, an explosion and the resulting fire destroyed a reactor in the nuclear power plant in Chernobyl, in northern Ukraine, in the former Soviet Union.[68] It unleashed an environmental catastrophe unparalleled in history. For nine days, gases containing fission products of uranium and plutonium, including the isotopes iodine 131, strontium 90, and cesium 137, were released into the atmosphere, carried by prevailing winds to the north and west, affecting countries near and far. Large tracts of land in Ukraine, Belarus, and Russia became uninhabitable and non-arable. Hundreds of thousands of residents were uprooted. Crops and milk in Eastern and Central Europe had to be destroyed. In northern Scandinavia, the traditional livelihood of the indigenous Saami (Lapp) people, based on the herding of reindeer, which had grazed on contaminated vegetation, was devastated. The political fallout from the disaster may even have hastened the demise of the Soviet Union itself.

The health effects, both immediate and long-term, are still being tallied. Acute radiation sickness affected 187 people, of whom 31 died. Most of the early casualties were firefighters sent to put out the fire. In the aftermath, 400,000 inadequately protected workers were sent to clean up and build a concrete and metal structure (dubbed the "sarcophagus") to envelop the reactor. About 30,000 of them subsequently reported a variety of health problems, and 5,000 had to be medically invalided from work.

Individuals become exposed to radiation by absorbing radionuclides deposited on the ground and from ingesting contaminated food. Potential long-term health problems include cancer, adverse reproductive outcomes, and psychological distress. The World Health Organization and the European Commission established various surveillance programs to monitor the health effects throughout Europe. Special attention was focused on thyroid cancer, since large quantities of the radioactive isotope ^{131}I were released. Iodine concentrates in the thyroid, one of the most radiosensitive organs in the body, and children under 10 are most at risk. Within five years, the incidence of thyroid cancer in the most contaminated areas increased by 5- to 10-fold. It should be recognized that some of the increase can probably be attributed to increased awareness and screening, and few of the cases had undergone histopathological examination. The rise in incidence was much earlier than expected, as thyroid cancer tends to have a latency of around 10 years. Clinically, the cancer appeared to be more invasive and faster-growing. Widespread iodine deficiency in the region may have been responsible for the earlier appearance of the cancer.

The graph on the following page shows the incidence of thyroid cancer in parts of Belarus, Ukraine, and Russia, based on data published in the 2000 report of the United Nations Scientific Committee on the Effects of Atomic Radiation (UNSCEAR).

There has been no increase in the other types of cancer, such as the leukemias and lymphomas, which have been shown to be associated with radiation exposure. Further afield, cancer surveillance in Scandinavia and other European countries also has not shown an increase.

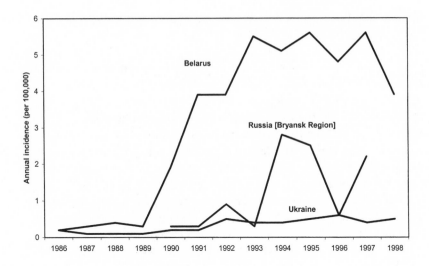

There is no evidence that the rates of adverse reproductive outcomes, including spontaneous abortions and congenital anomalies
such as Down's syndrome and neural tube defects, have increased
in Ukraine, Belarus, or Scandinavia.

Psychological distress affects the largest number of people, and
not just those exposed to high levels of radiation. Many are faced
with the uncertainty of not knowing if and when they might develop a radiation-induced illness. Many suffer from psychosomatic
symptoms.

Chernobyl offers valuable lessons. It illustrates what can go wrong
with modern technology. The causes of the disaster are technical as
well as political. It offers a glimpse into the standard of industrial
safety practices, of public accountability, and of timely disclosure of
health risks in totalitarian regimes. It sharpens the debate between
proponents and opponents of nuclear energy worldwide. From the
perspective of population health, it provides a rare opportunity to investigate the health effects of ionizing radiation. Much of what we
know comes from the survivors of the Hiroshima and Nagasaki
atomic bombs and some occupational groups at high exposures.
Chernobyl serves as a "natural experiment" to study prospectively
the effects of exposure to relative low doses of radiation by large,
widely distributed populations.

Two reactors in the Chernobyl plant continued to be operational
years after the fire, providing 5% of the power needs of Ukraine. The
physical condition of the hurriedly built "sarcophagus" containing
the burnt-out but still highly radioactive reactor was rapidly deterio-
rating. It was not until 2001 that the power station was completely
shut down. There are other, similar reactors, presumably with the

same design flaws that led to the Chernobyl disaster, scattered across the former Soviet Union.

Case Study 4.3.   Social Medicine in Pre–World War I Germany

Lest we think that the association between health and social conditions is a new discovery, historians of public health remind us that much research was conducted on the social origins of infectious diseases at the beginning of the twentieth century in Europe, when the germ theory was in the ascendancy.[69] In Germany, social medicine (*Soziale Medizin*) was both an academic discipline and social movement, pioneered by the eminent pathologist Rudolf Virchow (1821–1902), who was briefly mentioned in Chapter 1. After unification in 1871, the German Empire (the Second Reich) underwent rapid industrialization and economic growth, accompanied by increased urban migration and social disparities among the population. To forestall the growth of radical socialism, Chancellor Otto von Bismarck (1815–1898) instituted a series of welfare schemes that alleviated the misery of the laboring classes, including sickness insurance, disability benefits, accident insurance, and pensions. It was within this environment that social medicine emerged.

There were three main themes of social medicine or *social hygiene* (the terms were often used synonymously):

1. Social causation of disease;
2. National improvement through eugenics;
3. State responsibility for medical care.

The relative importance of these three "pillars" was the source of much dispute and academic rivalry. That eugenics was subsequently embraced by National Socialism and, combined with the theory of the superiority of the Aryan "race," ultimately led to the Holocaust obscured the fact that in the early part of the twentieth century, eugenic notions were widely subscribed to by both the left and the right of the political spectrum. Many social democrats and progressives in northern Europe saw a role for the state in influencing reproduction and improving the health of future generations.

An influential textbook of the era was *Krankheit und Soziale Lage* (Illness and Social Position), edited by Max Mosse and Gustav Tugendreich and published in 1913. It aimed to show "the influence of social circumstances on the prevention, origin, and causes of disease" and reviewed extensively the relationship between diseases such as tuberculosis and venereal diseases, major scourges at the time, and housing, nutrition, income, and occupation.

Among the data presented in the chapter on tuberculosis was the association between mortality and income in Hamburg from 1905–1910:

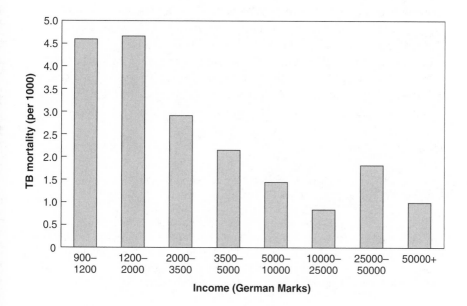

A French study was also cited, which correlated tuberculosis mortality with housing quality (as measured by the number of windows per resident) in 20 Parisian *arondissements* (districts):

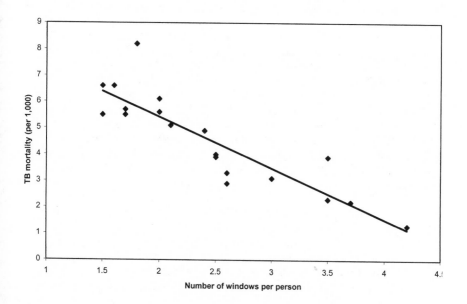

The book by Mosse and Tugendreich not only provided a state-of-the-art review of the subject circa 1910, but it also anticipated many issues that are now still being debated or have been resurrected. Thus the authors attributed the mortality decline from tuberculosis not to treatment in sanatoria or improved access to medical care through insurance, but to social reforms that led to an improved economic position of the workers. In the 1970s, Thomas McKeown (see Chapter 2) drew similar conclusions regarding the negligible role of medical care in reducing mortality in populations. Mosse and Tugendreich also emphasized the influence of early exposures on health later on in life, which today goes under the rubric of "life course."

Notes

1. This book, by Evans, Barer, and Marmor (1994), is a product of the Population Health Program of the Canadian Institute for Advanced Research.
2. See Morris (1975:177).
3. The document (Health and Welfare Canada 1974) is widely referred to as the Lalonde Report, after then Health and Welfare Minister, Marc Lalonde. While internationally acclaimed, the report is not without its critics. For a review of the responses, see Evans (1982). Terris (1984) called it "brilliantly conceived . . . one of the great achievements of the modern public health movement."
4. Evans and Stoddart (1990) generated considerable debate. For a retrospective more than a decade later, see Evans and Stoddart (2003), which also provides a succinct review of major advances in research into health determinants.
5. See Philippe and Mansi (1998) for an overview of nonlinearity in epidemiology, and Philippe (1993) on chaos theory. Discussion of nonlinear dynamics in infectious diseases can be found in Anderson (1994) and Koopman and Longini (1994).
6. Further information about the Human Genome Project can be obtained from its web site (www.genome.gov), which also contains a useful nontechnical glossary of genetics terms. The international project was launched in 1990 and achieved its goals two years ahead of schedule, in 2003. Khoury et al. (2000) provide an introduction to the interface between genetics and public health.
7. Mendel was an Augustinian monk (later abbot) at the monastery in Brünn, Austria (now Brno in the Czech Republic), who conducted pea hybridization experiments in the garden and developed the principles of segregation and of independent assortment, thus laying the foundation of the genetics of discrete characteristics. He reported his findings in 1866 to the local natural history society. His paper languished in the society's proceedings and was not rediscovered until 1900.
8. See Baird et al. (1988) and McKusick (1998). Information about the registry can be obtained from the web site of the British Columbia Vital Statistics Agency (www.vs.gov.bc.ca/stats/hsr/).
9. See King et al. (2003) for a discussion of the genetic bases of common diseases; and Andrieu and Goldstein (1998) for a review of genetic epidemiological methods.
10. Before Robert Koch's pioneer work on the tubercle bacillus in the late nineteenth century, tuberculosis was widely believed to be an inherited disease. Evidence is now accumulating of the role of polymorphisms in the human leukocyte antigen (HLA) loci, the vitamin D receptor gene, and the natural resistance-associated

macrophage protein gene (*NRAMP1*) in determining susceptibility to mycobacterial infections. See the reviews by Cooke and Hill (2001) and Bellamy (2003).

11. See the reviews by Cowan et al. (2002) and Raine (2002).

12. Polednak (1989) surveyed ethnic and racial variation in disease risk in a variety of populations. The correlation of Native American ancestry and diabetes prevalence in Native Americans and Mexican Americans is reported by Knowler et al. (1988) and Stern and Haffner (1990), respectively.

13. For a general overview of migrant studies in cancer epidemiology, see the chapter by Thomas and Karagas (1996) in Schottenfeld and Fraumeni (1996); for specific data on the Japanese, see Locke and King (1980). The Ni-Hon-San Study has generated many publications; see in particular the introduction by Syme et al. (1975) and the review by Benfante (1992). Note that the Hiroshima and Nagasaki cohort was part of a study of the effects of atomic radiation, while the Honolulu cohort became the Honolulu Heart Program.

14. For example, in a study of 1698 members of 409 families in Québec, including nine types of relatives by descent or adoption, Bouchard (1991) reported a heritability of 5% for the body mass index, a measure of overall obesity or excess body fat based on height and weight. For more direct measures of body fat, the heritability was higher, at 25%.

15. DNA polymorphisms include *restriction fragment length polymorphisms* (RLFPs); *variable number tandem repeats* (VNTRs); and *single-nucleotide polymorphisms* (SNPs). Table 4.1 is adapted from Potter (2001). The relevance of genomics to disease prevention is explored by Willett (2002). Note the convention of printing the names of genes in *italics*.

16. Godfrey Hardy, a Cambridge mathematician, and Wilhelm Weinberg, a Stuttgart physician, independently discovered the "law" and reported it in 1908. This law represents Hardy's only foray into genetics. Weinberg, on the other hand, made other important discoveries but suffered a similar fate to that of Mendel in not being recognized in his own time.

17. For further information on environmental health, see the introductory text by Yassi et al. (2001).

18. It should be clear that "pesthood" is in the eyes of the beholder. The poem is entitled "Reply to Comrade Kuo Mo-jo." The English translation of Mao's poem appears in *Away with All Pests* (Horn, 1969), not a treatise on environmental health, but the autobiography of Joshua Horn, an English surgeon who supported Mao and worked in China during 1954–1969.

19. Students should dig up their college-level physics and chemistry textbooks and refresh their memory of the atomic structure of matter. Periodic reports from UNSCEAR (e.g., the 2000 report, available from www.unscear.org/reports/2000_1. html, and the National Research Council's Committee on the Biological Effects of Ionizing Radiation (1999), known as BEIR-VI, provide state-of-the-art reviews. Physicists and chemists, unlike medical scientists, have physical units rather than diseases named after them. "Coulomb" is named after Charles de Coulomb (1736–1806), a French physicist, while "joule" is named after British physicist James Joule (1818–1889). Wilhelm Röntgen (1845–1923) was the German physicist who discovered X-rays in 1895, for which he was awarded the Nobel prize in 1901. Antoine Becquerel (1852–1908), a French physicist, shared the 1903 Nobel prize in physics with fellow countryman Pierre Curie (1859–1906) and his wife, Marie Curie (née Sklodowska, 1867–1934) for their pioneering work in radioactivity. Marie Curie went on to win a second Nobel prize in 1911, in chemistry. The Curies were a distinguished family indeed, as their daughter, Irène

Joliot-Curie (1897–1956), also won a Nobel prize for chemistry in 1935. Louis Gray (1905–1965) was a British radiobiologist, and R. M. Sievert a Swedish radiologist.

20. A biomarker can be a marker of exposure, effect, and susceptibility. See the IARC monograph by Toniolo et al. (1997).

21. See Blum and Feachem (1983) and Esrey and Habicht (1986) for critical reviews of the copious international literature on the impact of water and sanitation on health.

22. The continuing interest in housing and health is evident from a series of short reviews in the *British Medical Journal* (Lowry, 1989–90). See also the review by Krieger and Higgins (2002).

23. The APHA's housing standards have been updated periodically (see Wood, 1986) and widely used in many jurisdictions. WHO (1989) has also produced a set of health principles of housing.

24. For a review of the relevance of global environmental change to population health, see the report by the WHO Commission on Health and the Environment (1992). McMichael (2001) offers a sweeping, evolutionary perspective on the interrelationships between the human species and the environment.

25. Green and Kreuter (1991:433) provide the current definition from the perspective of the "health promotion movement." Coreil et al. (1985) traced the origins of the word to its nineteenth-century origins in sociology.

26. Data for the graphs in Figure 3.2 are obtained from Department of Health and Human Services (1991:130). Smoking prevalences for birth cohorts are reconstructed from cross-sectional data provided by the National Health Interview Surveys of 1970, 1978, 1979, 1980, and 1987.

27. See Jarvis et al. (1987) for a study comparing these methods with self-reports. Carbon monoxide combines with hemoglobin to form carboxyhemoglobin, which has a half-life of three to four hours and is hence sensitive to the time of day when the specimen is collected. Thiocyanate, on the other hand, has a half life of 10–14 days.

28. Data in this box are obtained from the 1989 Surgeon General report, reviewing 25 years of progress since the 1964 landmark report. See also the monograph on tobacco from the IARC (1986).

29. There is a substantial literature on the determinants of smoking: see the reviews by Fisher et al. (1990), Logan and Spencer (1996), and the manual on chronic disease control by the APHA (Brownson et al., 1998).

30. A 1947 full-page color advertisement in *Life* magazine was headlined "More Doctors Smoke Camels Than Any Other Cigarette." The ad claimed that this brand was most preferred by doctors. It showed a GP out on his rounds and an insert saying that after a hectic day of saving lives the doctor paused to enjoy the pleasure of a cigarette.

31. See the relevant sections in ICD-10 (WHO, 1992) and *DSM-IV* (APA, 2000). Rinaldi et al. (1988) conducted a Delphi survey (see Chapter 8) of a multidisciplinary group of experts and reached consensus on the definitions of 50 substance-abuse terms. See Morse et al. (1992) on the background of the National Council on Alcoholism's definition.

32. A succinct summary on alcohol and health is provided by Rehm et al. (1997). See also the 10th Special Report to the U.S. Congress by the National Institute on Alcohol Abuse and Alcoholism (2000), available from its web site: www.niaaa.nih.gov. Rimm et al. (1999) performed a meta-analysis of studies on the beneficial effects of alcohol on lipids and hemostatic factors. Rehm (1998) reviewed the measurement of quantity, frequency, and volume of drinking.

33. See Marlatt (1996) and Roche et al. (1997) for further discussion of harm reduction.

34. See the review by Petraitis et al. (1995). Theories such as Ajzen and Fishbein (1980) and Bandura (1986) are of course more generally applicable to a variety of health-related behaviors, discussed further in Chapter 7.

35. The literature on nutrition and health is immense. Comprehensive reviews have been provided by various expert committees, such as WHO (1990). The web site of the Food and Nutrition Information Center of the National Agriculture Library provides many resources (www.nal.usda.gov/fnic/).

36. Björntorp and Brodoff (1992) provide a comprehensive introduction to the voluminous literature on the pathophysiology and health implications of obesity. See WHO (2000) and NIH (1998) for their obesity criteria. See also the Surgeon General's Call to Action (DHHS, 2001). The CDC growth charts can be downloaded from its web site (www.cdc.gov/growthcharts/).

37. Eaton and Konner (1985) discuss the modern health implications of paleolithic nutrition. Trowell and Burkitt (1981) compare the health status of various populations undergoing "Westernization."

38. The *Dietary Guidelines for Americans* is available from the USDA's Food and Nutrition Information Center web site (see note 35), which also provides a table comparing the current with previous guidelines, as well as links to guidelines from other countries. Guidelines are also available from the American Cancer Society (www.cancer.org) and the American Heart Association (www.americanheart.org), from their specific disease perspectives.

39. For a comprehensive discussion of dietary assessment methods, see Willett (1998) and Gibson (1990).

40. The literature on physical activity is extensive. Useful reviews are provided by the Surgeon General's report (DHSS, 1996) and the text by Sallis and Owen (1999). Hardman (2001) discusses current research issues.

41. The determinants and consequences of STDs are reviewed by Aral (2001). Kotchick et al. (2001) arrgued for a multisystem approach to adolescent sexual risk behavior.

42. Wellings and Cleland (2001) discuss research issues under the demedicalized paradigm of "sexual health." Stein (1990) emphasizes the need for protective methods that empower women and are under their sole control.

43. For an overview of injury epidemiology, see the monograph by Robertson (1992). Barss et al. (1998) provide an international perspective. The importance of social factors such as single motherhood, unemployment, smoking, and absence of a sibling is demonstrated in the study of a birth cohort in Montreal (Larson and Pless, 1988). Eichelberger et al. (1990) surveyed parental attitudes and knowledge of child safety.

44. Chadwick was Secretary to the Poor Law Commission. Engels was a cofounder of "scientific socialism" and collaborated with Karl Marx in drafting the *Communist Manifesto* (1848). Engels lived mostly in England and was co-owner of a cotton factory in Manchester. See Hamlin (1997) for a history of public health and social justice in the Victorian era.

45. Krieger (2001) reviewed the history of "social epidemiology." She traced the first use of the term to a paper by Alfred Yankauer in the *American Sociological Review* in 1950. Cassel (1976) is a modern classic. For a guide to the rapidly expanding literature on social epidemiology, see the texts by Marmot and Wilkinson (1999) and Berkman and Kawachi (2000).

46. González et al. (1998) reviewed the epidemiological literature from 1960–1993 and found that the reversal occurred around 1970. Since then, the risk of ischemic heart disease among manual workers relative to non-manual workers has progressively increased.

47. Subramanian et al. (2002) reviewed the macroeconomic determinants of health. Data for Figure 4.3 are from the United Nations Development Program's *Human Development Report 2002*. (Chapter 3 introduced the UNDP's human development index). A spreadsheet of the key indicators for all countries in the world can be downloaded from the UNDP web site (www.undp.org).

48. Wilkinson's 1992 *BMJ* paper initiated a whole new area and direction of research. He elaborated his ideas further in his book (1996). For critiques, see Judge (1995) and Mackenbach (2002). North American data have been presented by Ross et al. (2000) and Kennedy et al. (1996). The latter used the "Robin Hood index," which measures the share of the total income that has to be taken from those above the mean and transferred to those below it to achieve equality in the distribution of income.

49. See the comprehensive review by Krieger et al. (1997). Wright's scheme can be found in his book on class analysis (1996).

50. As an example of SES index construction, see Mustard and Frohlich (1995). Mackenbach and Kunst (1997) reviewed the many indicators available on SES inequalities. Singh-Manoux et al. (2002) analysed the Whitehall Study and compared different approaches to modelling the data. The temporal ordering of variables is made possible using structural equation modelling.

51. See Kawachi et al. (1997, 1999).

52. Sir Douglas Black, Chief Scientist at the Department of Health and Social Services and later President of the Royal College of Physicians of London, chaired the Working Group on Inequalities in Health. It released its report *Inequalities in Health* in 1980. A Penguin edition is available (Townsend, Davidson, and Whitehead, 1992), which reproduces the original Black report, with an update by Margaret Whitehead entitled *The Health Divide*, and a new introduction detailing its public reception and the political controversy surrounding the report. See MacIntyre (1997) for a reevaluation of the report.

53. For a comprehensive treatise on the origin and evolution of the concept (or fallacy) of race, see Montagu's 700-page tome (1997). Lock (1993) provides a succinct review. Cavalli-Sforza et al. (1994) produced a massive encyclopedia and atlas. The concepts and methodological issues surrounding the use of race as a variable in epidemiological studies are extensively reviewed in Lin and Kelsey (2000). Mays et al. (2003) discussed the measurement of race and ethnicity by U.S. government agencies such as the census bureau and NCHS. The debate continues unabated—see Cooper (2003) and Karter (2003).

54. Power et al. (1996) followed the 1958 British birth cohort. For further background on the selection vs. causation debate, see West (1991), Dohrenwend et al. (1992), and Marmot et al. (1997).

55. The Whitehall Study has produced important insight into the determinants of health; see, for example, Marmot et al. (1991). Evans and Kantrowitz (2002) reviewed the evidence for the role of environmental exposure in mediating SES and health.

56. Much of the empirical data on social support and social networks are generated by the Alameda County Study in California. See the review by Berkman (1984). Jacobson (1987) cautioned about the need to be aware of the cultural context of social support.

57. The terminology is inconsistent and confusing. The scheme used by Morgenstern (1985:12) is followed here. For a review of the epidemiological literature, see Vernon and Buffler (1988).

58. Examples can be found in the review by Nations (1986).

59. For a detailed exposition of cultural determinants of health, see Corin (1994), who produces a matrix to indicate how political forces, economic constraints and the social environment interact with cultural *stressors* and *mediators* to produce the manifestations of ill health.

60. See the book (Kuh and Ben-Shlomo, 1997) and editorial (Ben-Shlomo and Kuh, 2002) on the life course approach to chronic disease epidemiology. Barker's research has been summarized in Barker (1998).

61. Harding (2001) reviews the basis for the nutritional hypothesis.

62. See Power et al. (1999) and Hertzman et al. (2001) on analyses of the British Birth Cohort Study. Mheen et al. (1998) reported on the Dutch study.

63. Martikainen et al. (2002) provided a conceptual framework to understand the macro, meso and micro levels where health determinants operate. For an application to real data, see Hertzman et al. (2001).

64. The model is reproduced from Brunner and Marmot (1999). Kelly et al. (1997) evaluated several PNE and PNI markers for their suitability in population surveys.

65. The data from the *World Health Report 2002* can be downloaded as a spreadsheet from the WHO web site. For a short summary of the analysis, see Ezzati et al. (2002).

66. See Beaglehole and Magnus (2002). They unkindly refer to the search for new coronary heart disease risk factors as occupational therapy for epidemiologists!

67. Data in this case study can be found in Allison (1954), Motulsky et al. (1966), and Paszol et al. (1978). Livingstone (1958) discussed the anthropological implications of sickle-cell studies in human populations. Linus Pauling (1901–1994) received two Nobel prizes: chemistry in 1954, for his work in molecular structures; and peace in 1962, for his advocacy of nuclear disarmament. In his later years he claimed that vitamin C could cure the common cold, among other ailments. James Neel, a prominent human geneticist, is associated with the "thrifty gene" hypothesis on the high prevalence of diabetes in many Native American populations.

68. An account of the disaster was provided by Shcherbak (1996), at the time of writing the ambassador to the United States from independent Ukraine. A physician, he founded the Green Movement in Ukraine and was elected to the Supreme Soviet of the USSR in 1989, where he initiated the first parliamentary investigation of the Chernobyl disaster. Comprehensive reviews of the health effects of Chernobyl can be found in Bard et al. (1997), Moysich et al. (2002), and the UNSCEAR 2000 report, from which the data in the graph are derived.

69. Data in this case study are obtained from Murphy and Egger (2002). See also Rosen's (1947) investigation into the origin of "social medicine." For a comprehensive history of public health, race, and politics in Germany from Bismarck to Hitler, see Weindling (1989).

EXERCISE 4.1.   Geographic and Social Class Variation in Infant Mortality

That social factors and health status measures are correlated has been known for many years. In the 1930s a study in England and Wales compared infant mortality rate (IMR) across social class and geographical region. The following table summarizes the data obtained. Social class categories are based on those of the Registrar-General (I is "highest" and V "lowest"). The regions are arranged roughly from south to north.

	Social class				
Region	I	II	III	IV	V
Southwest	35.0	43.7	45.4	54.4	58.6
Southeast	33.1	38.4	41.6	46.8	54.0
London	29.6	39.8	49.7	62.3	71.2
Wales I	43.1	52.2	70.0	73.0	77.4
Midland I	32.7	44.5	58.9	63.8	77.7
East	29.9	41.7	56.7	55.9	61.5
Wales II	38.6	54.5	61.7	69.6	70.3
Midland II	35.6	45.0	61.2	64.5	76.0
North IV	31.1	51.2	66.8	78.9	93.3
North III	34.4	46.9	67.8	74.7	84.6
North II	39.2	52.6	61.7	73.1	82.3
North I	37.8	50.3	71.9	86.8	100.6

(a)   What effect does social class have on IMR?

(b)   What is the relationship between geographical region and IMR?

(c)   What conclusions can you draw regarding the determinants of IMR, based on the available data?

(d)   Plot IMR, social class, and geographical region on a three-dimensional graph.

Source: Woolf and Waterhouse (1945)

EXERCISE 4.2.   Occupational Health Risks of Miners

An underground fluospar mine in Newfoundland was operational between 1936 and 1978. In the 1950s an increase in lung cancer deaths was noted. In 1960, a high level of radon "daughters" (radioactive decay products) in the air and ground water was detected. A retrospective cohort study (see Chapter 6) was launched to examine the association of occupational exposure in the mine and excess cancer deaths. The vital status of 1772 underground miners was determined over the period from 1950–1984. Exposure was measured in "working level months" (WLM), which combines concentration of radioactivity in the air and the duration of employment. The age-, period-, and cause-specific mortality experience of the total Newfoundland population was used in generating "expected" number of deaths from cancer and other causes.

Cause of death	Observed	Expected	SMR
All causes	445	369.9	
Infectious diseases	16	7.9	
All cancers	185	85.3	
Cancer of buccal cavity/pharynx	*6*	*2.2*	
Cancer of trachea/bronchus/lung	*113*	*21.5*	
Silicosis	6	0.1	
Injuries	43	33.8	

(a) Compute the SMRs for the causes of death listed.

(b) Is mining a hazardous occupation?

The SMRs corresponding to various exposure level are as follows:

Cumulative WLM	SMR
0	0.90
<50	1.81
50–100	1.55
100–400	2.14
400–1000	4.41
1000–1600	11.32
1600–2500	23.97
2500+	33.55

(c) How would you describe the relationship between exposure and cancer mortality risk? Plot a graph.

(d) Are there other factors that could have produced such a pattern?

Source: Morrison et al. (1988)

EXERCISE 4.3.   Childhood Determinants of Adult Diabetes

The birth weight and height and weight during childhood of babies born during 1924–1944 in the University Hospital in Helsinki, Finland, were monitored. Their records were then linked to the national registries of hospitalizations, medication use, and deaths to identify incident cases of chronic diseases such as diabetes, hypertension, and coronary heart disease, up to 1997. Data were available for some 13,500 individuals.

The following table cross-tabulates birth weight (BW) and the body mass index (BMI) at age 11 and shows the odds ratios (discussed in detail in Chapter 5) for diabetes later in life. The "reference category" (with odds ratio set at unity) comprises the individuals with birth weight greater than 4 kilograms and at the lowest quartile of BMI at age 11. An odds ratio of 2.0

means individuals in that category have twice the risk of disease compared to the reference category, whereas an odds ratio of 0.5 means that they have half the risk.

	BMI at age 11			
BW (kg)	1st quartile	2nd quartile	3rd quartile	4th quartile
≤3.0	1.3	1.3	1.5	2.5
3.0–3.5	1.0	1.0	1.5	1.7
3.5–4.0	1.0	0.9	0.9	1.7
>4.0	1.0	1.1	0.7	1.2

(a) Which category of individuals in this birth cohort is most likely to develop diabetes?

(b) What general trends regarding birth weight and childhood obesity as risk factors can be observed? (Never mind statistical significance!)

In addition, change in BMI during childhood also affects the risk of diabetes. The following table presents the cumulative incidence (%) of diabetes:

	Change in BMI between ages 3 and 11	
Tertile of BW	Decrease	Increase
Lowest third	3.1%	5.5%
Middle third	2.4%	4.3%
Highest third	1.5%	5.4%

(c) Plot a three-dimensional graph using the data in the table.

(d) Based on the information provided by the two tables, what conclusions can be drawn regarding the association of diabetes with birth weight and childhood obesity?

Source: Barker et al. (2002)

5

Assessing Health Risks in Populations

Risks in Population Health

The assessment of health risks is a central task of population health practice and research. Simply defined, *risk* is the probability that an event will occur, although in everyday usage *risk* implies the likelihood of harm rather than good fortune. Each year as many as 40,000 to 50,000 articles are published where the term *risk* appears in the titles and abstracts—this has led some observers to refer to a "risk epidemic" in the medical literature! It is not just health scientists and practitioners who are obsessed with risks. Indeed, risks are such an integral part of our modern social, political, and cultural life that some social theorists claim that we now live in a "risk society" or in a generalized "climate of risk."[1]

In population health, the word *risk* is used in a variety of ways. Thus we talk about the risk of developing lung cancer from smoking (either in absolute terms, say x% over a lifetime; or in relative terms, comparing smokers and nonsmokers). We refer to smoking as a risk factor of lung cancer. We sometimes also state that among the risks of smoking is lung cancer. In its 2002 *World Health Report*, which is devoted entirely to quantifying, comparing, and reducing health risks, WHO recommended restricting the definition of risk to the first two usages; i.e., "the probability of an adverse health outcome and the factor that raises this probability," but not in terms of a health consequence or effect.[2]

While the "causes" of many diseases may not be known, population-based health research has uncovered an ever-increasing number of *risk factors*, which are statistically associated with the development (or inhibition) of diseases. The hope is that even if the true cause of a disease is not yet known, removal of the risk factors will reduce the frequency of disease. Sometimes distinction is made between risk factors and *risk markers*, which are not causally related to the disease but only indicate its presence (e.g., blood groups and other genetic markers). Most risk markers are in fact non-modifiable. There are several other terms as well, such as *precursor*, *risk indicator,* and *risk multiplier,* all of which convey a somewhat different mode of action. The term *proximate determinants* is also popular among demographers. There is little consistency in the use of terms related to risk in the population health literature.

At the level of the individual, certain "lifestyles" such as smoking, physical activity, and alcohol use, and biochemical measures such as plasma cholesterol level, are considered risk factors as they have been shown to be associated with the development of specific diseases (see Chapter 4). The term *health risk appraisal* (HRA) is used to describe a quantitative procedure to estimate the risk of mortality and morbidity for an individual possessing a certain risk factor profile. HRA has in fact become a tool for health promotion and education. The recognition of risks, when followed by goal setting and appropriate counselling, can result in behavioral change and improved health.[3] As most of us are not blessed with the ability to see into the future, we can only extrapolate from population experience for individual prediction. The more specifically defined the group experience, the more accurately it will apply to an individual with the same characteristics. Large, long-term epidemiological studies such as the Framingham Heart Study have contributed the data upon which many HRA programs are based. Mathematical models are available, creating so-called Framingham risk functions for myocardial infarction and stroke. However, the validity of applying risk scores developed from one population to another needs to be tested before they are recommended for general use.[4]

A slightly different term, *health risk assessment,* is generally used in the context of environmental and occupational hazards, such as radiation, airborne pollutants, contaminants in the food chain, etc. The definitions and concepts of health risk assessment were formulated in a U.S. National Research Council committee report, issued in 1983 and entitled *Risk Assessment in the Federal Government: Managing the Process,* often referred to as the Red Book. It was highly influential and widely cited. Health risk assessment "entails the evaluation of scientific information on the hazardous properties of environmental agents and on the extent of human exposure to those agents." The NRC proposed a four-step process in health risk assessment (WHO adopted a similar approach, with a somewhat different terminology)[5]:

1. Hazard identification: Identify the agents suspected to cause harm, quantify their concentrations in the environment, and describe the forms of toxicity and the conditions under which they might be expressed in exposed humans.
2. Dose-response assessment: Model the relationship between the magnitude of the exposure and the size of the health effect, and assess the variation in response between population subgroups.

3. Exposure assessment: Specify the population that might be exposed, identify the routes of exposure, and estimate the intensity, duration, and timing of the doses received by the exposed.
4. Risk characterization: Integrate information from the previous steps to develop an estimate of the likelihood of harmful effects occurring in people exposed to the hazard, and the degree of uncertainty involved.

Risk assessment should be followed by *risk management*, the policy decisions and actions that need to be taken in order to reduce the health risk to the population. In establishing the acceptable level of risk, the decisions need also to take into consideration the risks caused by other agents or societal factors, and the benefits associated with the hazard. Once the acceptable limit is established, actions are required to reduce the exposure and to maintain it below the limit. Finally, there should be a continuing process of risk monitoring after exposure control has been instituted.

Risk assessment has been characterized as "sophisticated quantitative analysis of available 'real world' data and hypothetical models in the absence of such data."[6] The need for extrapolation of data, particularly from animal studies to human populations, and from high-dose acute toxicity in experimental situations to chronic, low-dose exposure in everyday life, is at the root of much disagreement among scientific experts. Because there are so many uncertainties and gaps in knowledge, the *precautionary principle* is often invoked as a safeguard—a potentially harmful hazard is best avoided if we don't know much about it. But an overzealous application of this principle can stifle industrial and technological innovations.

There are no certainties in life or in health. As individuals and collectively, we need to weigh risks against benefits to guide our individual behavior and social policy. The idea that risk can be assessed and managed emerged only when human beings believed that they were not ruled by fate. The probabilistic approach to risk assessment has a long history. The French mathematician and philosopher Pascal, who eventually abandoned science for religion, proposed his famous "wager" on the existence of God. Given that one cannot know for sure the existence of God, should one believe in God? Pascal argued that one should believe in God, because *if you win, you win everything; if you lose, you lose nothing.*[7] We can put this into our familiar 2 × 2 table:

	Believe in God	Do not believe in God
God exists	a	b
God does not exist	c	d

BOX 5.1.   Words and Origins

The origin of the word *risk* is somewhat obscure.[8] One version is that it comes from the Greek *rhiza*, meaning "a cliff." Clearly sailing around a cliff is not without risk. Risk assessment is thus of interest to those both providing and in need of maritime insurance. *Hazard* is of Persian origin, referring to the dice used in a game of chance. It came to Europe via the Arabs and Spain. While health risk assessment is considered within the domain of population health, the profession of *actuary* (Latin *actuarius*: one who writes in shorthand) may have a prior claim, at least in their concern for individuals' longevity. Actuaries are usually employed by the insurance industry, which operates on the basic principle that past experience (reflected in mortality statistics and life tables) can be used to predict the future.

Risks can be big or small. In law, the *de minimis* principle is often invoked to prevent litigation for trivial damages. It comes from the Latin dictum *de minimis non curat lex*—the law does not concern itself with trifles. It is also used by regulatory agencies to bar action against risks of little consequence to public health and safety.

The original meaning of *probability* is quite different from its modern usage. Its Latin root *probare* means "to test, to prove, or to approve," and when something is probable it is "worthy of approbation." One of the earliest works on probability was a book on games of chance by Girolamo Cardano (1500–1571), a physician and gambler in Milan, published posthumously in 1663. He was the first to use the $1/x$ format to express probability, where x is the total number of possible outcomes and 1 the desired outcome. Probability theory developed as a branch of mathematics under such pioneers as Blaise Pascal (1623–1662), Jakob Bernouilli (1655–1705), and Pierre-Simon Laplace (1749–1827), among others. Bernouilli conceived of probability *as degree of certainty*. Ignorance of probability theory and the use of vital statistics (students, take heed!) resulted in the massive bankruptcies of the English Friendly Societies (a prototype of life insurance) in the early nineteenth century. The economist John Maynard Keynes (1883–1946) also made contributions to the logical and philosophical aspects of probability in *A Treatise on Probability* in 1921.

Thus, if God does not exist, it clearly does not matter whether one believes in God or not (cells c and d). However, if God exists, then it is far better to be in cell a (blessed with eternal bliss) than in cell b (languish in damnation).

Such reasoning is an example of *dominance* in decision theory, that one choice is as good as all others and clearly superior to some. It can be applied in many of the uncertainties of population health. The public's demand for guaranteed safety and the certainty of "no risk" is clearly not achievable, yet there are means to quantify the risk and make decisions accordingly.

Concepts of Causation

Causation is one of the few theoretical concerns of modern epidemiology, which is often perceived to be preoccupied with methods and rather devoid of theories. Because of epidemiology's major task of studying why diseases occur, it has devoted much energy to the discussion of causation.[9] Causation is of course not an issue exclusively for epidemiologists, it has also been of interest to philosophers, scientists, and theologians through the ages. Theologians ponder about the "ultimate cause" and have invoked the concept of *causa sui*, which in Latin means "cause of itself," a property that only the Supreme Being can possess. In his book *Physics*, Aristotle (384–322 BC) distinguished between four types of causes: material, formal, efficient, and final. For a marble statue, which the Greeks were fond of, the marble is the material cause, the pattern or blueprint is the formal cause, the sculptor is the efficient cause, and the purpose art is created for is the final cause.[10]

The eighteenth-century Scottish philosopher David Hume (1711–1776) wrote: "We may define a cause to be an object followed by another . . . , where, if the first object had not been, the second never had existed." This is an early example of the *counterfactual* concept of causation, by determining what would have happened under conditions contrary to those that actually happened. A contemporary epidemiologist, Kenneth Rothman, defined a cause as "an act or event or a state of nature which initiates or permits, alone or in conjunction with other causes, a sequence of events resulting in an effect."[11]

Causes can be *necessary* and/or *sufficient*. A cause is necessary when it must be present for an effect to occur. A cause is sufficient when it alone will inevitably produce the effect. This can be presented in a 2×2 table (indeed, much of epidemiology can be explained using the 2×2 table!). Let X be the cause and Y the effect:

	Effect (Y)	
Cause (X)	(+)	(−)
(+)	a	b
(−)	c	d

If X is a necessary cause, then $c = 0$; i.e., all cases of disease (Y+) have been exposed to it (X+).

If X is a sufficient cause, then $b = 0$; i.e., all people exposed to it (X+) develop the disease (Y+).

If X is both necessary and sufficient, $b = c = 0$, all the diseased have been exposed, and the exposed always becomes diseased.

The tubercle bacillus is necessary for tuberculosis to develop, yet it alone is not sufficient for the disease to occur, as there are other factors such as nutritional status, overcrowding, etc. Most infectious diseases require microorganisms to act as necessary causes. Even to say that the tubercle bacillus is a necessary cause for tuberculosis is in some ways "circular"—tuberculosis is defined as a disease caused by the tubercle bacillus, which then, by definition, is a necessary cause of tuberculosis.

For chronic diseases such as ischemic heart disease or diabetes, it is hard to think of a necessary cause. It is even harder to think of an example of a sufficient cause for any health condition, apart from a bolt of lightning being sufficient to cause death or extensive burns without the need for anything else to help in the act!

Causes can be also *remote* or *proximate*. Thus, in a causal chain represented by A → B → C → D → E, D is the proximate cause of E, whereas C, B, and A are increasingly remote causes. For example, infection with the bacteria *Helicobacter pylori* can lead to chronic superficial gastritis, to chronic atrophic gastritis, and ultimately to gastric adenocarcinoma.[12]

An early attempt to formulate a systematic approach to causation was made by Hume, who proposed in his *Treatise of Human Nature* (1739) three criteria for causation: (1) spatio-temporal continuity; (2) temporal priority of the cause; and (3) necessary connection. For the first criterion, Hume wrote "Nothing can operate in a time or place which is ever so little removed from those of its existence." The second criterion refers to the fact that cause must precede effect. The concept of necessary cause is included under the third criterion.[13]

In the nineteenth century, another British philosopher, John Stuart Mill (1806–1873), published *A System of Logic,* which contained his famous *five canons of causal inferences.*[14] *Canon* as used in logic does not mean "law" (and definitely not "artillery"), but rather the basis for forming a judgment. In Mill's words, the canons are:

1. Method of Agreement: "If two or more instances of the phenomenon under investigation have only one circumstance in common, the circumstance in which alone all the instances agree, is the cause or effect of the given phenomenon";
2. Method of Difference: "If an instance in which the phenomenon under investigation occurs, and an instance in which it does not occur, have every circumstance in common save one, that one occurring only in the former; the circumstance in which alone the two instances differ is the effect, or cause, or an indispensable part of the cause, of the phenomenon";
3. Joint Method of Agreement and Difference: "If two or more instances in which the phenomenon occurs have only one circumstance in common, while two or more instances in which it does not occur have nothing in common save the absence of that circumstance, the circumstance in which alone the two sets of instances differ is the effect, or cause, or an indispensable part of the cause, of the phenomenon";

4. Method of Residues: "Subduct from any phenomenon such part as is known by previous inductions to be the effect of certain antecedents, and the residue of the phenomenon is the effect of the remaining antecedents";

5. Method of Concomitant Variations: "Whatever phenomenon varies in any manner whenever another phenomenon varies in some particular manner, is either a cause or an effect of that phenomenon, or is connected with it through some fact of causation."

The quaint nineteenth-century language in which these canons were phrased is rather hard to comprehend in the abstract. They can be explained using the example of a food-poisoning investigation. Thus terms used by Mill, such as "instances," "circumstances," and "phenomena," can be translated into modern epidemiological parlance as "cases," "exposures," and "outcomes."

Let there be eight cases, four of whom were sick and the other four well. Four foods—A, B, C, D—were eaten in various combinations by the eight cases:

Case	Exposure	Outcome
1	A, B, C, D	sick
2	A, C, D	sick
3	A, B, C	sick
4	A, B, D	sick
5	B, C, D	well
6	C, D	well
7	B, C	well
8	B, D	well

A is the cause of the food poisoning, according to the first canon (Agreement), since A is present in all four cases who are sick. Comparing pairs of sick and well cases (i.e., 1 and 5, 2 and 6, 3 and 7, and 4 and 8), they have exactly the same exposures except for A; hence, according to the second canon (Difference), A is also the cause. The third canon (Joint Method) combines the first two canons, thus confirming that exposure to A is the cause of the food poisoning. The fourth canon (Residues) can be represented as ABC → xyz. If B has been previously shown to cause y, and C is known to cause z, then A must be the cause of x. The fifth canon (*Concomitant Variations*) should be familiar to students of statistics, for it essentially describes correlation. If x ↑ when A ↑, and if x ↓ when A ↓, then A is the cause of x. Mill's inductive logic is intended for the experimental sciences, and Mill chose his examples primarily from physics and chemistry.

By the late nineteenth century, at the dawn of the golden age of bacteriology, the need to develop criteria to "certify" the newly discovered and isolated microorganisms as causative agents of the major killer diseases of the day became apparent. A set of postulates became associated with Robert Koch (1843–1910), the discoverer of the tubercle bacillus and Nobel laureate.

In his monumental 1884 paper *Die Aetiologie der Tuberkulose*, Koch stated:

> First it is necessary to determine whether the diseased organs contain elements that are not constituents of the body. . . . If such alien structures can be exhibited, it is necessary to determine whether they are organized and show signs of independent life. . . . It is also necessary to consider the relation of such structures to their surroundings and to nearby tissues, their distribution in the body, their occurrences in various states of the disease, and so forth. . . . Establishing the coincidence of the disease and the parasite is not conclusive. In addition, one requires a direct proof that the parasite is the actual cause. This can only be achieved by completely separating the parasites from the diseased organism and from all products of the disease that could be causally significant. If the isolated parasites are then introduced into healthy animals they must cause the disease with all its characteristics.

According to the historical review by epidemiologist Alfred Evans (1917–1996), Koch's postulates were first formulated by Jakob Henle (1809–1885) in 1840 and elaborated by Robert Koch, Henle's student, some 40 years later. Evans set the record straight and introduced the term *Henle-Koch's postulates*. Henle's role has also been disputed, however, as Koch's ideas were believed to have been influenced more strongly by another German pathologist, Edwin Klebs (1834–1913).[15]

These postulates can be simplified as follow:

1. The agent must be present in every case of disease;
2. The agent should occur in no other disease;
3. The agent must be isolated from the body of the diseased, grown in pure culture, and when introduced into another person or animal, cause the disease.

To put it in another way, the agent must be *necessary* (postulate 1), *specific* (postulate 2), and *sufficient* (postulate 3). These criteria are far too stringent even for infectious diseases (particularly viral diseases), let alone the noncommunicable, chronic diseases. As Evans pointed out, they are limited by the failure to accommodate such concepts as the carrier state (infected but not sick), multiple causation, immunological processes, and reactivation of latent agents as causes of disease.

The predominance of the germ theory in medical science may have hindered the development of causal thinking with regard to other diseases that are noninfectious in origin.[16]

The landmark 1964 United States Surgeon General's report *Smoking and Health* pulled together the evidence then in existence linking smoking and lung cancer. A set of criteria was used, which was later expanded by the British statistician Austin Bradford Hill (1897–1991).[17]

The much-quoted *Bradford Hill's criteria* are:

1. Strength of association
2. Consistency
3. Specificity
4. Temporality
5. Biological gradient
6. Plausibility
7. Coherence
8. Experiment
9. Analogy

Temporality, strength, coherence, consistency, and specificity were in the Surgeon General's original list. Hill added analogy, experiment, and biological gradient, and separated biological plausibility from coherence. Hill never intended that these be hard-and-fast rules. In fact, he declared that none of them were essential, although logically speaking, temporality—that cause must precede effect—is clearly required. There are indeed exceptions to all the other conditions.

If an observed association is "strong," as indicated by a "high" ratio of the incidence of disease among the exposed to that among the nonexposed ("relative risk"—discussed later in this chapter), it is likely to be causal. Yet weak associations are often causal, and there is no agreed dividing line between a high and low relative risk. *Consistency* refers to corroboration of one's study results by other studies using different research designs and conducted in diverse populations. However, the problem may not have been well studied in the past and there may be few reports in the literature. *Specificity* means "one cause, one disease," clearly not expected to hold true very often. *Temporality* (or temporal sequence) must be present, but it may be difficult to establish, particularly in studies involving the retrospective collection of data. *Biological gradient*, or *dose–response relationship*, if it exists, strengthens the case for causality. Yet a dose–response relationship may not be observed if there is a "threshold" or "saturation point" beyond which changing the dose has no effect on disease risk (Figure 5.1). Most carcinogens do not show a threshold effect.

Plausibility and *coherence* are similar concepts, and even Hill himself could not distinguish the two in clear and convincing language! "Plausible" means "believable," particularly in view of known biological mechanisms. In explaining "coherent," Hill cited the Surgeon General's report, which used it in the sense of "not seriously [conflicting] with the generally known facts of the natural history and biology of the disease." Most authors

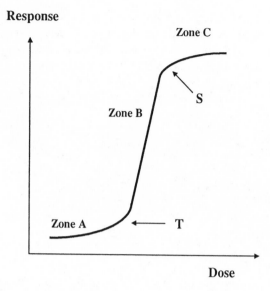

Figure 5.1. A dose-response curve. Zone A and Zone C: ↑ dose associated with little change in response; Zone B: ↑ dose associated with ↑ response; T: threshold; S: saturation point.

tend to lump plausibility and coherence together and ignore their subtle difference in meaning. At any rate, for a trailblazer and innovator working in a new field, existing knowledge cannot always be relied upon to support or refute a study's results. Experimental evidence, particularly involving human subjects, is the exception rather than the rule. Analogy, such as chemicals with similar molecular structure causing the same cancer, also cannot be relied upon.

Note that strength of association, temporality, specificity, and biological gradient are internal to a particular study, whereas the others require placing the results of that study in the context of existing knowledge and similar studies reported in the scientific literature. Some researchers encouraged the use of causal criteria to avoid bias in assessments of weak associations, while others considered such criteria scientifically invalid. In reviewing the practice of causal inference in the epidemiological literature, Douglas Weed found that, at least in the examples chosen, the criteria used most often were consistency, strength of association, dose–response, and biological plausibility. There was, however, no consensus on the definitions of the criteria and the rules for their use. For example, at what proportion of studies with "positive" results would consistency be deemed to exist—a simple majority, 80%, 100%? With regard to biological plausibility, its use ranged from merely hypothesizing a reasonable mechanism without any supportive evidence, to applying it only where a well-defined mechanism already existed. The use of meta-analysis (see Chapter 8), which is a quantitative procedure of aggregating data from different studies, would be helpful in the application of the strength of association and dose–response criteria. Its test of heterogeneity (which if "significant" should deter one from lumping the studies together) would be helpful in assessing consistency.[18]

Conspicuous by its absence is statistical significance, which is an indication of the role of chance. Its presence or absence has no bearing on whether a relationship is causal or not. Indeed, an over-reliance on statistical significance may lead to false-negative conclusions about causal associations.

Mervyn Susser reorganized and reduced to five the criteria of causation and provided clear definitions for them[19]:

1. Strength: size of estimated risk;
2. Specificity: "precision with which one variable, to the exclusion of others, will predict the occurrence of another, again to the exclusion of others." *Specificity* can refer to cause and to effect;
3. Consistency: "persistence of an association upon repeated tests." This can be subdivided into *survivability*, referring to the rigor of the tests, and *replicability*, referring to the diversity of tests;
4. Predictive performance: "ability to predict an unknown fact that is consequent on the initial association";
5. Coherence: the extent to which the causal association is "compatible with preexisting theory and knowledge." This can be subdivided into *theoretical, factual, biological*, and *statistical*.

A theoretical advance on causation as applied to diseases was Kenneth Rothman's concept of sufficient causes. He envisioned sufficient causes as complexes consisting of component causes, some of which are necessary.[20] For a hypothetical disease, there may be three sufficient causes; say, I, II, and III, each with component causes represented by letters A, B, C, etc.

Sufficient Cause I: A, B, C, D, E
Sufficient Cause II: A, B, F, G, H
Sufficient Cause III: A, C, F, I, J

Because A appears in all three sufficient causes, it is a necessary cause for this disease.

Causal models like Rothman's have been criticised for their excessive (and indeed exclusive) focus on individual-level determinants. In Rothman's model, each sufficient cause can be conceived of as a single individual or a group of individuals sharing the same component causes. A population is thus merely the sum of individuals, ignoring dynamic interactions between individuals that may produce a pattern of exposure only observable at the population level.[21]

As "health" and not "disease" is supposed to be the central focus of population health research and practice, it is worth noting that Alfred Evans directed our attention to the *causation of health* with his own postulates:[22]

1. "The preventive factor must be consistently present in persons of good health or free of a particular disease."
2. "The factor must be isolatable in a pure form (i.e., can be identified as causal)."
3. "The extent to which the factor is effectively applied must parallel an increase in good health and/or freedom from that disease."
4. "Experimental application of the factor to one segment of a population should significantly increase their good health as compared with matched controls."
5. "Withdrawal of the preventive factor should be associated with an increase of disease associated with that factor."
6. "The effect of the factor shall be measured in terms of lower morbidity and mortality, longer life, and lower medical costs."

Despite the importance of causation in the epidemiologist's rather sparse chest of theories, Nancy Krieger pointed out that there was something glaringly missing. Of all the talk about the "web of causation," a metaphor to represent the interconnectedness of risk factors and multifactorial etiology of disease, the "spider" is noticeably absent. What are the real origins, as opposed to interactions, of such multiple causes? Krieger identified the prevalent worldview of epidemiology as one of "biomedical individualism," which emphasizes biological factors of disease amenable to health care interventions and downplays social and political determinants. Krieger proposed an "ecosocial" framework, which directs attention not only to the social production of disease, but also to the social production of science—how a society's predominant worldview influences the way scientists develop their theories. It should encourage a reformulation and more careful consideration of such much used but loosely defined terms as class, race, lifestyle, and environment.[23]

Measures of Association and Effect

In quantifying the *strength of association* between a risk factor (or exposure) and a disease (or outcome), various measures of association are commonly used in population health research. There are three major types:

1. Ratio measures: relative risk, risk ratio, rate ratio (RR), and odds ratio (OR);
2. Difference measures: risk difference (RD) or attributable risk (AR);
3. Correlation coefficients (r): well known to students of statistics, such as Pearson's product-moment and Spearman's rank correlation coefficients.[24]

Types (1) and (2) will be discussed in detail here. In population health, the outcome of interest is often binary or dichotomous—diseased/not

---

BOX 5.2.   An Ethnomedical View of Disease Causation

Inherent in any culture's medical system are ideas about how diseases are caused and what types of treatment are required. Such beliefs form part of the coherent, rational understanding of the world and people's place within it. One culture's rational thought is not necessarily the same as another's; for example, the Western biomedical scientific culture.

William H. R. Rivers (1864–1922), a physician and anthropologist who is considered to be one of the founders of medical anthropology, listed three major groups of disease causes in his 1924 classic *Medicine, Magic and Religion*: human agency, supernatural agency, and natural causes. In a 1932 ethnographic survey of North American Indians, Forrest Clements distinguished between sorcery, taboo violation, disease-object intrusion, and soul loss.[25] Some of these causes were more important in some tribes than in others. The distinction between "natural" and "supernatural" causes is not always made in the worldview of many cultures, nor is the dichotomy of psychological and somatic diseases recognized. The mind, body, and spirit are considered an integrated whole, and disease is seen as serious disruption in the balance that exists between human beings and various spirits that cohabit the world.

Ethnomedical concepts of disease causation are very much alive in contemporary cultures, and not just among indigenous aboriginal peoples, but are present in "folk" systems of medical beliefs within industrial societies.

---

diseased, where the use of correlation coefficients is not appropriate. The use of types (1) and (2) represents an attempt to take into account the "background" risk; i.e., the risk of disease among the unexposed (even nonsmokers can get lung cancer).

The ratio of the incidence of an outcome in the presence of an exposure to the incidence without the exposure is the *relative risk*. The larger the relative risk, the stronger the association between exposure and outcome. Depending on the type of study (see Chapter 6) and the data available, the RR can be obtained in a variety of ways. If incidence densities (which are true rates with person-time in the denominator—see Chapter 2) are being compared, the ratio that results is more properly called a *rate ratio*. If cumulative incidence is used, the ratio is referred to as *risk ratio*.[26] This can be illustrated as follows:

	Diseased	Not diseased	Total
Exposed	a	b	(a + b)
Not exposed	c	d	(c + d)
Total	(a + c)	(b + d)	(a + b + c + d)

The cumulative incidence of disease among the exposed,

$$I_1 = a / (a + b)$$

The incidence of disease among the nonexposed,

$$I_0 = c / (c + d)$$

The risk ratio,

$$RR = I_1 / I_0 = \frac{a/(a+b)}{c/(c+d)}$$

An alternative way is to compare odds. The odds of something happening is the ratio of the number of times an event happened to the number of times it did not happen. Thus: the odds of exposure among the diseased is a/c; and the odds of exposure among the non-diseased is b/d. The ratio of these two odds is then:

$$\frac{a/c}{b/d} \text{ or } \frac{ad}{bc}$$

This is the odds ratio, computed by the cross-product in a 2×2 table. It is particularly useful in a type of epidemiological study called the case-control study (discussed in detail in Chapter 6).

It can also be shown that, instead of comparing the odds of exposure between the diseased and non-diseased, one can also compare the odds of disease among those exposed and not-exposed. The odds of disease among the exposed are a/b, and the odds of disease among the nonexposed are c/d. The ratio of these two odds is then:

$$\frac{a/b}{c/d} \text{ or } \frac{ad}{bc} \text{, which is also the cross-product.}$$

An odds ratio (OR) of 2.0 can mean that the diseased are twice as likely to have been exposed as the non-diseased, and that the exposed are twice as likely to be diseased as the nonexposed.[27]

While the RR and OR provide a measure of how many times more likely it is that disease will occur among the exposed compared to the nonexposed, it should be recognized that the additional risk being incurred by exposure may actually be quite small. Let I_0 be 1/100,000 person-years and I_1 be 5/100,000 person-years. The RR is 5.0, which is quite strong. The rate difference (RD), on the other hand, is 4/100,000 person-years. While exposure to a risk factor is associated with a fivefold increase in the risk of disease, the absolute increase in risk is only 4/100,000 (or 0.00004), which is still a relatively rare occurrence. (As an analogy: would you rather I give you five times what I have in my wallet, or whatever I have in my wallet plus $10?). Similarly, one can refer to a difference in two cumulative incidence as the *risk difference*. The term *attributable risk* is sometimes used as well, but it should be avoided because it is also used to refer to completely different entities (see below).

Clinical epidemiologists interested in the efficacy of clinical treatment also use the reciprocal of the risk difference (1/RD), termed *number needed to treat* (NNT), to denote the amount of effort required to achieve a desired clinical outcome. It is usually used in the clinical trials setting (see Chapter 6), where the RD is the difference between the incidence in the control group (i.e., not treated) and the treatment group.[28]

A population consists of individuals who are exposed or nonexposed to any given risk factor, and those who become diseased or do not become diseased. Given that some individuals are exposed, what proportion of the cases of the disease is due to, or attributable to, their having been exposed? Such a measure is called *attributable risk among the exposed*, or AR(E). Since nonsmokers can develop lung cancer, when smokers develop lung cancer, only a proportion of the cases can be "blamed" on the smoking. Computationally, $AR(E) = (I_1 - I_0) / I_1$, where I_0 is the incidence among the nonexposed, and I_1 the incidence among the exposed. $(I_1 - I_0)$, as we have just seen, is the risk difference.

At this point the literature becomes thoroughly confusing, as other terms meaning the same thing are used, including *attributable fraction*, *attributable proportion*, and *attributable risk percent*.

In the total population, each year a certain number of new cases of disease occurs. What proportion of them can be attributed to the exposure? This measure is called *population attributable risk* (PAR), and is conceptually similar to the AR(E), with the difference that we are now concerned with the total population and not just those exposed to the risk factor. It can be computed using the formula

$$PAR = (I - I_0)/I$$

where I_0 is the incidence among the nonexposed and I the incidence in the total population, consisting of both exposed and nonexposed. Confusion again sets in, as PAR is also variously called *population attributable fraction*, *population attributable proportion*, and *etiological fraction*.

A note of caution: Although the population is composed of exposed and unexposed people, the population incidence rate (I) is not simply the sum of I_0 and I_1. It must be adjusted according to the proportion of exposed and nonexposed in the total population. (As an analogy: Room A has 50% women, and Room B has 80% women: the combined proportion of women in Room A and Room B is not 130%! One has to first find out the number of women in Room A and Room B, then divide the sum by the total number of people in the two rooms.)

In computing AR(E) and PAR, it may not be possible to know the actual incidence of disease among the exposed and nonexposed. There are, however, alternative formulae to compute these measures using the relative risk (RR) instead.[29] The derivation of these formulae is rather complex and need not concern us here.

$$AR(E) = (I_1 - I_0)/I_1 = (RR - 1)/RR$$

$$PAR = (I - I_0)/I = [P(RR-1)]/[P(RR - 1) + 1]$$

where P is the proportion of the population exposed; i.e., the prevalence of the risk factor.

Note that the quantity $(RR - 1)$ is sometimes also referred to as the *excess relative risk* in the literature.

The alternative formula for PAR illustrates the point that the public health importance of a risk factor depends on both how common it is in the population and the strength of its causal association with a particular disease. Public health action directed at a risk factor with a high relative risk and prevalence is unlikely to be disputed (smoking and lung cancer). Comparing ozone depletion and the BRCA1 gene as risk factors for skin and breast cancer respectively, the former has a low RR (around 1.15) but affects almost everybody on earth, while the latter is extremely strongly associated with breast cancer (RR in the range of 15–130) but is a rare gene affecting few people (estimated to be 0.07%). The PAR for the ozone depletion/skin cancer association is about 0.13, whereas that for BRCA1 gene/breast cancer link is in the range of 0.01–0.08. On the basis of the PAR, remedying ozone depletion should take priority. This is, of course, a very simplistic approach—many other factors should also be taken into consideration when adopting and implementing population health interventions (see Chapter 7).[30]

Quantities such as RR, AR(E) and PAR are used to describe and compare risks in populations. It is one thing to say that 40% of deaths each year are "attributable" to smoking. It is another to say that Mr. X, a smoker, died of cancer caused by the smoking. Yet law courts and compensation boards are constantly asked to determine precisely that. If a specific individual who had been exposed to a certain occupational or environmental hazard (e.g., toxic chemicals, radiation) subsequently died or became sick, what is the probability that the harm was caused by the exposure? Legal and quasi-legal institutions are not primarily interested in population risks, but liabilities in individuals. Yet, in determining the *probability of causation* (PC) in specific individuals (sometimes also called the *assigned share*), they have increasingly relied upon epidemiological evidence that is population-based and statistical (probabilistic) in nature.

BOX 5.3.   Estimating Tobacco Deaths

Many public health agencies, national cancer societies, and anti-smoking groups routinely publish data on the number of deaths attributable to smoking. Since "smoking" is not an ICD code used in death certificates, how are such estimates made? It involves the computation of population attributable risk (PAR), which is in turn derived from estimates of smoking prevalence (P) and the risk of death among smokers compared to nonsmokers (RR). In a study of mortality attributable to smoking in Canada in 1985, data on P were obtained from the 1985 General Social Survey (the percent of ever-smokers was used), and RR from the 10-year followup of the Nutrition Canada Survey cohort aged 35–79:[31]

	P	RR	RR − 1	P(RR − 1)	P(RR − 1) + 1	P(RR − 1)/ P(RR − 1) + 1
Men	0.776	1.74	0.74	0.57424	1.57424	0.36477
Women	0.401	1.65	0.65	0.26065	1.26065	0.20676

From Vital Statistics, the total number of deaths in the 35–79 age group in Canada in 1985 was obtained. Multiplying these number by the PAR results in the number of deaths "attributable" to smoking:

	Total no. deaths	PAR	No. deaths due to smoking
Men	66,855	0.36477	24,386
Women	42,548	0.20676	8,797

To find out the proportion of deaths among smokers that can be attributed to smoking, one can compute the attributable risk (exposed), or AR(E), which is (RR− 1)/RR. For men this is 0.74/1.74 or 42.5%, and for women this is 0.65/1.65 or 39.4%.

A common rule of thumb is that the suspected exposure should be "more likely than not" to have caused the outcome. There is a tendency to extrapolate population data, particularly the use of AR(E). If RR > 2 (a "doubling dose"), then (RR − 1) > 1, and AR(E) > 50%. The court will then conclude that the "more likely than not" condition has been satisfied and make the award accordingly. This approach has been severely criticized by Sander Greenland, including its inability to account for the acceleration of disease occurrence, thus underestimating the probability of causation.[32]

BOX 5.4. 95% CI for RR and OR

To calculate 95% confidence intervals for relative risks and odds ratios, the same notation as that used in the text above can be used, with a 2×2 table with four cells, a, b, c, and d.[33]

$$RR = \frac{a/(a+b)}{c/(c+d)} \text{ and } OR = \frac{ad}{bc}$$

The procedure involves the use of the natural logarithm (log to the base e)

The standard error (SE) of $\log_e RR = \sqrt{1/a - 1/(a+b) + 1/c - 1/(c+d)}$

Let $L = \log_e RR - n(SE)$ and $U = \log_e RR + n(SE)$,

where $n = 1.96$, the critical value from the standard normal distribution for the 95th percentile.

The 95% confidence interval of RR is obtained by exponentiating e^L and e^U

The SE of $\log_e OR = \sqrt{1/a + 1/b + 1/c + 1/d}$

Let $L = \log_e OR - n(SE)$ and $U = \log_e OR + n(SE)$,

where $n = 1.96$, the value from the standard normal distribution for the 95th percentile.

The 95% confidence interval of OR is obtained by exponentiating e^L and e^U.

Competing Risks

Human beings die only once. While many diseases may contribute to a person's ultimate demise, there is usually one major underlying cause of death. If someone dies from heart disease, that person cannot then die from cancer or a motor vehicle accident. However, during her lifetime, a person is continuously exposed to many competing risks of death, one of which eventually "wins." The issue of competing risks is different altogether from the problem of coding multiple causes of death in death certificates. Even if there is a single, unequivocal, direct cause of death ("struck by lightning"), when there is no need to code other causes, the deceased would still have been prevented from dying from some other competing cause.

Competing risks need to be taken into account when describing and explaining long-term health trends. The decline of infectious diseases as a major killer in childhood means that the survivors are now "eligible" to die from other causes later in life, such as cancer. Indeed, in studies of disease causation, if smoking causes both lung cancer and heart disease and if heart disease occurs first and kills the smoker, there is no probability that the smoker can die from lung cancer. Looked at perversely, smoking has "prevented" a death from lung cancer!

Competing risks are important considerations in population health, since it would be a useful aid to public health policy to be able to estimate the impact of eliminating a certain disease on the overall mortality from all causes as well as the mortality rate from another disease. Note that before death, a disease or health problem is a *risk*; after death it becomes a *cause*. (People die of causes, not risks—as long as you are still at risk for dying, you have not died yet! Once you are dead, you are no longer at risk.)

Statisticians have tackled competing risks for some time—in fact, the concept can be traced to the Swiss mathematician Daniel Bernoulli (1700–1782) in the mid–eighteenth century, who attempted to estimate the improvement in life expectancy had smallpox been eliminated. In the 1950s, Jerome Cornfield, of odds ratio fame, pointed out that, in the context of an epidemiological study of Disease A, if a person dies from Disease B, he has no probability of dying from A. By designing a type of life table, it is possible to find out what would happen to his risk of dying from A if he had not died from B. Those who die from B, however, might have had a chance of dying from A, and they may differ in some systematic ways from those who actually die from A. Competing risks are also critical in the evaluation of the long-term effectiveness of therapies—the true benefits of a drug would be obscured if a substantial proportion of participants in a clinical trial were killed in car crashes!

Demographer Chin Long Chiang developed formulae based on age-cause-specific mortality rates routinely available from vital statistics agencies to determine the probability of dying from a specific cause in the presence of all other competing risks (*crude probability*), the probability of dying if a specific risk is eliminated from the population, or if there is only one risk acting on the population (*net probability*), and the probability of dying from a specific cause if some risks are eliminated (*partial crude probability*).[34] Figure 5.2 examines the impact on the mortality experience of the U.S. population if cardiovascular diseases are eliminated.

Measures of premature mortality such as potential years of life lost (see Chapter 2) do not take into account competing risks. One that does is the *potential gain in life expectancy* (PGLE), which is the number of added years of life expectancy for a population if deaths from a certain cause are removed. The probabilities shown in Figure 5.2 can be converted into life expectancy in years. With cardiovascular disease eliminated from the United States, a white male at birth can be expected to live an extra 8.3 years, and at age 65, 7.7 years.

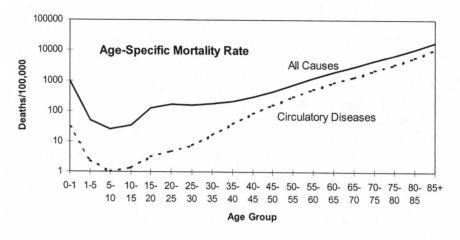

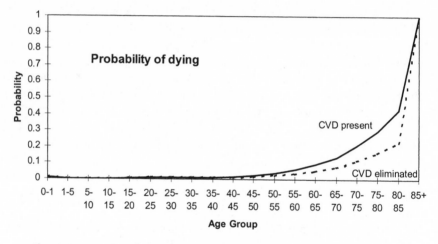

Figure 5.2. Impact of eliminating cardiovascular diseases on mortality.

An alternative approach to the rather unrealistic scenario of a competing cause being completely eliminated is to calculate the impact on mortality from all causes, or of a specific cause, if the competing cause is kept at a constant, historical level. Case Study 5.2 investigates the impact of a declining cardiovascular mortality on cancer mortality, using both the "elimination" and the "constant" models.

Risk Perception and Communication

In health risk assessment, the population health researcher believes that he or she is engaged in a strictly scientific and technical activity, and is often surprised to find out that the general public, or subsections of it, may have a totally different perception of what constitutes risk and what

BOX 5.5.   Betting On Your Odds

We live in a world full of hazards. The risks of death from these hazards, however, vary substantially. The graph below compares the mortality risk for various diseases, occupational groups, and recreational activities, expressed as deaths per 100,000 person-years at risk, primarily derived from U.S. statistics toward the end of the twentieth century, except when otherwise specified.[35] Note that one axis is logarithmic, to accommodate the wide range in mortality rates.

There are clearly some surprises—e.g., that dying in the line of duty is more likely among presidents than policemen in the United States.

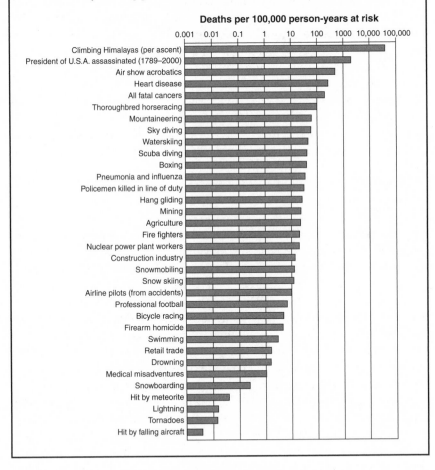

actions should be undertaken. Part of the job of a population health practitioner is to interpret and communicate the myriad risks in our lives to the public.[36] There is a fine line between inciting mass hysteria and engaging in a cover-up.

The community's judgment about risk should not be assumed to be inferior to that of the experts; they are only different. Community involvement in environmental health issues is a relatively recent social phenomenon (even movement), which poses a challenge to the traditional scientific approach to risk analysis.

Earlier in this chapter, the distinction between risk assessment and risk management was made. Among scientists and technical experts, there is a strong conviction that the former is objective and neutral, whereas the latter is subject to prevailing social, cultural, and political considerations. Mary Douglas and Aaron Wildavsky, in their influential 1982 book *Risk and Culture*, advanced the view that risk is socially and culturally "constructed." According to them, risk assessment is not free from societal values but is the outcome of socially determined methods and judgments. Risk assessment is by nature biased, and scientists disagree among themselves anyway. Educating the public and reasoning with them about risks is unlikely to make people more rational in their approach to environmental hazards.[37]

Why are some risks accepted by the public and others not? The technical issue of level of risk is only one consideration. The public is more likely to accept a certain risk if it is perceived to be fairly distributed, if it provides some benefit (e.g., economic) to those exposed, if no alternative is available, if it is not imposed on them, and if they can exert some control.

Many hazards are hidden from public awareness for a variety of reasons. Hazards that are too complex, diffuse, and occur in faraway places (e.g., global climate change, destruction of the Amazonian rain forest) often do not rate highly in the public consciousness. Ideological positions may downplay adverse effects and elevate the benefits, or vice versa. Historically, the capitalist profit motive has been associated with attempts to downplay industrial hazards. On the other hand, the relentless drive to industrialization in the socialist economies has resulted in some of the world's most horrendous environmental degradations. Marginal groups in society (such as the poor and ethnic minorities) may be more likely to be exposed to hazards and less likely to receive attention from the "mainstream." Hazards that threaten cherished societal values (e.g., the "right to drive cars and to own guns") tend to be resistant to change.[38]

Risks are expressed as probabilities, which may be the reason why risks are often poorly understood by non-mathematicians. Psychologists Amos Tversky and Daniel Kahneman identified three common biases in interpreting and assessing probabilities of uncertain events, which they attributed not to the lack of intelligence, wishful thinking, or deliberate distortion, but to people's use of information in problem-solving (heuristics): (1) representativeness—a small class of events is assumed to be representative of a larger class; (2) anchoring—a first estimate is progressively adjusted to fit subsequent events; and (3) availability—more memorable events are perceived to be more frequent.[39]

BOX 5.6.   A Matrix of Dread and Unknown Risks

A body of literature on risk perception is derived from psychological research based on surveys of attitudes and opinions, using psychometric
scaling techniques and multivariate modelling. In a study of 81 hazards, Paul Slovic used factor analysis to distinguish two axes, one called
"dread risk" and the other "unknown risk."[40] At one extreme of the
dread risk axis are risks perceived to be uncontrollable, have global cat-
astrophic consequences, fatal, not equitably distributed, pose a high
risk to future generations, not easily reduced, increasing in magnitude,
and involuntary. The "unknown risks" are those that are not observable, unknown to those exposed, new and unknown to science, and associated with delayed effects. The two intersecting axes produce four
quadrants.

   In quadrant 1 are such risks as nuclear reactor safety and electromagnetic fields; in quadrant 2 are such risks as general aviation and
mining safety; in quadrant 3 are such risks as smoking and alcohol use;
and in quadrant 4, water fluoridation of the water supply and using
oral contraceptives.

Factor 2: Unknown Risk

Not observable, etc.

	4	1	**Factor 1: Dread Risk**
Controllable,			Uncontrollable,
etc.	3	2	etc.

Observable, etc.

Risks remain personal and localized issues unless they are communicated to others. Under the *social amplification of risk* model, developed by
R. E. Kasperson and others, risk events interact with psychological, social,
institutional, and cultural processes, which may attenuate or intensify the
perception of risk and ultimately change behavior. Through this process,
certain hazards and events judged low-risk by experts can be intensified
as they are transmitted to, and received by, the general public, and become
a major scare, while serious hazards may be attenuated to such an extent
that they are virtually ignored. In the language of communication theory,
risk signals (images, signs, and symbols) are received, interpreted, and
transmitted by a variety of social agents. They are filtered through amplification stations where the signals become transformed—the volume of
information can be increased or decreased, certain messages selected for

special attention, and the signals reinterpreted. Amplification stations can be individuals or institutions, such as scientists, research institutes, the media, politicians, and government agencies. Transformations of the risk signals can be predicted from the prevalent sociodemographic characteristics, cultural patterns, institutional structure, personal attitudes, and so on.[41]

Given the complexity of the technical issues underlying risk assessment and the social, cultural, and political bases for the public's perception of risks, risk communication is by necessity a very difficult and sensitive task. Risk communication may be a statutory requirement to inform the public and other bodies, particularly for large-scale projects. It can be used to transfer technical information among scientists, policy-makers, managers, and stakeholder groups to inform decision-making. It also provides information that allows individuals to make informed decisions about whether to accept a risk or not and to take risk-reducing actions.[42]

The risk communicator not only has to understand the strengths and weaknesses of the methodology used in risk assessment, its assumptions, biases, and uncertainties, but also to arbitrate and integrate conflicting scientific data in a manner that can be easily understood. Vincent Covello and others offered a seven-point guide to risk communication:[43]

1. Accept and involve the public as a legitimate partner;
2. Plan carefully and evaluate performance;
3. Listen to the audience;
4. Be honest, frank, and open;
5. Coordinate and collaborate with credible sources;
6. Meet the needs of the media; and
7. Speak clearly and with compassion.

Trust, liability, fairness, and accountability are key to successful risk communication. It needs to recognize and respect different forms of view, be transparent and accessible. It thus bridges scientific research, public policy, and community action.

Summary

Assessing health risks is a central task of population health research and practice. Risk is a probabilistic concept, and its uses extend from risk factors and risk markers of diseases to formalized procedures such as health risk appraisal, a tool in individual health promotion, and health risk assessment, generally applied to environmental and occupational health hazards.

Guidelines for the establishment of causation have attracted the attention of philosophers such as Hume and Mill. In the nineteenth century, the revolution in bacteriology led to the development of Koch's postulates. The requirement that an agent must be necessary, specific, and sufficient is too stringent for the chronic, noninfectious diseases. In the 1960s, Bradford Hill's criteria had a major influence in epidemiological research and have been used in establishing the link between smoking and lung cancer. Apart from temporal sequence, exceptions to these criteria abound, and they are not meant to be followed blindly. Other theoretical contributions to the theory of disease causation have been made more recently by Susser, Rothman, Evans, and Krieger.

The strength of association between a risk factor and a health outcome can be quantified in a variety of ways, including the relative risk, odds ratio, and risk difference. It is also important to know the effect or impact of a risk factor on the population at large and those who have been exposed to the factor, using measures such as the population attributable risk and attributable risk among the exposed, respectively. These measures can be used in the decision to select health problems for public health action by estimating the potential gain in cases of disease averted if the risk factor is successfully removed from the population.

Public health action can also be informed by mortality analyses involving competing risks; for example, in estimating the impact of eliminating a disease on the overall risk of death and life expectancy.

Finally, it must be recognized that the perception of risk is determined by social, cultural, psychological, and political factors, which add to the complexity of the scientific and technical aspects of risk assessment and the task of communicating health risks to the general public.

Case Study 5.1. Is British Beef Safe?

"But I am a great eater of beef, and, I believe, that does harm to my wit."

Sir Andrew Aguecheek, in Shakespeare's
Twelfth Night, Act I, Scene 3

In 1996, the entire British beef industry faced collapse and millions of cattle, wholesale slaughter. In March, the Minister of Health announced that Creutzfeldt-Jakob disease (CJD) might be linked to a similar disease found in cattle called bovine spongiform encephalopathy (BSE), popularly known as "mad cow disease." It was based on a review of 10 recent cases of CJD with unusual clinical features, especially the much younger age of onset. The possibility of contracting a dreaded, incurable neurological disease from eating a widely available food was most disconcerting to the public and politicians. Apart from milk and beef, there is a whole range of beef byproducts. Gelatin derived from beef can be found in chicken stock, medicine capsules, soap, shampoo, and creams. While the absolute risk may be low, the size of the population exposed is very large. The European Union imposed a worldwide ban on the export of British beef, countries around the world banned its import, and leading fast food chains, schools, and other institutions in Britain stopped serving British beef altogether. Beef prices plummeted while farmers and workers faced economic ruin. Political parties accused each other of reckless disregard for the public's health and coverup on one hand, and of scare-mongering and whipping up mass hysteria on the other.

BSE is a chronic, progressive, degenerative disease of the central nervous system, first diagnosed in 1986 in Britain and reported in several other European countries. The disease is characterized by change in temperament, uncoordination, weight loss, and eventual death. There is no cure and no diagnostic test other than postmortem examination of brain tissues, which shows the characteristic "holes." BSE developed into a major epidemic among British cattle, which peaked in 1992 with over 35,000 confirmed cases reported in that year. By 2003, the annual number of new cases had dwindled down to around 1,000. The cumulative total since the beginning of the epidemic was 180,000 cases in Britain, compared to only several thousands in the rest of the world combined.[44]

BSE belongs to a group of diseases called transmissible spongiform encephalopathies (TSE), which include scrapie in sheep and goats, CJD and kuru in humans, and several varieties in other species. CJD has been recognized since the 1920s. It is named after two German physicians, Hans Gerhard Creutzfeldt (1885–1964) and Alfons Jakob (1884–1931). It is extremely rare, with an incidence of about one case per million per year. A small proportion of cases are familial. Some cases are iatrogenic in origin, where the infection is acquired from medical procedures such as neurosurgical instrumentation, corneal implant, and the injection of pituitary-derived human growth hormone and gonadotrophin. To distinguish it from the "classic" and sporadic form of CJD, the cases suspected to be caused by exposure to BSE are called variant CJD, or vCJD. Since the first case reports, the number of definite or probable cases has exceeded 130 (by 2003).

The infectious agent responsible for the TSEs, at one point called a "slow virus" or "unconventional virus," is now generally believed to be prions (from "proteinaceous infectious particle"), discovered by Stanley Prusiner in the early 1980s, for which he was awarded the Nobel prize in 1997. While self-replicating, prions do not contain DNA (and cannot really be called "organisms") but are composed of an abnormal form (PrP^{SC}) of a normal cellular protein called PrP^C.

Kuru has a distinguished and fascinating history. It was first recognized among the Fore people in the highlands of Papua New

Guinea. Carleton Gajdusek, of the U.S. National Institutes of Health, discovered that the disease was transmitted through the cannibalistic rituals of the tribe. A deceased person was honored by being eaten. While men received the choice meats, women and children got to eat the brains and were at highest risk for the disease. Gajdusek received the Nobel prize in 1976. His detective work provides a classic case of how ethnographic knowledge contributes to the understanding of disease causation.[45]

The cause of BSE in cattle is unknown, but it is believed that exposure probably occurred in the early 1980s. The practice of feeding cattle proteins from rendered carcasses of sheep infected with scrapie (a form of forced cannibalism among herbivores) may have started the epidemic. While the practice of rendering animal carcasses into cattle feed is not new, in the 1970s the technique of solvent extraction and steam heat treatment (which could have destroyed the infectious agent) was substituted by a low-temperature method. There is little evidence of spread from cattle to cattle by contact or of vertical transmission from mother to newborn.

To stop the BSE epidemic in cattle, the practice of including ruminant-derived proteins in cattle feed was prohibited, and all potentially infected animals were destroyed, although noncompliance by some farmers and abattoirs was suspected. The British government also instituted epidemiological surveillance of human CJD in 1990, with a national surveillance unit based in Edinburgh. Since the BSE epidemic began, British agriculture ministry officials had maintained that the risk to the public was minimal—the Minister of Agriculture even fed his young daughter a hamburger in a public show of confidence. The Minister of Health's announcement in Parliament in March 1996 admitting to uncertain and possible risk to human health, based on a report from the national surveillance unit, thus represented a reversal of the government's position and sparked the public panic.

The case of mad cow disease provides many valuable lessons in risk assessment, perception, and communication—topics discussed in this chapter. Indeed, it touches on almost every important issue in population health:

- What constitutes an "epidemic"—are 130 human cases of vCJD in a decade enough? Is this burden of disease "too high"—how does it compare to AIDS, traffic accidents, etc.? Are these cases the tip of the iceberg, and are more cases still to come from the unknown number of people already exposed and infected?
- Can one contract vCJD from eating beef which may have been contaminated with BSE—what criteria of causation have been satisfied? What is the extent of BSE contamination in beef sold in the

market? What is the extent of BSE infection in apparently "healthy" cattle, and what is the chance of infected but asymptomatic cattle finding its way into abattoirs and the human food chain?

- Why is BSE prevalent only in Britain and not in other countries with a large cattle population? Is it a matter of different diagnostic and coding practices? Could the reluctance to affix the BSE label to sick cattle in some countries be influenced by economic interests?
- How should one communicate a health risk associated with high uncertainty and great fear to the public? What type of advice should be given to consumers?
- How should the BSE epidemic in cattle be controlled and a vCJD epidemic in humans prevented or aborted? Should all cattle be slaughtered, or only some; and how many is enough? How should one balance economics and public health?

BSE is still very much alive as a public health, political, and economic issue. In 2003 one case was diagnosed in a cow in an Alberta farm. An export ban of cattle and beef was invoked and maintained for months, resulting in severe economic dislocations for the cattle and related industries. Later that year, an infected cow was also discovered in Washington State.

Case Study 5.2.   Do Heart Attacks Prevent Cancer Deaths?

"Do more people die from cancer today because fewer people now die from heart attacks?" This is not a frivolous question. In evaluating whether there had been progress in the "war on cancer," it is important to determine that any change in cancer mortality that is observed is not simply because mortality from a competing cause has changed.

In a study of mortality among women over the age of 40 in Spain, it was found that between 1981 and 1994, mortality for ischemic heart disease (IHD) had declined in all age groups, whereas for cancer, mortality had increased among women over the age of 75.[46]

From the sets of age-specific mortality rates, the lifetime probability of death from cancer in 1981 was computed to be 8.2%, which increased to 10.7% in 1994, due to the increase among the older age groups. Using computer modeling, the probability of death from cancer would increase to 11.1% if IHD were eliminated, but it would decrease slightly to 10.4% if the IHD rate for 1981 were maintained. Thus it can be seen that the observed increase in cancer mortality among Spanish women between 1981 and 1994 was not produced by the competing effects of a declining IHD mortality. The cause

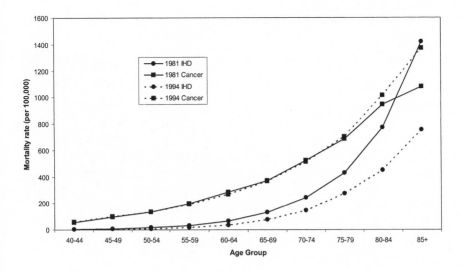

of the increase must be sought elsewhere: perhaps in changes in risk factor profile, cancer screening practices, and effectiveness of treatment.

Case Study 5.3.   Communicating SARS Risk with Numbers

Early in 2003, an apparently brand-new disease emerged from southern China, from which it spread to over 30 countries around the world. Named *severe acute respiratory syndrome* (SARS), the disease is characterized by high fever, coughing, and respiratory distress. A newly identified coronavirus is believed to be the causative agent. There is no effective treatment other than supportive care. Close household members and hospital workers are particularly vulnerable.

Among the countries affected was Canada, primarily its largest city, Toronto. As the epidemic evolved, the issue quickly became not just one of epidemic control, but also risk perception and risk communication. At the height of the epidemic, daily press conferences with leading government officials were held, and there was saturation media coverage. In communicating the progression of the epidemic, the provincial government relied heavily on the number of active cases (under treatment, both in hospital and at home), the number who died and recovered, and the cumulative number of cases diagnosed since the beginning of the epidemic. The following graph shows the cumulative number of cases.

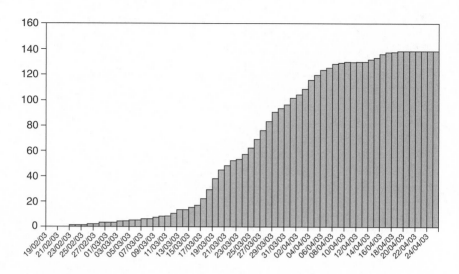

The conclusion drawn by the media and the public was one of a relentless, progressing epidemic that was getting worse as time went on. But, little attention was paid to the one number that would truly indicate the rise (and fall) of the epidemic—the number of new (i.e., incident) cases:

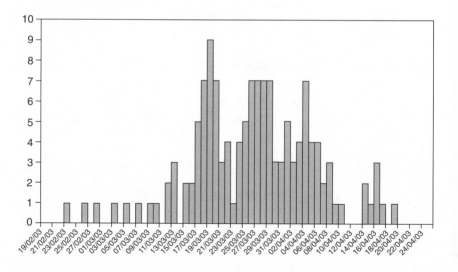

A different picture emerges—the epidemic had passed its peak, and was tapering off towards the end of April. Interestingly, WHO imposed a travel advisory for Toronto on April 23, 2003, the day after the last case was reported!

The first graph was most alarming to the public—it could only go up (except when a case was reclassified and removed from the cumulative list). The second graph—the classic epidemic curve (see Chapter 3)—gave hope to the public that the end was in sight. Although the number of deaths and the number of people in hospital are useful information, they convey the clinical severity of the cases and the effectiveness of treatment, but not whether more people are getting infected, a measure of the effectiveness of the epidemic control measures.[47]

Notes

1. Skolbekken (1995) coined the term *risk epidemic* in medical journals. Much of what is written suffers from a lack of conceptual coherence and theoretical limitations (Hayes, 1992). Beck (1992) and Giddens (1991:123) wrote about risk society and modernity—I was led to their work by Miller (1999).

2. See WHO (2002:11). The entire report, including statistical annexes, can be downloaded from the WHO web site.

3. There is a large amount of HRA literature. See the review by Spasoff and McDowell (1987). The modern origin of HRA is often traced to the book on prospective medicine by Robbins and Hall (1970). Computer programs for HRA have been developed; for example, by the Carter Center and the CDC. Their predictive accuracy was evaluated by Gazmararian et al. (1991).

4. See Wilson et al. (1998) for the prediction of coronary heart disease using the Framingham risk scores. The American Heart Association's web site (www.americanheart.org) offers a risk assessment tool that computes a 10-year risk of coronary heart disease when an individual enters the relevant data for age, sex, total cholesterol, HDl-cholesterol, systolic blood pressure, current smoking status, and treatment for hypertension. Thomsen et al. (2002) cross-validates Framingham data with those from a Danish population study in estimating coronary risk.

5. See National Research Council (1994:4–5), which updates the 1983 document. The terminology used by WHO can be found in *A Dictionary of Epidemiology* (Last, 2001:159). They are derived from *Assessment and Management of Environmental Health Hazards* (unpublished document no. WHO/PEP/ 89.6.)

6. The quotation is from Short (1984). Hertz-Picciotto (1995) called for more use of epidemiological studies and less reliance on toxicological studies in risk assessment and proposed a framework to determine and classify the adequacy of studies for use in dose–response extrapolation.

7. Pascal's wager was discussed in Fragment 418 of his *Pensées*, first published posthumously in 1670. Various English translations are available. The quotation is from the Penguin Classic edition (Krailsheimer, 1966:149–153). Pascal was a prodigy. Besides the theory of probability in mathematics, his legacies include Pascal's law of hydrostatic pressure in physics (and the barometric unit "kilopascal" is used in meteorology). He even invented a calculating machine to help his father, a tax collector! The modern PASCAL computer programming language was not invented by him but was named in his honor.

8. See Covello and Mumpower (1985) and Jasanoff (in Mayo and Hollander, 1991:34–35). Hacking (1975) and Bernstein (1996) provide fascinating accounts of the historical development of the concepts of risk and probability.

9. The Epidemiology Resources, Inc., published two collections of papers on causal inference (Greenland, 1987; Rothman, 1988).

10. Students without a background in the humanities should consult reference works such as *An Encyclopedia of Philosophy* (Parkinson, 1988) and the *Oxford Dictionary of Philosophy* (Blackburn, 1994). A succinct review of the more recent contributions to the discussion of causation in the philosophy of science literature can be found in Schaffner (in Mayo and Hollander, 1991:204–17).

11. The quotation from Hume's *An Enquiry Concerning Human Understanding* (1748) is cited in Maldonado and Greenland (2002). There are, of course, many other definitions. The definition cited here, from Rothman (1976), is aimed at epidemiologists.

12. Chronic superficial gastritis also gives rise to peptic ulcer and lymphoproliferative disease of the stomach. Indeed, Koch's postulates (discussed later in this chapter) were satisfied in this case as the final proof was furnished by Barry Marshall in Perth, Australia, who ingested the bacteria and developed severe (but brief) gastritis in 1985. Two years later, a volunteer in New Zealand also developed gastritis, which ran a prolonged course. See Blaser (1996) for the story of the bacterial cause of peptic ulcer and stomach cancer. See also Exercise 5.4.

13. See Parkinson (1988:282–83).

14. Mill's treatise on logic was first published in 1856 and underwent many editions, well into the 1940s. The five canons appeared in Volume 1, Book III, Chapter VIII. The quotation is from the 6th edition (1865; vol. 1:427–50). An introductory textbook of logic, for example, Copi and Cohen (1990), should be consulted for further explanation and additional examples. It is interesting that Mill's canons are rarely mentioned in textbooks of epidemiology, although they can be found in Last's *Dictionary*.

15. While Evans (1978) rehabilitated Henle, Carter (1985) championed Klebs. Jakob Henle is best remembered for "the loop of Henle," part of the renal tubule. Since the third edition, the *Dictionary of Epidemiology* has listed the postulates under Henle-Koch rather than Koch. Klebs is noted for a few discoveries of his own, and his name is associated with the bacterium *Klebsiella*, the Klebs-Loeffler bacillus (an earlier name for diphtheria), and Klebs' disease (glomerulonephritis).

16. Carter (1977) argued that the germ theory may have actually set a new standard for the understanding of noninfectious diseases and contributed to a revival of research interests in the "deficiency diseases" such as scurvy, beriberi, pellagra, and rickets. (See Case Study 1.4 in Chapter 1 on Goldberger's studies on pellagra.)

17. Hill's classic paper (1965) was preceded by earlier attempts at formulating causal criteria by Yerushalmy and Palmer (1959) and Sartwell (1960). Hill's many contributions to medical research were reviewed by Richard Doll (1992), his longtime collaborator. Hill had been professor and dean at the London School of Hygiene and Tropical Medicine and pioneered the randomized control trial in the 1950s, especially in the MRC trial of streptomycin in tuberculosis therapy. His cohort study with Doll on lung cancer and smoking among British doctors is one of the most important studies in modern epidemiology. His textbook *The Principles of Medical Statistics* was first published in 1937. The 12th edition (Hill and Hill, 1991) appeared in the year of his death.

18. See Weed (1997) and Weed and Hursting (1998) on the practice of causal inference. Weed (2000) discussed the potential uses of meta-analysis.

19. Susser (1991) also provided a succinct historical review of both the philosophy and epidemiology literatures. See also Renton (1994), who emphasized the need to incorporate the full scope of medical science, especially knowledge of pathogenetic mechanisms, in deciding causes and public health action. For

a Popperian approach (discussed in Chapter 1) and use of deductive logic in establishing causation, see Weed (1986).

20. Rothman's ideas can be found in his 1976 paper as well as his textbook (Rothman and Greenland, 1998:7–16). The concept is considerably more complex than described here, as it can be quantified and discussed in terms of the various measures of effect.

21. See particularly Koopman and Lynch (1999) and McMichael (1999).

22. Quoted from Evans (1978).

23. See Krieger (1994). One of the earlier uses of the "web" metaphor can be found in the now-classic epidemiology text by MacMahon and Pugh (1970:23–25), who used it to correct the oversimplification of the traditional, linear view of a "chain of causation." Tesh (1981) pointed out the political implications of theories of disease causation (e.g., germs vs. lifestyles vs. the environment), which differ in how they place the responsibility for disease prevention and how they view the role and proper organization of society.

24. Greenland et al. (1986) argued against the popular use of standardized regression coefficients (*beta*), correlation coefficients, and "percent of variance explained" as measures of effect.

25. Clements's paper "Primitive Concepts of Disease" was published in the *University of California Publications in American Archaeology and Ethnology*, vol. 32, 1932. For a general introduction to North American Indian medical systems, see Vogel (1970), and, with special reference to Canada, Waldram et al. (1995). North American Indians have also developed theories of causation for relatively "new" diseases such as diabetes and hypertension—see the work of Garro (1988) among the Ojibwa of Manitoba.

26. Risk is thus defined in terms of the cumulative incidence—the probability that an individual will develop a disease (or change in health status) over a specified period, conditional on not dying of some other disease (Morgenstern et al. 1980).

27. According to Greenland (1987) the risk ratio and risk difference are the measures of choice as summary expression of impact or risk. The odds ratio is interpretable in so far as it is an estimate of the risk ratio.

28. See Laupacis et al. (1988). Steiner (1999) provides a short description of the analog of the RR, AR(E), and RD in terms of therapeutic efficacy rather than disease causation.

29. These formulae are based on the "cohort study," which will be discussed in Chapter 6. For a review of the estimation of PAR in case-control studies, see Coughlin et al. (1994). Advanced students should consult Greenland and Robins (1988) for a discussion of the conceptual problems in the definition and intrepretation of PAR.

30. This example is adapted from Northridge (1995), which contains references to the various estimates of RR, P, and PAR.

31. The data are obtained from Collishaw et al. (1988). More recent estimates for the 1990s are provided by Illing and Kaiserman (2004), using different sources of smoking prevalence and relative risks.

32. See Greenland (1999); and for the statistically competent, Robins and Greenland (1989). Brennan and Carter (1985) offer a legal perspective.

33. The formulae are obtained from Morris and Gardner (1988).

34. See the comprehensive (but highly mathematical) review of the concept of competing risks by Chiang (1991). Cornfield's (1957) paper is not quite as classic as the one on odds ratio published in 1951. For a comparison of YPLL and PGLE, see Lai and Hardy (1999).

35. The data were based on those compiled by Wilson and Crouch (2001).

36. The ideas in this section are based on the collection of papers in Johnson and Covello (1987), Mayo and Hollander (1991), and Bennett and Calman (1999). An entire issue of *Daedalus*, the journal of the American Academy of Arts and Sciences, is devoted to "risk" (vol. 119, no. 4, 1990; see especially Wildavsky and Dake).

37. For a critique of Douglas and Wildavsky (1982), see Shrader-Frechette (1991), who steered a middle road between their "cultural relativist" stance and the "naïve positivists" among technical and scientific experts in risk assessment.

38. For further discussion on "acceptable" risks and "hidden" risks, see Kasperson and Kasperson (1991) and Covello et al. (1991).

39. See the classic paper by Tversky and Kahneman (1974).

40. See Slovic (1987, 1991) for details of the factor analysis.

41. See Pidgeon et al. (1999), and the original paper by Kasperson et al. (1988).

42. See Green et al. (1999:59).

43. See Covello et al. (1991). Slovic (1991) also pointed out the importance of the choice of risk measures for comparisons in public discourse. For example, statements such as "the risk of cancer from the nuclear waste facility is infinitely smaller than the risk of being run over by a car on your way to this public meeting" are unlikely to win the trust of the public.

44. For the latest statistics and access to background documents on BSE and vCJD, go to the web sites of the U.K. Department for Environment, Food, and Rural Affairs (formerly Ministry of Agriculture, Fisheries and Food): www.defra.gov.uk/animalh/bse/index.html, and the Department of Health: www.doh.gov.uk/cjd/. Coulthart and Cashman (2001) reviewed the relevant literature in animal and human health. Prusiner (1998) reviewed the role of prions in his Nobel lecture. For a dissection of the interface between science and public policy during the BSE crisis in the United Kingdom, especially the role of the mass media and government information management, see Miller (1999). For a dissenting view on the link between BSE and vCJD, see Venters (2001).

45. Gajdusek shared the 1976 Nobel prize with Baruch Blumberg, discoverer of the hepatitis B antigen, originally called the "Australia antigen" as it was found in an Australian aborigine. For a review of Gajdusek's work on kuru and the "unconventional viruses," see his Nobel lecture (1977).

46. Based on data presented in Llorca and Delgado-Rodriguez (2001).

47. For archived statistics on SARS in Canada, go to the Health Canada web site (www. hc-sc.gc.ca) and search under "SARS." There was a second epidemic peak in mid-May of 2003. WHO provides a global perspective (www.who.int).

EXERCISE 5.1.   Impact of Cardiovascular Risk Factors

The Nutrition Canada Survey was conducted during 1970–1972 and collected a large amount of data related to health and nutritional status. This survey was linked to the National Mortality Database for the years 1970–1980 and thus allowed the analysis of the risks of death from various causes according to different levels of risk factors in the original cohort. The following table summarizes the results relating to cardiovascular mortality risk for ages 35–64:

Factor	Sex	Prevalence	PAR
Smoking > 20 cigarettes/day	M	35.5%	37.6%
	F	7.9%	43.1%
Serum cholesterol > 240 mg/dl	M	18.9%	8.8%
	F	21.6%	16.0%

Based on the information provided, at which risk factor would you target your health promotion program (smoking or cholesterol)? Why?

Source: Semenciw et al. (1988)

EXERCISE 5.2.   Investigation of an Epidemic of Murders

During a nine-month period in a major Canadian university–affiliated children's hospital, the mortality rate for patients on the cardiology ward was 43.1 deaths/10,000 patient-days. The average mortality rate on that ward over the preceding four years was only 11.0 deaths/10,000 patient-days.

(a)   What is the risk of death during the nine-month "epidemic period" relative to the "usual" experience on that ward?

The duty schedules of the nurses were examined. The number of deaths occurring during the shifts of four nurses were as follows:

Nurse	No. deaths while on-duty	No. hours on duty	No. deaths while off-duty	No. hours off duty
A	31	1,278	2	5,323
B	22	1,293	11	5,308
C	21	1,330	12	5,270
D	18	1,204	15	5,397

(b)   Calculate separately for nurse A and D the risks of death occurring when they are on-duty and off-duty.

Nurse	On-duty death rate	Off-duty death rate
A		
D		

(c)   How many times was a death more likely to occur when nurse A was on-duty, compared to when she was off-duty?

(d)   How many times was a death more likely to occur when nurse A was on-duty, compared to when nurse D was on-duty?

Source: Buehler et al. (1985)

EXERCISE 5.3.   Sexual Behavior and Cancer of the Cervix

The association between sexual behavior and cervical cancer has been investigated in many epidemiological studies. Can you indicate for each of the following statements if there is support for a causal relationship between exposure (sexual behavior) and outcome (cervical cancer), and name the Bradford Hill criterion that would have been satisfied or not satisfied?

(a)   The relative risk for cervical cancer is 2.8 for women with 10 or more partners, compared to those with only one.

(b)   The risk of cervical cancer increases as the lifetime number of sexual partners increases.

(c)   Similar results were obtained from a study among women in five U.S. cities, a study in four Latin American countries, and various studies in other parts of the world.

(d)   The investigators were unable to convince you that the exposure had in fact preceded the outcome.

It is now well established that cervical cancer is caused by a virus, the human papillomavirus (HPV), which is sexually transmitted. Sexual behavior is thus a risk marker for HPV infection. The relative risks for the association between HPV infection and cervical cancer are in the 20–70 range, greater than that between smoking and lung cancer, and comparable to that between chronic hepatitis B and liver cancer. There are over 100 types of HPV, of which types 16 and 18 are the most carcinogenic. The use of highly sensitive polymerase chain reaction (PCR) techniques has shown that almost 100% of cervical cancer specimens contain HPV DNA. Epidemiological studies have also shown that nonsexual factors such as smoking, diet, and parity are coexisting factors that may influence the acquisition and persistence of the infection and the progression from infection to invasive cancer.

(e)   Can one conclude that HPV is a necessary and sufficient cause of cervical cancer?

(f)   What type of evidence is needed in order for Koch's postulates (or Henle-Koch's postulates) to be satisfied?

Source: Muñoz et al. (1992); Franco et al. (2001)

EXERCISE 5.4.   Evidence for an Infectious Cause of Peptic Ulcer

Peptic ulcer disease was once generally believed to be caused by excessive production of stomach acid brought on by psychological stress and dietary factors. In 1982, two Australians, Robin Warren and Barry Marshall, isolated a bacteria (subsequently identified as *Helicobacter pylori*) nestled in between the cells lining the stomach and the layer of mucus gel. The following facts are known:

- The bacteria can be found in almost all cases of gastritis (inflammation of the stomach), a precursor of peptic ulcer.
- The bacteria can be found in healthy people also—it has a worldwide prevalence with considerable variation between geographical areas and socioeconomic groups.
- Eradication of the bacteria with antibiotics hastens the healing of the ulcers and reduces recurrence.
- *H. pylori* does not cause other infectious diseases in other organs of the body. It is, however, associated with certain forms of cancers of the stomach.
- Three human volunteers to date have deliberately been infected with the bacteria who then developed acute gastritis.
- Laboratory mice were infected with bacteria from humans, and developed a disease that mimics gastritis and ulcer in humans.
- It has been hypothesized that *H. pylori* infection induced an immune response in the host, which affects gastric physiology, including the production of mucus, which protects the stomach from acid.

Based on the above information, answer the following questions:

(a)   Is *H. pylori* a necessary cause?

(b)   Is *H. pylori* a sufficient cause?

(c)   Is there specificity of cause and effect?

(d)   Is the hypothesis biologically plausible?

(e)   Is there support from experiment?

Source: Blaser (1996); Sauerbaum and Michetti (2002)

EXERCISE 5.5.   Mad Cows and Englishmen: A Play in Three Acts

This exercise does not involve calculations. Instead, the class will engage in role-playing.

Act I: House of Commons, London

In which the Leader of the Opposition asks Government Ministers impertinent and embarrassing questions about the safety of British beef and the threat to public health, and what "they are going to do about it." The cast includes the Minister of Agriculture, the Minister of Health, and the Leader of the Opposition. Remaining students in the class will act as

Members of Parliament and should behave accordingly—i.e., heckle from time to time and interject with "Hear! Hear!"

Act II: Parliament Press Gallery

In which the Minister of Agriculture, the Minister of Health, the Chief Scientific Advisor, a lobbyist for the beef industry, and a representative of the farmers' union hold a joint press conference to reassure the public that "all is well." Students playing these roles should prepare short (one to two pages) press releases to be read during the press conference. These statements must reflect the level of scientific understanding and the biases expected of the speakers. The Chief Scientific Advisor is allowed five pages of scientific jargon and to be totally incomprehensible to the general public. The press conference is infiltrated by a consumer activist who disrupts the proceedings by shouting slogans. Remaining students in the class will act as members of the press, some from the "quality dailies" and others from the tabloids, or "gutter press." These students will each write a newspaper story of the press conference, complete with screaming headlines as appropriate. One student will play the role of a television reporter, who must summarize all the complex issues in 30 seconds.

Act III: A Court of Law

In which the family of a vCJD victim sues a supermarket for selling beef supposedly contaminated with BSE. Two students will act as lawyers representing the litigants and a third student, the judge. Remaining students in the class will act as members of the jury, who shall decide on the "winner."

The class will decide whether this play is a tragedy or comedy. In preparation, students should review thoroughly the scientific literature and the popular press related to the "mad cow disease" affair.

6

Designing Population
Health Studies

A Matter of Measurement

In Chapter 1 it is stated that the purpose of studying the health of populations is to describe, explain, predict, and control health problems. In this
chapter, some of the key methodological issues in designing studies to
achieve these objectives are discussed. This chapter will not deal with the
management, analysis, or presentation of research data, as excellent resources at a variety of levels are available.[1]

Research studies require the collection of data, which usually involves
some sort of measurement. Epidemiology, a core discipline in population
health research, is a *quantitative* science where measurement is of primary
importance. It must be recognized that for certain research problems, *qualitative* methods, which originate from within the tradition of the social sciences, offer a superior or alternative approach. Much of this chapter deals
with the quantitative aspects of research design. A brief discussion of
qualitative methods is also presented.

Biomedical scientists tend to view measurements and data as inherently objective. Many social scientists, on the other hand, do not regard
them as merely a neutral collection of empirical facts, but as a social product. Their form and content are based on decisions made by individuals
and institutions, which reflect their beliefs and values. This is particularly
evident in data relating to social class and ethnicity. Indeed, "if you don't
ask, you don't know, and if you don't know, you can't act."[2]

Research data can be primary or secondary. Data collected specifically
for the purpose of a study are referred to as *primary data*. Sometimes data
collected for other purposes may be reorganized and reanalyzed for a different purpose or research question—such data are referred to as *secondary
data*. In population health studies, *administrative data* are often used because of their ready availability—examples include health insurance
claims data, and employment records. Data collected by other people may
be accessed to address new questions or test hypotheses not covered by the

original studies. Large national health surveys (discussed in Chapter 3) are excellent sources of secondary data.

Because the phenomena, attributes, or events that are measured in a study tend to vary, they are referred to as *variables*. Much of data collection and analysis is organized around variables. Variables can be defined according to the *level* or *scale of measurement*.[3]

Basically a variable may be *categorical* (also called *discrete*) or *continuous*. For categorical variables, if there are only two possible values (e.g., male/female, dead/alive), then the variable is *dichotomous*; and if there are more than two values, *polytomous*. When the categories are merely names, the categorical variable is called a *nominal* variable—sex, ethnic group, blood type. Numbers need not even be involved, but when they are used, they do not imply any type of ranking. Thus even if "male" is coded as "1" and female as "2," the equality of sexes is implied!

When the information measured is ranked or ordered, one speaks of an *ordinal* level or scale of measurement. In health surveys, respondents are often asked to report their perceived health as "excellent," "good," "fair," or "poor." While these are still names or labels, there is a ranking of preference: "excellent" is better than "good," "good" is better than "fair," and so on. If categories are assigned numbers (say, 1 for "excellent," 2 for "good," and so on), then these numbers are not of equal rank. Moreover, it does not mean that 4 is twice as preferable as 2, or that the amount of preference between 3 and 2 is the same as that between 2 and 1.

Continuous variables can be defined in terms of a potentially infinite number of fixed and equal units—for example, height, weight, or blood pressure. This may be measured on the interval scale or the ratio scale. In an interval scale, there is a constant change across the range of the scale. For example, the difference in weight between 30 and 20 kilograms (kg) is the same as that between 20 and 10 kg. A ratio scale requires a true zero such that one unit can be expressed as so many times another unit. Body weight is also a ratio scale in that zero kg means there is no weight whatsoever. A person weighing 20 kg is twice as heavy as one weighing 10 kg (the distance on the scale between zero and 20 kg is twice that between zero and 10 kg); a person weighing 40 kg is also twice as heavy as one weighing 20 kg (the distance on the scale between zero and 40 kg is also twice that between zero and 20 kg). Body temperature in degrees Celsius is an interval but not a ratio scale, since zero degrees does not mean there is no heat. While +10 degrees is warmer than −10 degrees, and there are 20 degrees difference between the two points on the scale; +10 degrees cannot be expressed as so many times warmer than −10 degrees ($+10/-10 = -1$).

Note that while one can analyze a continuous variable such as blood pressure as millimeters of mercury, one can also reduce all possible values into categories such as "high," "medium," or "low," converting the variable to an ordinal, or even a nominal one. The reverse, however, cannot occur.

Measurements can be obtained from individuals or aggregates of individuals. An *ecological study* is one in which the unit of observation and analysis is the aggregate rather than individuals. For example, in Chapter 8, Case Study 8.2 shows that localities with high fluoride content in its water supply have lower dental caries rates. (The unit of observation is the city—each city has a mean water fluoride content, obtained by testing the city's water supply which goes to all citizens, and a mean caries rate based on a survey of many individuals). This observation is then applied to the individual level, namely, that an individual consuming water with high fluoride will be less likely to suffer from dental caries, and in fact studies have been done to demonstrate just that. The association between smoking and lung cancer holds true at both the individual and ecological levels. Smokers are more likely to get lung cancer, and countries with a higher prevalence of smokers also have a higher incidence of lung cancer. Note that even at the individual level of observation, the comparison is always between groups of individuals (smokers vs. nonsmokers, not Mr. Smith vs. Mrs. Chan). Ecological studies compare groups of groups of individuals (groups of countries consisting of varying concentrations of smokers).

Sometimes an association observed between variables on the ecologic level may not represent the association that exists at an individual level—it may disappear, be reduced, or even be reversed. A numerical example is provided in Box 6.1. An *ecological fallacy* occurs when one concludes incorrectly that an association found at the group or aggregate level also applies at the individual level.

Ecological studies have been much maligned, and many textbooks take great lengths to warn students against it, although some efforts have been made by many researchers to "rehabilitate" them. Traditionally they are considered useful only in generating hypotheses to be tested at the individual level. Often aggregate-level data are used as inferior substitutes for individual-level data because the latter are not available (e.g., using neighborhood mean income obtained from the census and assigning it to all participants of a survey who live in that neighborhood, if the surveyor is too embarrassed to ask individuals about their income). Many population health issues, however, such as those involving environmental exposures (air pollution, water hardness), community infrastructure (availability of public transportation, universal health care insurance), and interpersonal and social relationships (income inequalities, democratic government), can only be studied using aggregate-level data. It is increasingly recognized that causal models need to take into account determinants measured at both the individual and ecological levels. Analyses of such studies are complex, but have been eased by the development of newer statistical techniques for multilevel analyses, such as hierarchical modeling.[4]

One message that this chapter wishes to reinforce is that no research design or method is inherently superior (be it quantitative vs. qualitative,

BOX 6.1.   Ecological Fallacy: A Numerical Demonstration

Let there be three classrooms of 10 students each, all taking the same course. Classroom A has 8 women and 2 men, B has 6 women and 4 men, and C has 4 women and 6 men. After the final examination, the average grade for each classroom is (A) 79%, (B) 78%, and (C) 77%. One can conclude that the more women there are in a classroom, the higher the average grade. This would be an ecological-level observation, and it is correct (ignoring the issue of statistical significance). Yet if one were to also conclude that women on the average have higher grades than men, which is an individual-level observation, one would run the risk of an ecological fallacy.

Suppose the sex and grades of all students in the three classrooms are distributed as follows:

	Classroom A	Classroom B	Classroom C
	F 70	F 65	F 65
	F 70	F 70	F 70
	F 70	F 70	F 80
	F 75	F 75	F 80
	F 70	F 80	**M 70**
	F 80	F 85	**M 75**
	F 80	**M 80**	**M 75**
	F 80	**M 80**	**M 80**
	M 95	**M 85**	**M 85**
	M 100	**M 90**	**M 90**
Class Mean	F 74	F 74	F 74
	M 98	M 84	M 79
	F, M 79	F, M 78	F, M 77

With all classes combined, the female (F) average is 74% and the male (M) average 84%.

It can be seen that the M average grade is higher than the F average grade in all three classrooms, whether separately or combined. The reason we observe classrooms with a higher proportion of women doing better is not because women perform better, but because men, when put in a minority situation amid a larger number of women, tend to perform better than when men are in the majority. (This is a hypothetical example.)

experimental vs. observational, or ecological vs. individual-level studies)—it depends on what question is being addressed and the purpose of the research.

Types of Research Design

There are many ways to classify study designs in epidemiological research. Indeed, the terminology is often confusing and inconsistent.[5] To understand the different study designs, it is helpful to think in terms of E and D, or exposure and disease. "Exposure" can be a risk factor (working in a mine, smoking, drinking, not wearing a seatbelt) or an intervention (drugs, exercise program, sewage plant, ultrasound screening). "Disease" can mean not just a disease, but any other health outcome (injury, obesity, death, survival). E_0 and D_0 represent individuals who do not have the exposure or disease, while E_1 and D_1 are the exposed and diseased.

Research designs differ in terms of several key features: purpose, investigator control, directionality, sample selection, and timing.

Purpose

Some studies are descriptive, while others are analytical. A descriptive study establishes the burden of disease or the extent of exposure to a risk factor. Analytical studies test hypotheses about disease causation or the effectiveness of interventions. A study that determines the proportion of smokers in a population (E) and a separate study that estimates the incidence of lung cancer (D) are descriptive. A study that investigates whether smokers develop more lung cancer than nonsmokers is analytical. In analytical studies, information on E and D are collected from the same individuals.

Investigator control

Studies can be distinguished by whether the investigator controls the allocation of exposure status. In an interventional study the investigator determines who gets E and who does not, whereas in an observational study, the investigator has no control on the exposure status of study subjects. If one were to conduct an interventional study on whether smoking causes lung cancer, one would need to assemble people who have never smoked, and then order some to start smoking (E_1) and others to remain nonsmokers (E_0). It is obvious that most studies of disease causation in humans are observational. A further distinction can be made between a truly experimental study, exemplified by the randomized controlled trial (RCT), where subjects have an equal chance of being selected to become E_1 or E_0, and a quasi-experimental study where there is no such random allocation (but the process of allocation is still in the hands of the investigator). Laboratory scientists are most familiar with experimental studies. Clinicians do RCTs to evaluate drugs and other therapies (in which case the "C" in RCT may stand for *clinical*). In population health, community trials of preventive and curative interventions are conducted. Many program or policy studies are quasi-experiments wherein the interventions are allocated on the basis of convenience and sometimes political expedience.[6]

Directionality

Directionality refers to the time sequence in collecting information on E and D in a study. Cross-sectional studies collect information on E and D in the same individuals concurrently (i.e., at a point in time, a "snapshot") whereas longitudinal studies do so in separate time periods. A longitudinal study, whereby study subjects are followed forward from E to D, is called a *cohort* study. If the directionality is backward, i.e. from D to E, then it is called a *case-control* study. Again using the smoking–lung cancer example, in a cross-sectional study, smoking status and disease status are determined at the same point in time in a survey. In a cohort study, smokers and nonsmokers are followed forward, and the development of lung cancer over time is observed. In a case-control study, one starts with lung cancer patients and goes backward to determine their smoking status in the past. Note that a cohort study is sometimes also called a prospective or incidence study, while a case-control study is also called a retrospective study. Such usage should be avoided as it only adds to the confusion. Terms such as "prospective" and "retrospective" should be applied to *timing* (see below), whereas "forward" and "backward" are used for *directionality*.

Sample selection

Any study requires subjects (or participants)—and there are different ways in how they are recruited. Subjects can be selected on the basis of their exposure status, their disease status, or neither. In cohort studies, subjects are selected on the basis of their exposure status (E_0 or E_1); in case-control studies, it is on the basis of disease status (D_0 or D_1); whereas in cross-sectional studies, it is neither E or D, but usually some sort of representative sampling of the target population without regard to their E and D status initially. It is only after the sample has been assembled that the exposure and disease status are determined. In studying the smoking-lung cancer association, a cohort study will set out to recruit smokers and nonsmokers, whereas a case-control study will identify lung cancer cases and another group of people without lung cancer.

Timing

Timing refers to the time relationship between when the study begins (which is "now") and the occurrence of exposure and outcome. When the study starts today, but exposure and disease status refer to occurrence in the past (although it may not have been discovered until the time of the study), the timing is "retrospective." When the study starts today, and the subjects' current exposure status is determined as they are recruited into the study, and disease status is observed into the future, then it is "prospective." Case control and cross-sectional studies are retrospective.

There are two types of cohort studies—prospective cohort and retrospective cohort studies. In a retrospective cohort study (also called "historical" cohort), one starts the study today, but assembles the cohort based on whether someone was a smoker or nonsmoker 10 or 20 years ago. The two groups are then followed forward from the past to the present and their disease incidence rates during the intervening period compared. In a prospective cohort study (also called "concurrent" cohort), the investigator decides to start the study and collects information on smoking status today. She then follows the subjects forward in time into the future and tracks the appearance of new cases.

Table 6.1 summarizes how the five basic types most relevant to population health—cross-sectional, case-control, retrospective cohort, prospective cohort, and randomized controlled trial—differ in terms of these basic features. These study designs are now discussed in more detail.

Cross-sectional studies

Cross-sectional studies (CSS), also called prevalence studies, collect information on E and D concurrently. Although the purpose of CSSs may only be descriptive (e.g., the proportion of high school students who smoke), they can also be analytical (e.g., are high-school smokers more likely to come from poor families?). If a CSS is used only to find out the prevalence of E or D without any attempt to link the two together, it is only descriptive, not analytical. Usually, a representative sample of the population is chosen regardless of their exposure status or disease status. In determining exposure status, subjects may be asked to recall events from the past (e.g., age when first started smoking), or measured at the time of the survey (e.g., plasma cholesterol level). Disease status is determined at the time of the study (e.g., scores on the McGill Pain Questionnaire).

A major problem of CSS as an analytical study is that temporal sequence cannot always be established. Which comes first, E or D (do alcoholics drink themselves into poverty or are poor people driven to drinking to escape their misery)? Any association established between E and D only demonstrates that a risk factor is associated with *having* the disease, rather than *developing* the disease. Because a CSS makes observation at a point in time, only survivors of D can be sampled. For example, a CSS that measures respiratory function among firefighters exposed to smoke may miss out on those who were forced to retire because of poor health, and may lead to an incorrect conclusion that smoke exposure has little effect on firefighters' lungs.

CSS are also not appropriate for studying rare diseases or diseases of short duration (or with poor survival rates). If one determines from a CSS that certain factors are associated with the prevalence of a disease, it may be difficult to decide if these factors affect incidence or duration or both.

Table 6.1 Characteristics of Different Research Designs in Population Health Studies

	Purpose	Investigator control	Directionality	Sample selection	Timing
Cross-sectional study	Descriptive or Analytical	Observational	Concurrent (E, D separately)	Representative sampling	Retrospective
Case-control study	Analytical	Observational	Backward (E←D)	Based on disease status	Retrospective
Retrospective cohort study	Analytical	Observational	Forward (E→D)	Based on exposure status	Retrospective
Prospective cohort study	Analytical	Observational	Forward (E→D)	Based on exposure status	Prospective
Randomized controlled trial	Analytical	Interventional	Forward (E→D)	Based on exposure status	Prospective

**BOX 6.2.   Obtaining a Representative Sample from
a Population**

Key elements in sampling from a population are the target and study populations, the sampling frame, and the choice of sampling units. The target population is the population to which results of the study will apply and the study population the population that is actually sampled. The sampling frame is usually a list, either of names of individuals or of communities (or other larger units such as city blocks), which provides a means of access to the defined target population. Assembling such a list is one of the first tasks of a sample survey. Sampling units may be households or individuals or both.

There are different sampling strategies, all of which are intended to result in a sample that is "representative" of the target population.[7] Simple random sampling requires that all eligible individuals in the population constitute a single list. Using a process of generating random numbers from a computer, or a table of random numbers available in the back of most statistics textbooks, the required number of individuals can be selected. Each member on the list has an equal chance of selection. A more convenient method is systematic sampling, which involves simply selecting every nth person on the list, depending on the required sample size, after randomly selecting the first person. Stratified sampling requires the division of the population into groups or strata based on some characteristic (e.g., age and sex), and then selecting simple random samples from each of the strata. This process ensures that population subgroups are adequately represented in the final sample. Certain subgroups may even be oversampled (e.g., the elderly) if their proportion in the total population is small; alternatively, the subgroups can be proportional to size; i.e., in proportions that reflect their actual size in the population. Cluster sampling involves first sampling from a list of communities, and then interviewing either all individuals or simple random samples of individuals within the selected communities. The latter situation is referred to as 2-stage or multistage sampling.

It should be recognized that most statistical procedures assume a simple random sample. Complex surveys (those involving stratification, multiple stages of selection, and unequal probabilities of selection of respondents) tend to inflate the estimates of variance above that calculated by standard methods based on a simple random sample. The design effect is the ratio of the variance of the estimate for a particular design to the variance calculated from a simple random sample of the same size. The derivation of population prevalence from complex surveys is no simple matter of dividing the numerator by the denominator, but involves the use of weighting, re-scaling, and adjustments.

There are situations where non-probability sampling is used for convenience, economy, or in exploratory research, especially in "hard-to-reach" populations where sampling frames cannot be established

(continued)

(e.g., drug addicts, the homeless). A convenience sample, as its name implies, is nothing more than a "grab" sample of passersby and can least lay any claim to representativeness. The investigator may try a purposive sample, based on his or her subjective ideas of what the study population's characteristics are in order that different types of individuals be selected. A more quantitative approach is the quota sample, which presets a target number of individuals in specified subgroups to reflect their distribution in the study population. For example, if the census indicates that a 30% of a region's adults are college graduates, the researcher will recruit subjects who are college graduates until the required quota has been reached.

A low response rate is the bane of all surveys. Furthermore, in mailed surveys, the eligibility of the recipient may not be known until the questionnaire has been returned, resulting in many mailings being wasted. One technique that can be used to improve response rate and cost-effectiveness of surveys is so-called snowball sampling. Participants who are not eligible or refuse to participate are asked to forward the questionnaire to someone else who is eligible and willing. This method, however, does not eliminate potential bias between responders and nonresponders and is not a solution to non-response.

By using a non-probability sample, one can only hope that the sample is representative of the population, but the probability of each sampling units being selected is unknown.

Case-control studies

While sample selection in a case-control study is based on disease status, one can use either incident cases or prevalent cases. Incident cases are preferred, since to find prevalent cases one would have to do a cross-sectional study first, with the disadvantages of missing those with short duration of illness or poor survival. Incident cases can be obtained from a disease registry that records new cases as they appear in the population.

For each case chosen, one or more controls are selected. Statistical power tends to increase with a higher control-to-case ratio, but beyond 4 : 1 the gain is minimal while the study becomes unwieldy. In general, controls should come from the same population at risk for the disease and selected with comparable accuracy as cases. If bias is to occur (e.g., with recall of specific past exposures), then there should be a roughly equal chance of bias in both cases and controls.

Controls can be chosen from among hospital patients with diseases other than those that the cases have. If cases have died from the disease, the controls may be chosen from those who have died of some other diseases. Controls can be sampled from the general population of healthy people, or be restricted to the same neighborhood as cases in order to have subjects of comparable socioeconomic status. Sometimes controls are nominated by the cases, and may include their friends or relatives who are free from the disease.[8]

In a case-control study, one cannot compute directly the relative risk or rate ratio (RR), since the marginal totals—the number of cases $(a + c)$ and controls $(b + d)$—are fixed by the investigator:

	D_1	D_0	
E_1	a	b	$(a + b)$
E_0	c	d	$(c + d)$
	$(a + c)$	$(b + d)$	

In a cohort or cross-sectional study, the RR can be computed from the 2×2 table as follows:

$$\frac{a/(a+b)}{c/(c+d)}$$

In a case-control study, the odds ratio (ad/cb) can be used. (The odds ratio was introduced in Chapter 5.) In a major breakthrough in biostatistical theory, Jerome Cornfield in 1951 demonstrated that, in a case-control study, $OR \cong RR$. Note that as long as there is a 2×2 table, one can compute an OR, even in a cohort or cross-sectional study. Just that RR is more accurate and is preferred if it could be directly computed.[9]

The strengths of a case-control study are:

1. It is relatively quick and inexpensive;
2. It is optimal for studying rare diseases or diseases with long latent period;
3. It allows multiple risk factors for a single disease to be studied.

The limitations of a case-control study are:

1. It is inefficient for studying rare exposures;
2. It allows only one outcome to be studied;
3. It does not permit the direct computation of incidence rate, and one can only estimate the relative risk by computing the odds ratio;
4. It is difficult to establish temporal sequence;
5. It is particularly prone to certain bias (recall by respondents, inadequate medical records, etc.).

The extensive use of case-control studies of disease causation since the 1950s is responsible for the great advances in epidemiological methods in the post–World War II period. Moreover, the case-control study is very versatile and has been used for a variety of purposes, not just in the etiological

BOX 6.3.   Don't Get Your Odds Confused

The odds ratio assesses association between exposure and disease. There are two categories of exposure (E_1 = present, and E_0 = absent) and two categories of disease (D_1 = present, and D_0 = absent). To avoid confusion, it is best to construct your 2×2 table with D_1 and E_1 in the left upper corner, or alternatively, with both D_0 and E_0 in the left upper corner, as in the following example:

	D_1	D_0
E_1	4	2
E_0	3	6

OR $= (4 \times 6)/(2 \times 3) = 4.0$

	D_0	D_1
E_0	6	3
E_1	2	4

OR $= (6 \times 4)/(3 \times 2) = 4.0$

Both tables will get you the same conclusion that being exposed is associated with four times the risk of being diseased. In many studies where both E and D have "yes or no" responses, the interpretation is straightforward. Thus, in a case-control study of smoking and lung cancer, it is obvious that smokers are E_1, nonsmokers E_0, lung cancer cases D_1, and non-cases D_0. Using the numbers above, we can say that smokers are four times as likely as nonsmokers to have lung cancer.

	Cases	Controls
Smokers	4	2
Nonsmokers	3	6

OR $= (4 \times 6)/(2 \times 3) = 4.0$

	Controls	Cases
Nonsmokers	6	3
Smokers	2	4

OR $= (6 \times 4)/(3 \times 2) = 4.0$

There is nothing to prevent one from saying that "not smoking" is the exposure of interest, and assigning it E_1, in which case, the tables will now look like this:

	Cases	Controls
Nonsmokers	3	6
Smokers	4	2

OR $= (3 \times 2)/(6 \times 4) = 0.25$

	Controls	Cases
Smokers	2	4
Nonsmokers	6	3

OR $= (2 \times 3)/(4 \times 6) = 0.25$

It can be seen that the OR now is the reciprocal ($0.25 = \frac{1}{4}$) of the previous one. The conclusion will then be: nonsmokers are associated with one-fourth the risk of lung cancer, compared to smokers. This is still the same conclusion, which is to be expected, since the numbers have not changed, only their position in the table. It is therefore very important to be clear about what E_1, E_0, D_1, and D_0 are and that to avoid

(*continued*)

confusion, always put like and like (D_1 and E_1, or D_0 and E_0) together in the left upper corner of the table.

In many studies, variables are not expressed as "yes/no". Let's say the E of interest is "gender" (male vs female) and D is "intelligence" (stupid vs. smart). Four 2×2 tables can be constructed:

(A)	Stupid	Smart
Male	4	2
Female	3	6

$OR = (4 \times 6)/(2 \times 3) = 4.0$

(B)	Smart	Stupid
Female	6	3
Male	2	4

$OR = (6 \times 4)/(3 \times 2) = 4.0$

(C)	Stupid	Smart
Female	3	6
Male	4	2

$OR = (3 \times 2)/(6 \times 4) = 0.25$

(D)	Smart	Stupid
Male	2	4
Female	6	3

$OR = (2 \times 3)/(4 \times 6) = 0.25$

There are four different ways to express this association:

A. Males are four times more likely to be stupid, compared to females

B. Females are four times more likely to be smart, compared to males

C. Females are one-fourth as likely to be stupid, compared to males

D. Males are one-fourth as likely to be smart, compared to females

It is crucially important to be clear about what E_1, E_0, D_1, and D_0 are and what the odds ratio is referring to. A statement that "smoking is associated with lung cancer with an odds ratio of 4.0" is unlikely to lead one astray, whereas a statement that "gender is associated with intelligence with an odds ratio of 4.0" is entirely uninformative and could even be misleading.

studies of diseases. For example, it has been used in the evaluation of preventive and therapeutic interventions, including vaccines (e.g., BCG, pneumococcal), screening tests (Pap smear), pharmacological agents (antibiotic prophylaxis, anticoagulants), health services (intensive care units, emergency trauma care), and safety measures (bicycle helmets).[10]

Cohort studies

A cohort study starts off with a group free of the disease to be studied—some exposed to the risk factor of interest, and some not exposed. They are then followed and observed for the occurrence of disease. Thus sample selection is based on exposure status, and directionality is forward. A cohort should be distinguished from an experimental study in that the

---

BOX 6.4.   Words and Origins

The term *control*, unfortunately, is overused and has accumulated several distinct meanings:

1. The "control" of a disease or an epidemic;
2. To "control" for confounding (see below), as in "age has been controlled for in the analysis";
3. An experimental "control," the study subject who is not given the intervention or treatment; and
4. As in a case-"control" study, the subject who does not have the disease or outcome.

Meanings (3) and (4) are most often confused. In an experimental study, a control is the one who does not get the exposure (E_0), while a control in a case-control study is the one who does not get the disease (D_0).

Cohort is another source of confusion. It comes from the Latin *cohors*, meaning warriors. A Roman legion consisted of 10 cohorts, each with 300–600 soldiers. In epidemiology, *cohort* was initially used to refer to a *birth cohort*, a group of individuals born at the same time (usually same year) whose health experience can be followed as the group ages. This usage has been broadened so that "a cohort" is now used to describe any group followed over time, as is done in a *cohort study*. *Cohort effect*, also called *generation effect*, refers to the unique set of environmental conditions a particular generation or birth cohort may have been exposed to during some time in its lifespan. Thus, adolescents who were born in wartime may suffer a higher prevalence of malnutrition than a similarly aged group born 10 years later. A *cohort analysis* attempts to tease out the effect of age and of birth year on disease rates. (An example is shown in Case Study 6.1.) It is not to be confused with the analysis of a cohort study. For clarity, *age-period-cohort analysis* is often used.

In an attempt to replace the confusing term *case-control* study, Alvin Feinstein, a clinical epidemiologist, suggested *trohoc* study, which is *cohort* spelled backward! This neologism has not been widely adopted. Other contenders to replace case-control include *case-compeer* and *case-referent*, but so far *case-control* seems to be able to hold its ground.

---

investigator does not determine or allocate exposure status, which is chosen by the subjects themselves.[11] (They either already smoke or do not smoke, and are not told to smoke or not smoke by the investigator.) The distinction between a prospective and retrospective cohort study lies in timing. It is possible to have a mixed design, where the study begins today, based on exposure status determined in the past, but disease status will be monitored from the past, through the present, and into the future.

The strengths of a cohort study are:

1. It provides an opportunity to observe the natural history of disease;
2. It is of particular value when the exposure is rare;
3. It allows multiple outcomes of a single exposure to be examined;
4. It assures that temporal sequence can be established;
5. It allows direct measurement of incidence of disease in the exposed and nonexposed and determination of relative risk.

The limitations of a cohort study are:

1. It is inefficient for studying rare diseases;
2. It allows only one or a few exposures to be studied;
3. It is usually expensive and time-consuming;
4. It is difficult to maintain the cohort and reduce loss to follow-up.

There are hybrid designs, which combine features of case-control and cohort studies. One can have a case-control study nested within a cohort study. In the course of a cohort study, new cases that emerge are entered into the case-control study, with the controls sampled from the cohort. Detailed measurements can then be obtained only from the limited number of cases and controls and not the entire cohort.

Randomized controlled trials

In an RCT, the purpose of random allocation is to apportion evenly between E_1 and E_0 all known and unknown factors that might affect the study outcome. In clinical trials, this is often done at the individual level. In studies of population health interventions, often an entire community (e.g., a geographic region, a school, a city block) is assigned the exposure, while another is not. Allocation of intervention to individuals within a community is not possible for studies such as water fluoridation or mass media campaigns.

Clinical trials often use blinding to avoid bias in favor of an anticipated effect. A study is "double blind" if neither the study subject nor the investigator is aware of the exposure status of the subject. In drug trials, a placebo, an inert substance that looks and tastes like the drug being tested, is given. Often the "code" listing the names of those given the placebo and those given the drug is not broken until the study is completed. Blinding is difficult if knowledge of the exposure can be clearly recognized by the subject (e.g., a surgical procedure, exercise program, or type of health care provider).

Clinical trials can be divided into four phases. Although they give the impression that they are different types of clinical trials, in reality, only a "phase III trial" constitutes a true experiment with random allocation of treatments. Phase I "trials" are preliminary studies of drug safety on human subjects, usually healthy volunteers. It is neither randomized nor controlled, simply a case series. Phase II trials are small-scale studies to establish efficacy of different doses and frequencies of administration. They tend not to be randomized, although controls are used. Phase IV trials refer to surveillance for adverse reactions after the drug has been put on the market.

An experimental study offers the investigator the most control, but this is a rather artificial situation and does not represent the "real life" experienced by most "free-living" populations. Also, many research questions cannot be answered by this method because of ethical concerns or logistical problems. The need for placebos has been challenged on methodological, ethical, and legal grounds. Many RCTs do not compare treatment with no treatment (where a placebo will be used), but a new treatment and an existing treatment, or an intervention program and "usual care." Some researchers tend to regard experimental studies as the gold standard against which observational studies are judged. The closer they resemble experimental studies, the more rigorous the design. While their call for better quality of data, freedom from bias, and cogency of methods (e.g., no "data dredging" and retroactive alteration of hypotheses) are valid, these principles apply to all study designs.[12]

Validity and Reliability

The term *validity* has two contexts: One relates to the measurement of exposure or disease status—a measurement is valid if it measures what it is supposed to measure. The second relates to the study's overall results and inferences: How close to the truth in terms of estimation of effects or establishing causal relationship?

There are different types of validity in the context of measurement. At the most basic (and least scientific) is *face* validity—a measure has face validity if it "looks reasonable." One would be surprised to find that in much of the research literature, this is all there is for many "standard" measures. Traditionally, textbooks on research methods distinguish between the three "Cs"—construct, criterion, and content validity. *Construct* validity refers to the extent to which a measurement corresponds to some theoretical concepts. For example, since diabetes is a disorder of carbohydrate metabolism, measuring blood glucose has construct validity. Constructs such as intelligence, on which intelligence tests are based, are far more complex and indeed controversial. *Content* validity is the extent to which a measurement incorporates the full scope of the phenomenon studied (e.g., a health index should be composed of measures of mortality, morbidity, disability, and other attributes of health or ill health). *Criterion* validity is the extent to which the measurement correlates with an external criterion or standard. It may be concurrent, when both the measure and its criterion are compared at the same point in time (a self report of arthritis in a survey can be compared with a physician's diagnosis in the subject's medical records); or predictive, when the measure is able to predict the value of the criterion (a high score for suicidal risk in a multiple-item mental health questionnaire is predictive of future suicide).[13]

In the context of the overall study, one can distinguish between internal and external validity. The former refers to the degree to which inferences drawn from the study are correct for the actual group of subjects being studied. External validity is sometimes also called *generalizability*; i.e., can inferences drawn from the study be applied to some other groups not actually studied? Internal validity is clearly the more important issue: without it, external validity has no meaning.

For example, a study on the association between oral contraceptives and myocardial infarction among young female nurses was properly designed, executed, and analyzed—it should have internal validity.[14] If an association was found, should we conclude that this association only applies to nurses and not to other women of the same age? Clearly the study was not meant to be an occupational health study of the hazards of the nursing profession. Nurses were chosen because they represent a large pool of women who are knowledgeable about health issues and likely to be cooperative over a long period of followup. Doll and Hill's cohort study of smoking and lung cancer (Case Study 6.3) used physicians for similar reasons. External validity is often a judgment call. There is nothing within the study that can make it externally valid, and there is no statistical test to determine if external validity exists. One must base one's judgment on the results of other studies, on known biological factors, and on a theoretical understanding of the disease process. External validity is also subject to much controversy—how often should one repeat a study in a different group?

Validity needs to be distinguished from reliability, which may also refer to the study overall or a particular measurement. It is also called "repeatability, stability, consistency, reproducibility, and precision." For measurements obtained by different observers, the inter-observer reliability can be assessed; reliability of measurements obtained by the same observer at different times is referred to as intra-observer reliability. An "observer" can refer to an interviewer administering questionnaires or a laboratory performing biochemical tests. Test-retest reliability refers to the concordance of results when the same test is administered to the same individual/group on separate occasions.

An analogy commonly used to distinguish between reliability and validity is the shooting target (Figure 6.1). If one hits the bull's eye consistently, there is both validity and reliability; if one misses the bull's eye but hits the same wrong spot all the time, there is reliability but not validity; if one hits a different spot each time but misses the bull's eye, there is neither validity nor reliability. Strictly speaking, it is not possible to have validity without reliability, although if the fluctuations are centered around the true value, the mean of the measurements may indeed be valid.

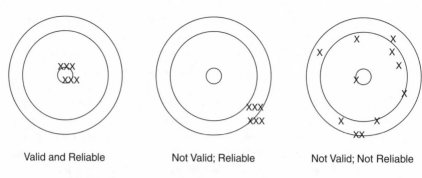

Valid and Reliable   Not Valid; Reliable   Not Valid; Not Reliable

Figure 6.1. Distinguishing between validity and reliability.

Most of us have experience of being pestered by unsolicited telephone surveys conducted by commercial polling firms. Such firms usually report their sample size but rarely the response rate, and for good reason. While the sample size is usually large enough to give a stable estimate of the prevalence of a specific attribute, the response rate can be pitifully low. Such "studies" have good reliability but little validity, as they suffer from serious selection bias (see below).

Error and Bias

In epidemiological research, an error is said to exist if there is any deviation of results from "true" values. Errors can occur either through sampling (when it is called *random error*; i.e., due to chance), or because of some design flaws (when it is called *systematic error*, or *bias*).

Random or sampling error affects the reliability of the measurement and the precision of the estimate, a problem that can be reduced by increasing the sample size. Systematic error, on the other hand, affects validity. It can be avoided by careful design, and to a lesser degree, compensated for by the analysis. A simple system of classifying biases recognizes three major types: selection bias, information bias, and confounding bias.[15]

Selection bias occurs from the manner in which subjects are selected to be studied. There are some systematic differences between those who are selected and those not selected in terms of their exposure status or outcome status. Many situations can give rise to selection bias.

A survey with a low response rate cannot ensure that responders do not differ from nonresponders in a systematic manner. People who fail to respond to a questionnaire may be ashamed of their socially unacceptable lifestyle. Conversely, people who respond may be more health conscious. People lost to followup may differ from those who can be tracked in terms of health outcomes. Volunteers may be a self-selected group with unique characteristics. Workers who suffer from symptoms may retire from the workforce, and those that remain appear to be a healthy lot—the "healthy-worker" effect. Those who are selected for referral for specialist care tend to be sicker than those treated at the primary care level. People who are exposed may be more likely to be more closely watched, tested, and thus diagnosed as being diseased. The use of prevalent rather than incident cases tends to favor "survivors."

Information bias results from errors in measurement, which may result in a misclassification of subjects into E_1 and E_0, or D_1 and D_0. It occurs after subjects have been included in the study and is thus unrelated to the selection process. Examples include invalid survey instruments, faulty lab equipment, incorrect diagnostic criteria, recall bias in responding to questionnaires, inadequacy of old medical records, an interviewer who is aware of the exposure or disease status of the subject may use a different tone of voice (or body language) which may influence the response, the early sign of a disease may cause a subject to change its exposure status (e.g., coughing during the early stage of lung cancer may cause someone to stop smoking, thus misclassifying him from "smoker" to "ex-smoker" category).

Confounding and Confounders

The third type of bias is called *confounding*. Unlike selection and information bias, confounding can, to some extent, be corrected by analysis. Confounding is said to occur when the observed association between exposure and outcome is mixed up with a third factor.[16] A confounder is a variable that is:

1. associated with and predicts the disease; or a surrogate of some unknown or unmeasurable factors causally related to the disease;
2. associated with the exposure; but
3. not a consequence of the exposure (an intermediate or intervening variable, or part of the causal pathway).

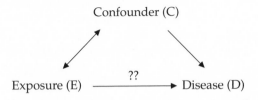

(Note: → refers to causal association, while ↔ refers to non-causal association.) Situations where confounding is not present include:

- If there is no arrow between C and D, condition (1) is not satisfied;
- If there is no arrow between E and C, condition (2) is not satisfied;
- If E causes C (i.e., E→C), condition (3) is not satisfied.

BOX 6.5.   A Long List of Biases

There are different ways of classifying bias. A classic paper by clinical epidemiologist David Sackett lists over 50 types of biases![17] Bias can creep in every step in the research process:

- *In reading-up on the field*: biases of rhetoric, controversy avoidance, one-sided reference, positive results, and current fad;
- *In specifying and selecting the study sample*: popularity, centripetal, referral filter, diagnostic access, diagnostic suspicion, detection signal, mimicry, previous opinion, wrong sample size, admission rate (Berkson), prevalence-incidence (Neyman), diagnostic vogue, diagnostic purity, procedure selection, missing clinical data, non-contemporaneous control, starting time, socially unacceptable disease, migrant, membership, non-response, and volunteer biases;
- *In executing the experimental maneuver*: contamination, withdrawal, compliance, bogus control and therapeutic personality biases;
- *In measuring exposures and outcomes*: insensitive measure, rumination, apprehension, end-digit preference, unacceptability, family information, obsequiousness, recall, expectation, substitution, exposure suspicion, attention, and instrument biases;
- *In analyzing the data*: post-hoc significance, data dredging, scale degradation, tidying-up, and repeated peeks biases;
- *In interpreting the data*: mistaken identity, cognitive dissonance, magnitude, significance, correlation, and under-exhaustion biases; and
- *In publishing the results*.

In practice, any risk factor, the control of which results in changing the strength of the exposure–disease association, can be considered a confounder.

Several methods are available to control confounding. This could occur either in the design stage or at the analysis stage.

At the design stage, one can use (1) randomization, (2) restriction, and (3) matching. At the analysis stage, one can use (4) stratification, and (5) multivariate modeling.

Randomization (or random allocation) is used in experimental studies, which ensures that all potential confounders are equally distributed between the experimental group and the control group.

Restriction means that only people with certain attributes are studied. For example, to avoid age being a confounder, one can restrict the study to only a rather narrow age group, say 20–45.

One can use *matching* to ensure that potential confounders are evenly distributed between the two comparison groups. If one wants to control for age in a case-control study, for every case of a certain age, a control is found who is of the same age or within a relatively narrow range. Matching makes a study more complicated, especially if the matching criteria are too strict (e.g., exact age, down to the same birthday) or too numerous (same age, sex, level of education, sexual orientation, etc.).

Stratification involves breaking the subjects into different levels or strata of the confounding variable. One can inspect the association between E and D either separately, at each level, or use some statistical procedure to summarize the association. A well-known procedure, named after Nathan Mantel and William Haenszel, produces a summary odds ratio from odds ratios of all the different individual strata.[18] The age-standardized procedures discussed in Chapter 2 are one examples of stratified analysis that produces a summary measure—the ASMR or SMR—from which the effect of a confounder, age, has been removed.

The statistically sophisticated, with the aid of computers and software packages, use *multivariate modeling*, which can control for many potentially confounding variables all at once. Examples include multiple logistic regression and Cox proportional hazards, two of the more popular multivariate techniques found in the epidemiological literature.[19]

The Mantel-Haenszel summary or adjusted odds ratio can still be computed using nothing more sophisticated than a hand calculator, provided that there are reasonably few strata (see Exercise 6.1 for an example). Its formula is relatively simple:

$$\frac{\Sigma(ad/n)}{\Sigma(bc/n)}$$

Suppose in a case-control study, there are two age strata:

Stratum 1:

	D	D_0	
E	a_1	b_1	
E_0	c_1	d_1	n_1

Stratum 2:

	D	D_0	
E	a_2	b_2	
E_0	c_2	d_2	n_2

The OR_{M-H} will then be:

$$\frac{[(a1d1/n1)+(a2d2/n2)]}{[(b1c1/n1)+(b2d2/n2)]}$$

Stratification is often limited by the study size. Even for large studies, after stratifying for several variables (e.g., 2 sexes, 3 age-groups and 2 races would yield $2 \times 3 \times 2 = 12$ strata), the effective cell size could become quite small.

Uncontrolled confounding is manifested in a biased estimate of the relative risk or odds ratio, whose size depends on the strength of association between the confounder and the exposure, and between the confounder and the disease. Multiple, small confounders, when aggregated, can have a substantial effect.

The detection and control of confounding has become the central pre-occupation of epidemiology. One introductory textbook of epidemiology introduces its readers to the concept of confounding in the first paragraph of Chapter 1! An editorialist in the *International Journal of Epidemiology* made the following wry but apt observation:

> Our best friend in epidemiology, it seems, is the confounder. The confounder preoccupies our thinking, we respect its omnipresence, and we are endlessly entertained by attempting to identify one in someone else's study. As epidemiologists we spend our days chasing the confounder like detectives, anticipating its disturbing appearance when designing a study, considering potential confounders in our analysis, and trying to illuminate unconsidered confounders in our analysis when the results of our study do not conform with the expected.[20]

Interaction or Effect Modification

In real life, few diseases are caused by a single risk factor. When two or more risk factors are involved, they may combine their effects either syn-ergistically or antagonistically. In statistical terms, *interaction* may occur. It is sometimes also called *effect modification*. It is not to be confused with confounding. In studying the relationship between exposure (E) and dis-ease (D), the confounder (C), by virtue of its being associated with both E and D (as well as satisfying the other two conditions mentioned earlier), is the reason why E appears to be associated with D when it fact it is not. In interaction, the effect modifier (M) affects the association between E and D in such a way that the association is different (stronger or weaker) at different levels of M.

The concept of interaction can be illustrated graphically (Figure 6.2):

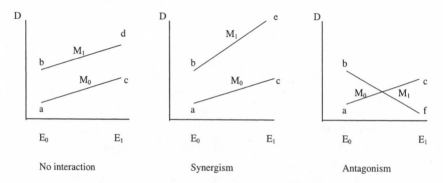

Figure 6.2. Graphical illustration of interaction.

We can consider the level of D when neither M nor E is present ($M_0 E_0$) as the baseline reference level, represented by (a). When only E is present ($M_0 E_1$), the level of D is raised above that of the reference point to a higher level, to (c). When only M is present ($M_1 E_0$), the level of D is also raised above that of the reference point to a higher level, to (b). The line (a–c) represents the association of E and D when M is absent, and the line (b–d) represents the association of E and D when M is present. When there is no interaction, the two lines are parallel (they have the same slope). The level of D when both E and M are present ($M_1 E_1$) is (d), which is higher than (a), (b), and (c). When there is synergism, the two lines diverge. The level of D at ($M_1 E_1$) is now (e), which is higher than (d). When there is antagonism, the two lines cross. The level of D at ($M_1 E_1$) is now (f), which is not only lower than (d), but also lower than (c). In other words, the presence of M has reversed the relationship between E and D, changing E from a risk factor to a protective factor.

We can also describe the interaction between E and M in terms of the relative risks when one or both of them are present in a 2×2 table. The baseline reference level, when neither is present (E_0, M_0), is set at 1.0.

	E_0	E_1
M_0	1.0	RR_E
M_1	RR_M	RR_{EM}

There are two basic models of interaction, the additive and multiplicative.

Under the additive model, there is no interaction if $RR_{EM} - 1 = (RR_E - 1) + (RR_M - 1)$, which simplifies to $RR_{EM} = RR_E + RR_M - 1$. If there is interaction, then $RR_{EM} \neq RR_E + RR_M - 1$ (> if synergistic, or < if antagonistic). Under the multiplicative model, there is no interaction if $RR_{EM} = RR_E \times RR_M$. If there is interaction, then $RR_{EM} \neq RR_E \times RR_M$ (> if synergistic, or < if antagonistic).

A well-known interaction is that between asbestos and smoking, both of which can independently cause lung cancer, but when present together in the same individual, increase the risk of lung cancer considerably.[21] Exercise 6.2 provides a numerical example.

Interaction is an important concern in population health research. Deviation from a multiplicative model is relevant to the understanding of etiology, while deviation from an additive model has implications for public health action. This is reminiscent of the use of attributable risk to assess the size of the health problem and relative risk as a measure of the strength of causal association (discussed in Chapter 5).[22]

Qualitative Methods

In population health research, there is no single method that is suitable for all situations. Indeed, the nature of the research problem dictates the method to be used. Since the health of populations is influenced by many social and cultural factors, not all of which can always be neatly quantified, there is a place for *qualitative* methods to supplement, complement or replace the more familiar *quantitative* methods.

The goal of qualitative research is "the development of concepts that help us understand social phenomena in natural settings, giving due emphasis to the meanings, experiences, and views of all the participants." Qualitative research is thus interpretative and naturalistic. It is also more closely linked to theory. A major influence is grounded theory, developed by sociologists Barney Glaser and Anselm Strauss in the 1960s. It is primarily an inductive approach to generating explanatory theory from gathering and analyzing data, which in turn informs further data collection as the study progresses.[23]

Much discussion of qualitative methods in the health research literature tends to contrast it with quantitative methods. Quantitative scientists have a tendency to criticize qualitative research for being too subjective, too value-laden, not replicable, not generalizable, too novelistic or journalistic, too descriptive, lacking in validity, and not empirical, rigorous, or systematic. Yet quantitative methods, by treating numbers as self-evident "facts," tend to ignore meaning, purpose, experience, and context. Theory is generally shunned, design is rigid, and thinking becomes mechanical. "Critics of qualitative research operate from a scientific or positivistic tradition that has idealized investigative models borrowed from the natural sciences . . . Qualitative research is criticized for not being something it never intended to be, and is not given credit for its strength."[24]

Unfortunately, practitioners of qualitative research have a penchant to define, and defend, themselves according to a proliferation of ideological labels, such as Marxist, feminist, constructivist, post-positivist, or any one of many "-ists." Indeed, a standard handbook on qualitative research states: "qualitative research is defined primarily by a series of essential tensions, contradictions, and hesitations . . . among competing definitions and conceptions of the field."[25]

There are several specific examples of how qualitative methods complement quantitative research:

1. As preliminary to quantitative research—to provide a description and understanding of a situation or behavior, such as appropriate wordings for use in a survey questionnaire;
2. As validation, part of a process of *triangulation*, comparing results from several methods to check for convergence, or studying the same phenomenon at different levels;

3. As an alternative to quantitative methods in studying complex issues;
4. To help explain quantitative results.

As an example, in a comprehensive regional-health-needs-assessment exercise, one may combine the collection and analysis of demographic and epidemiological data with the use of key informants and focus groups (see below) to seek data specifically on community perception of health problems, the causes of ill health, and the adequacy of health services. The qualitative data provide further insight into the meaning of mortality, disease incidence, and health care utilization rates; while the use of quantitative methods "improves the generalizability and inferential strength of the qualitative data."[26]

In a cross-cultural setting, the integrated design allows one to combine the *emic* perspective of ethnomedicine and the *etic* means of biomedical science. (These terms have been explained earlier in Chapter 3.) One approach to cross-cultural research on ethnomedical systems would involve identifying the phenomenon in emic terms, determining the extent to which the phenomenon described can be understood in terms of bioscientific concepts and methods, and finally identifying areas of convergence and divergence between the two.[27]

There are three basic types of qualitative methods: direct observation, interviews, and document analysis. Regardless of the data source, there is a common focus on talk and action, rather than numbers. In many ways these methods are not very different from the everyday experience of people, and they should look familiar, particularly to clinicians. However, the key difference is that qualitative research involves the systematic collection of data and rigorous analysis. It requires skill and experience, which can only be acquired through training.

A commonly used form of observation is participant observation. As the name implies, the researcher observes people and events in their natural settings, describing and analyzing what has been observed. Observation is particularly useful in distinguishing what people say from what they do. The degree of participation varies. Sometimes the research takes the form of a covert operation (e.g., posing as a motorcycle gang member); this may well be unethical and dangerous, especially if the researcher, impatient to see things "happen," becomes an *agent provocateur*. In other situations, the researcher stays aloof from the study subjects, with the outsider role clearly recognizable. The presence of the researcher may actually induce behavioral change in the subjects. Many anthropologists have been led astray when the "natives" decided to "put on a show" for their benefit. Another well-known phenomenon goes under the name of *Hawthorne effect*, whereby the behavior of study subjects changed as a result of being included in a study, and is named after the Western Electric plant in the Illinois town of that name.[28]

An interview may be *structured, semi-structured,* or *in-depth.* A structured interview involves administering in a standardized manner a structured questionnaire, usually with a limited number of responses. Semi-structured interviews involve open-ended questions. Responses to a particular question may be pursued further. In-depth interviews involve a very limited number of issues for discussion, but they are explored in much greater detail. The dynamics between interviewer and interviewee may determine the course, duration, and outcome of the interview. Interviews are particularly useful in discovering experience, opinions, beliefs, and feelings, which are difficult to express in the context of simple answers to a preset questionnaire. Thus surveys have long documented the discrepancy between health knowledge and behavior—it remains for qualitative research to discover why.[29]

A focus group is also a form of interview, except that it is conducted with a group rather than an individual. There is the added bonus that the observed interactions among members of the group become part of the data. This method is well used by marketing firms to test consumer preferences, and also by political parties to see which way the wind is blowing! The constitution of the group is up to the investigator, who may pick an existing group (e.g., a class of students) or create one based on some shared characteristics. The focus group is more than a tool to extract what people think, but also how opinions are formed. The group process may generate new questions and provide answers. Because a number of individuals are involved, some sort of norm can be established for the group, especially if the group is homogeneous and "typical" of the occupation, ethnicity, or whatever characteristic for which they are chosen.[30]

Qualitative research rarely uses random sampling, with the intent of creating a representative sample from which one can generalize to the total population. Sampling is often purposive, to ensure that a full range of opinions or experiences of the phenomenon being studied is included. Generalization is possible, but not by statistical inference. Rather, it is by demonstrating common links shared by the observed setting and others. Individuals may be chosen for interviews because of their particular knowledge, which is useful to the researcher. These are often called *key informants,* and may be local community health workers, senior bureaucrats, etc.

A document is not just a written record, but can include visual and audio media. Many are found in public archives or private collections, and encompass government reports, personal papers, correspondence and diaries, newspapers, magazines, videos, tapes, photographs, etc. These are all rich sources of qualitative information about a community, its members and institutions. Research by historians and policy analysts relies heavily on documents, creating narratives from data extracted from these sources. Some documents are amenable to *content analysis,* which can also be a quantitative exercise involving identifying, categorizing, and counting specific features that are of interest.

Ethical Concerns

Many ethical issues associated with human health research have been recognized and addressed by the scientific community for some years. A variety of international declarations and guidelines have been proposed, such as the *Declaration of Helsinki* of the World Medical Association, first adopted by the 18th World Medical Assembly in 1964 and amended in subsequent meetings, and the *International Guidelines for Biomedical Research Involving Human Subjects* proposed in 1982 by the Council of International Organizations of Medical Sciences (CIOMS), a WHO-affiliated organization. Much of this laudable effort, however, has focused on basic biomedical and clinical research. Because of the vastly different design and methods used in population health research, with its unique ethical problems, attempts to develop more relevant guidelines have been made by such organizations as CIOMS and the International Epidemiological Association.[31]

Population health research uses a variety of methods, each of which is associated with different levels of "invasiveness" (in terms of pain, discomfort, and inconvenience, as well as threats to confidentiality and privacy). In one extreme, entire communities may be subjected to drugs, vaccines, screening procedures, or health education campaigns. Other research may only require people to answer questions by mail, by telephone, or face-to-face. Some research does not involve any direct contact with the "subject" but involves medical record review and electronic data linkage of large databases. All these different approaches have their associated ethical concerns.

The *Shorter Oxford Dictionary* (1993) defines *ethics* as "moral principles by which any particular person is guided; and as rules of conduct recognized in a particular profession or area of human life."

There are four basic principles of bioethics:

1. *Autonomy*: the respect for self-determination and voluntary action; individuals with diminished autonomy (e.g., the mentally deficient) must be protected against abuse;
2. *Beneficence*: acting to enhance/maximize potential benefits;
3. *Non-maleficence*: doing no harm, a principle epitomized by the physicians' pledge of *primum non nocere*;
4. *Justice*: the equitable distribution of benefits and risks.

These principles are applicable in population health. Some adaptation is needed, however, because of the need to balance the interests of the individual and the interests of the population (e.g., individual responsibility vs. collective action in health promotion; the balance between the rights of individuals vs. protecting the public's health and security). In some studies, especially those dealing with large databases or archives, individuals may not even be directly involved.

An individual giving consent to participate in a study must understand the purpose and nature of the study and the risks and benefits involved. This is referred to as *informed consent*. This is not as simple as it seems. An individual seeking health care usually does not give specific consent that his particular hospitalization or physician visit will be analyzed by researchers to determine, say, the appropriateness of surgical procedures. An individual giving consent to take part in a health survey and have his blood tested for, say, cholesterol, is unlikely to have given a "blanket" consent that five or 10 years later, a researcher can use the stored specimen for some other test, like HIV.

In population health studies, particularly those conducted in communities, an additional requirement to individual consent may be collective or community consent through its representatives, usually some political leaders. How this is done will depend on the power structure within the community, its traditions and practices of decision-making. Consent given by a community's leaders should not replace individual consent; yet without community consent, access to the community may well be denied. The definition of a "community" can also be problematic, particularly if it is not defined in geopolitical terms (e.g., an ethnic community scattered throughout a city) and if there is no clearly identifiable hierarchy. Some communities are also stratified with underrepresented and underprivileged groups, whose consent may readily be given away by others in power to whom their interests are clearly not of concern. Population health studies cannot be conducted in a vacuum, without preliminary groundwork in understanding the characteristics and dynamics in a community.

The full disclosure of relevant information may sometimes have to be compromised. An example is the administration of a placebo in an RCT, where recipients of the placebo are not aware of what they are receiving, as full disclosure will have invalidated the study. Indeed, some would argue that not doing an RCT to determine the best treatment for the population at large is itself not ethical. Selective disclosure of information is justifiable, provided that it does not induce subjects to do what they would not otherwise consent to do.

Undue influence must be avoided: for example, an implied threat of withdrawal of health services for non-participants (if a study is identified with, or perceived to be allied with, an official source of health care). Those in authority in a community who support the study may sometimes apply subtle pressure. The other side of the coin—inducement to participate—may also pose a problem. Extravagant monetary compensation beyond reimbursement of expenses and loss of income may actually create inequity within a community and breed resentment, especially if only a sample is selected for participation (the technical rationale of sampling—"why him and not me?"—can be and must be explained). What is appropriate can only be determined in the light of cultural traditions and social norms.

Many individuals will gladly participate in a study even if there is no direct personal benefit, provided that there is some perceived benefit to the common good—such as "advancing scientific knowledge," "finding a cure for cancer," and so on. If only such indirect benefits will accrue to an individual or a community, then it is incumbent upon the investigator to ensure the study results are communicated back to the individual or community. Research communication and dissemination—the last link in the research chain—is often totally neglected by researchers. Often, publication in a scientific journal and/or presentation at a conference is all that is anticipated. (Studies that do not even make it to the attention of the scientific community are a gross misuse of limited research funds.) Research results need to be reported to the community in a form that is comprehensible.

Conflict sometimes arises over the issue of public release and dissemination of research results. Funding agencies and sponsors, especially governments and commercial enterprises, may claim power of veto over the release of "unfavorable" data. Communities may want to censor results that show them in a bad light—for example, a high prevalence of health conditions associated with social stigma. Clarification of the right to release data must be negotiated at the beginning, and may be a legal and political as well as ethical issue.

A form of benefit is the provision of health care during a study. In areas where there is no universal coverage of health care insurance, the United States being a prime example, the availability of a free "check-up" in the context of a health survey can be a form of benefit. Participants should be notified of any conditions uncovered by a study (e.g., hypertension). Whether such information should automatically be passed on to health care providers for follow-up should be agreed to by the participant.

Researchers should consider the impact and legacy of research when it is completed. Are communities strengthened as a result of the research, in terms of training opportunities, the transfer of research skills and equipment, etc. It is important that there is equitable distribution of benefits in whatever form. Since the aim of population health is to improve the health of the population, a study should demonstrate relevance to the health needs of the population being studied.

The research procedures themselves may sometimes pose a physical risk to participants (e.g., venipuncture, test of physical endurance, administration of drugs, vaccines, and other agents). More subtle harm comes in the form of interference with other normal activities in the community (e.g., time away from harvest or regular employment, resulting in economic loss), harmful publicity, social stigmatization, loss of self-esteem and prestige, etc. If risks are unavoidable, the researcher must demonstrate that the benefits outweigh the risks. Above all, the nature and extent of potential risks must be communicated frankly with participants. A study must also respect local social mores and be sensitive to cultural traditions.

A major concern of research is to ensure *privacy* and *confidentiality*. Privacy in the research context means the respect of the right from unwanted intrusion and divulgence of personal information. Confidentiality is a contract with the study participant that there will be no disclosure of information without the participant's consent.

It is customary in surveys and other data collection processes to delete personal identifiers so that it becomes impossible afterwards for the researcher or another user to link any particular set of information to a specific individual. Because population health is primarily concerned with the population, results are often presented in aggregates where the risk of individuals' being identified is very low. Census bureaus, in fact, have taken great pains to avoid even this small risk—often the data are "randomly rounded"—so that for small "cells," a "4" can be randomly assigned to "0" or to "5" (to make it well nigh impossible to do multiple cross-tabulations to identify specific individuals).

Data protection has become a major issue in many developed countries, where new laws have been enacted that severely restrict access of researchers to large, publicly maintained databases, including health care databases; others extend to all personal health information in whatever format. Some stipulate that individual consent must be obtained even for anonymous records in data linkage studies. The low consent rate is likely to severely threaten the validity and feasibility of many studies. Such developments affect, not only research, but also many routine population health practices such as disease surveillance. The situation is evolving, and the full impact is difficult to predict.[32]

Investigators should have no undisclosed conflict of interest with collaborators, sponsors, or study participants. Commercial sponsors (e.g., pharmaceutical firms) may wish to use a study to promote a particular product. In occupational health studies, unions and management may have different agendas, and a researcher hired or financially supported by one of the parties may deliberately or subconsciously alter the results to "toe the party line." Similar conflicts may arise in studies sponsored by governments or special interest groups (e.g., environmental activist groups, anti-poverty groups, animal rights groups).

There are additional ethical dimensions if the research is conducted in a cross-cultural setting, or in situations where those being researched perceive themselves to be in a disadvantaged power relationship vis-à-vis the researcher (socially, economically, and politically marginalized groups). The ethical "imperialist" can be contrasted with the ethical "relativist." The former assumes that the Western mode of scientific and ethical standards applies to all societies, and insists on their adherence; the latter takes the position that each society has the right to decide what is ethical and what is not—even human rights are then "relative." Regardless of the stance, the practice of doing in another country what one could not do in one's own country is not considered to be ethical.

Anthropologists are familiar with working in cross-cultural settings. The rights, interests, and sensitivities of the peoples and cultures being studied take precedence over the acquisition of new knowledge. Ethical principles are influenced by the values, interests, and demands of diverse societies.[33]

There is a school of thought, espoused by some community activists and not universally shared by researchers, that sees little difference between ethical and political issues. Research ethics is seen in a much broader light, and includes such issues as setting research priorities, and the ownership and control of the research process and outcomes.

Finally, ethical principles need to be translated into action. Most research institutions have established review procedures, which usually involve review committees (under the name of human subjects committees, institutional review boards, etc.). Such committees review projects at the proposal stage. Most funding agencies will not release research funds without an official letter of approval from such a committee. The composition of the committee varies, with some consisting exclusively of scientists, while others include professional ethicists and so-called lay members from the community-at-large.

Summary

This chapter reviews the various quantitative and qualitative research methods in population health. Research requires the collection of data, which may be primary or secondary. Different levels of measurement result in nominal, ordinal, and continuous variables. The unit of data collection and analysis may be the individual, or aggregates of individuals, when it is referred to as an ecological study.

Different research designs are used for different purposes, depending on the nature of the research problem. Studies may be descriptive or analytical. Among the latter, studies may be experimental or observational, depending on whether the investigator manipulates the exposure variable. The randomized controlled trial is a type of experimental study used in both clinical and population health research. Longitudinal and cross-sectional studies differ in terms of whether the exposure and outcome variables are measured at different times or concurrently. Longitudinal studies can be divided into cohort and case-control studies, which differ primarily in the directionality (from exposure to outcome, or vice versa) and in sample selection (based on exposure or outcome status). Timing determines if a cohort study is retrospective or prospective.

A study must be both valid and reliable, and be free from random and systematic error, or bias. There are three major types of bias: selection bias, information bias, and confounding. The control of confounding is a key task of study design and data analysis, and various options are available. Two or more causal variables may also interact synergistically or

---

BOX 6.6.   Participatory Research

Traditionally research is done on individuals or communities by the researcher. The very term research *subject* is indicative of an imbalance in power relationship. *Participatory* research (sometimes also called *action* research) represents a new approach to research that addresses this imbalance and has particular relevance for population health. Lawrence Green and his colleagues offered one definition, in the context of health promotion, which states that participatory research is "a process of developing new knowledge by systematic inquiry, with the collaboration of those affected, for the purposes of education and taking action or effecting social change."[34] The key elements are thus *collaboration, education,* and *action,* which are usually absent in the traditional style of health research. Its proponents believe that the knowledge, expertise, and resources of the involved community actually improve the validity, efficiency, and sustainability of the research project. The communities gain from empowerment and are in a better position to benefit from the research. Collaboration entails partnership, which needs to be mutually respectful, between equals with complementary expertise. Much participatory research has been conducted in, although not restricted to, disadvantaged or marginalized populations.

Although the principles are worthy and will not be disputed by most researchers, participatory research is not easily implemented in practice. The North American Primary Care Research Group suggested that the researcher and the community decide clearly their respective roles, responsibilities, and contributions. There are also ethical and managerial issues that may need to be negotiated, for example, over the ownership, control, access, and possession of research data; the dissemination of results; the terms of the partnership, and methods of conflict resolution.

---

antagonistically in producing an effect. The statistical relation may be described in terms of an additive or multiplicative model.

A multidisciplinary approach offers the best solution to research problems. Such qualitative methods as participant observation, interviews, and focus groups can supplement, complement, or replace quantitative methods. Research must be ethical. Because of different methods and topics of research, population health is associated with its unique ethical concerns. While basic ethical principles long established in laboratory and clinical research—such as autonomy, beneficence, non-maleficence, and justice—still apply, they need to be modified.

Case Study 6.1.   Age-Period-Cohort Analysis of Traffic Accident Mortality

Any time period defined by calendar dates reflect three dimensions—age, period, and cohort (or generation). Whenever a health outcome is seen to change with time in frequency and age distribution, these three interrelated effects need to be considered, and disentangled. *Age* is obtained by the difference between the year of observation and the year of birth. It represents the intrinsic, mostly biological, effect of maturation and resilience of the organism (e.g., starvation has different effects on different age groups). *Period* is bounded by the dates of observation of the outcomes. It reflects the prevalent environmental effect experienced by people of all ages living at the time (e.g., starvation experienced by Dutch citizens under German occupation during World War II). *Cohort* is defined by the dates of recruitment (usually birth) of those who share common environmental conditions as they age together (Dutch children born in the late 1920s experienced starvation during their adolescence in the early 1940s and the postwar economic boom as young adults).

The classic example of age-period-cohort analysis is the study of the decline of tuberculosis mortality in the United States by the pioneer epidemiologist Wade Hampton Frost (1880–1938).[35] The method can be applied to any health problem, provided that appropriately arrayed statistical data are available. As an illustration, mortality rates for motor vehicle traffic accidents (MVA) among Canadian males since 1921 can be used. The mortality rates (per 100,000 population) can be arranged according to the age at death and the year of death as shown in the table next page.

In the table, the rows represent the *secular trend* in MVA mortality, while the columns represent the *cross-sectional rates*. The mortality experience of each *birth cohort* can be observed diagonally: the 1921–1925 and 1941–1945 cohorts are shown in boldface. Thus those born during 1921–1925 who died from MVA within the first five years of life had a mortality rate of 5.7; as this cohort aged, the mortality rate increased to 13.0 by ages 5 through 9, etc.

Looking at secular trends, there has been a general increase in MVA mortality since the 1920s. For the youngest and oldest (0–9, 70–79), it peaked during the 1950s. For young adults (15–24), the peak rates occurred during 1971–1975. For all age groups, mortality rates dropped sharply after 1975. The energy crisis in the early 1970s may have reduced the usage of motor vehicles and hence exposure. Improved car safety features and highway engineering may have also contributed to the decline.

Looking at cross-sectional rates, it can be seen that MVA was primarily a problem for old people prior to the 1940s. Since then, MVAs

Period of death

Age at death	1921–25	1926–30	1931–35	1936–40	1941–45	1946–50	1951–55	1956–60	1961–65	1966–70	1971–75	1976–80
0–4	5.7	9.0	9.3	12.4	13.4	15.0	15.0	12.0	13.3	13.9	11.8	9.0
5–9	8.1	13.0	12.3	13.9	18.2	20.1	20.5	18.7	19.7	18.9	16.5	12.5
10–14	5.3	8.8	6.7	10.7	10.1	11.3	12.8	12.5	12.5	14.7	14.9	13.0
15–19	4.5	12.0	11.8	17.6	16.6	22.4	32.2	41.6	46.8	62.2	78.7	67.0
20–24	7.0	17.3	16.8	22.4	20.6	33.3	50.2	59.0	78.3	86.1	88.4	71.2
25–29	6.2	14.5	16.8	19.9	18.1	27.2	35.3	42.1	48.9	49.3	46.6	41.5
30–34	6.5	13.8	14.9	19.9	15.8	22.1	29.4	34.0	36.2	38.9	37.4	28.6
35–39	6.5	15.2	16.6	20.4	17.1	20.0	26.5	29.0	33.6	32.6	33.4	23.4
40–44	5.7	15.3	15.7	17.8	18.6	21.2	25.2	27.4	33.6	32.8	29.6	24.4
45–49	5.7	16.0	18.9	22.0	21.1	21.4	27.2	27.8	32.5	33.5	31.1	23.3
50–54	8.0	18.0	20.5	24.2	19.5	22.7	28.2	38.7	34.2	36.2	32.6	23.1
55–59	8.8	20.2	22.3	27.2	24.5	25.9	34.1	35.5	37.9	38.7	34.1	25.5
60–64	9.2	24.8	25.3	32.2	31.6	32.1	36.5	38.8	44.7	40.1	35.9	27.1
65–69	11.0	27.1	30.2	38.4	36.5	38.5	44.1	43.7	51.5	49.2	44.6	30.2
70–74	11.2	32.7	33.8	49.1	43.1	45.6	49.9	55.6	53.5	46.9	47.5	33.7
75–79	15.0	45.1	48.1	46.7	51.5	66.4	65.5	66.6	59.0	63.2	53.8	37.0

began to affect the age group 15–24 more and more. In the 1950s and 1960s two peaks can be seen, at ages 15–24 and 70–79. Since the 1970s, the highest rates are observed among the 15–24 age group only. This is probably the result of increased access to cars and acquisition of driver's permits in this age group.

The age-specific mortality rates for selected birth cohorts can be shown graphically:

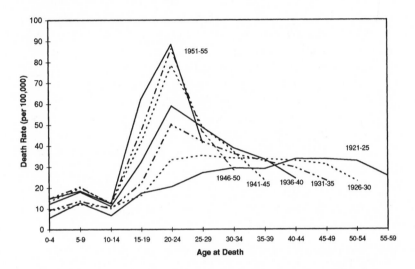

With each successive birth cohort, it can be seen that the shape of the curve has changed, with a general upward tendency. Beginning with the 1931–1935 cohort, a peak at age 20–24 is evident. The peak becomes more and more pronounced in the subsequent cohorts. The sharp decline since 1975 cannot be seen in the graph but is evident from the table: thus for the 1921–1925 cohort, mortality declined from 32.6 to 25.5, and for the 1941–1945 cohort, from 37.4 to 23.4. The postwar birth cohorts are generally much better off economically than the prewar generation, and are more likely to have access to cars and opportunity for driving when they reach the legal age for driving.

An age-period-cohort analysis of MVA mortality is a descriptive rather than analytical study. While it shows changes in the pattern of mortality with time, it does not actually study the causes of the change. Data on possible causes such as changes in car manufacturing, highway construction, and gasoline prices are not internal or linked to this study, but must be acquired elsewhere. One risk factor—age—can be clearly identified, however, so that some commentary on causation is not out of place even in a descriptive study. From a policy perspective, a descriptive study can be a powerful tool. Opportunities for further analytical studies may not arise, and policy decisions often cannot wait for definitive proof of cause and effect.

Case Study 6.2.   Durkheim's Studies on Suicide

A classic ecological study is the one performed by French sociologist Emile Durkheim (1858–1917), who published his *Le Suicide* in 1897 (English translation 1951).[36] Durkheim showed that, among Prussian provinces in the late nineteenth century, the suicide rate increased with increasing proportion of Protestants in the population (or decreased with decreasing proportion of Catholics in the population, as shown in the graph below). Interestingly, in Switzerland, predominantly Protestant cantons also had higher suicide rates than predominantly Catholic cantons, even when French-speaking and German-speaking cantons were considered separately.

Durkheim suggested that suicide varied inversely with the degree of social integration and regulation. He viewed suicide not only as an isolated, individual tragic event, but as socially patterned conditions experienced by the group. Protestantism was less rigid with regard to personal life, whereas Catholicism imposed stronger bonds on the individuals with the group.

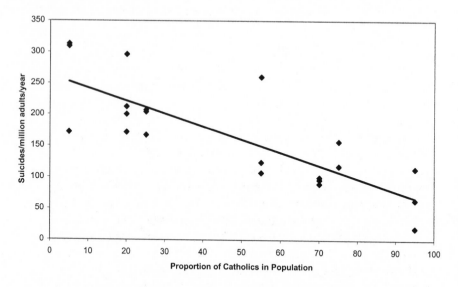

Suicide in Bavarian and Prussian Provinces, Late Nineteenth Century

Were Protestants more likely to commit suicide? Durkheim's study is often cited as a potential case for ecological fallacy. An alternative explanation for the ecological-level observation is possible: that it was predominantly Catholics, living in Prussian provinces or Swiss cantons where they were increasingly marginalized, who committed suicide (same idea as the male/female difference in examination scores in Box 6.1). However, there is no ecological fallacy in this particular case—Protestants did commit suicide more often than Catholics in nineteenth-century Europe:

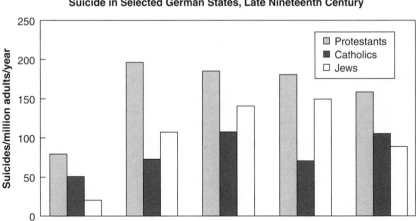

Whether in the whole of Europe or only in German-speaking states, the suicide rate among Protestants was higher than that of Catholics. Thus the association between suicide and religion in nineteenth-century Europe at the ecological level—that jurisdictions with a high proportion of Protestants had higher suicide rates— is corroborated by evidence at the individual level—that Protestants had higher suicide rates than Catholics.

Durkheim is today revered as one of the founders of modern sociology, especially as a pioneer social researcher. His other major work is *Les Règles de la méthode sociologique*, published in 1894. His work

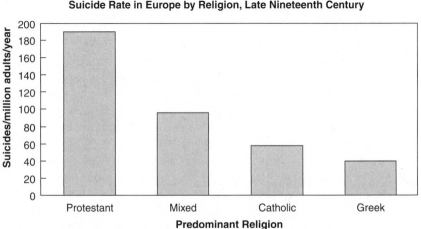

also anticipated much of the "upstream" rhetoric of population health in the 1990s, by explaining individual pathology as a function of social dynamics.

Case Study 6.3.   The Causal Trail: Cigarette Smoking and Lung Cancer

One of the most important discoveries in the history of population health research in the twentieth century is the association between cigarette smoking and lung cancer. Tobacco is indigenous to the Americas, where the plant was cultivated and gathered wild. The ceremonial use of tobacco was integral to the cultures of many Native American tribes, and it was traded far and wide. Tobacco was introduced to Europe in the mid–sixteenth century when it was touted as possessing medicinal value (a claim still made by tobacco companies in advertisements as late as the 1950s). Its addictive properties were soon evident, and King James I of England (famous for the King James version of the Bible) condemned it as a vice, and even published a diatribe against it in 1604. The first inkling of a cancer link appeared in 1795, when a German report suggested that cancer of the lip resulted from pipe smoking. In the 1920s German pathologists were the first to recognize a new lung cancer epidemic, and case series were published showing that lung cancer victims were mostly smokers. Among the competing candidates for the cause of the lung cancer epidemic were road tar, automobile exhaust, and the 1919 flu epidemic. In 1939 Franz Müller published what would be called today a case-control study, which showed that a higher proportion of cases than healthy controls were smokers. It should be recognized that the Nazi regime instituted strong anti-tobacco campaigns (including banning it in public places) and supported epidemiological research on the hazards of tobacco use.[37]

Trend data on per capita cigarette consumption and lung cancer mortality during the first half of the century are highly suggestive of a link. Data for the United States are shown on the next page.[38]

In 1950, five case-control studies were published linking smoking and lung cancer mortality, two of which appeared in the same issue of one journal. In the study by Ernest Wynder and Evarts Graham, they obtained information on histologically confirmed bronchogenic carcinoma cases in men from hospitals in 12 states across the United States. From among the "general hospital population" in St. Louis, Missouri (i.e., patients with non-cancer diagnoses), 780 controls were selected. Cases and controls were administered the same questionnaire on smoking history by personal interview or by mail. In a small number of deceased cases the information was obtained by proxy.[39] The main results of this study can be summarized in the following 2×2 table.

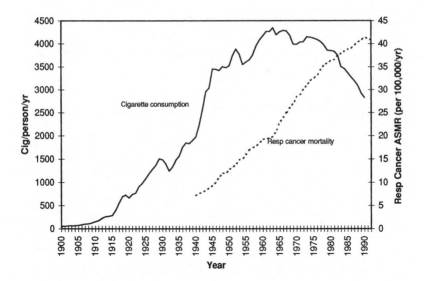

	Cases	Controls
Smokers	597	665
Nonsmokers	8	115
Total	605	780

The odds ratio is 12.9, which indicates an astoundingly strong association. Note that the authors did not use the OR—it was not then the popular thing to do. By breaking down smokers into categories based on the number of cigarettes per day, with nonsmokers as the reference category (OR set at 1.0), a dose–response relationship can be observed:

Smoking category	Number of cigarettes/day	Odds ratio
Light	1–9	2.5
Moderately heavy	10–15	6.0
Heavy	16–20	11.2
Excessive	21–24	27.3
Chain smoker	25+	27.6

In 1951, having published their case-control study the year previously, Richard Doll and Austin Bradford Hill launched a prospective cohort study of British physicians. They mailed out questionnaires on smoking habits to 59,600 physicians on the Medical Register, 68% of whom responded. Over the next decade, deaths were recorded, based on information obtained from death certificates and other sources. Person-years of exposure and mortality rate/1,000 PY/year were computed.[40] The mortality rates for lung cancer among the cohort of 34,000 male doctors can be shown in this graph:

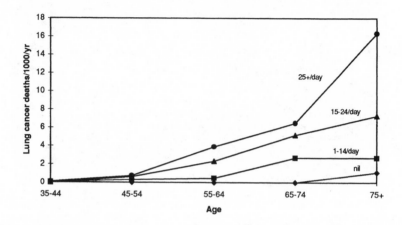

It is evident that mortality, as expected, increases with advancing age. The higher the daily consumption of cigarettes, however, the steeper the gradient. Because it is a cohort study, it is possible to study many outcomes other than lung cancer. The published data are reanalyzed in the form of relative risks (rate ratios):

Cause of death	RR	Cause of death	RR	Cause of death	RR
Lung cancer	13.3	Pulmonary tuberculosis	2.5	Other cancers	0.92
Chronic bronchitis	10.2	Coronary heart disease	1.3	Violence	0.84
Other upper respiratory/digestive tract cancers	3.8	Stroke	1.2	All causes	1.28

Doll and Hill were also able to investigate the effect of stopping smoking:

Number of years since stopping	RR
Did not stop	18.3
Stopped <5 years	9.6
Stopped 5–9 years	7.0
Stopped 10–19 years	2.6
Stopped 20+ years	2.7

Compared to nonsmokers (RR set at 1.0), the risk of lung cancer mortality declines sharply with increasing number of years since stopping smoking. In 1964 the Surgeon General of the United States published the landmark *Smoking and Health* report, which is often credited with reversing the trend in smoking consumption in North America. By that time some 29 case-control and seven cohort studies had been reported. The Surgeon General concluded that "cigarette smoking is a health hazard of sufficient importance in the United States to warrant appropriate remedial action."[41] Research continues on the health consequences of smoking. A substantial body of experimental evidence has been accumulated. Many mutagenic and carcinogenic substances have been isolated and identified from tobacco tar, and whole tobacco smoke and extracts have induced tumors in experimental animals. Molecular biology points to a genetic basis for modulating individual susceptibility to the action of tobacco carcinogens. More and more health effects of smoking are being identified. Lung cancer has also been found to be caused by other environmental, occupational, and dietary factors such as asbestos, radon progeny, and low intake of beta-carotene found in leafy green vegetables. Several large-scale, randomized controlled trials are underway to test beta-carotene and other cancer prevention agents, although smoking cessation remains the most effective strategy.[42]

At least in North America, a substantial change in social attitudes towards smoking has occurred. Smoking is now socially unacceptable and legally restricted in public places in many cities. Smoking prevalence and consumption have declined substantially. Among women, however, the trend for lung cancer is still rising, and smoking remains a prevalent health problem among adolescents and youths. In developing countries, smoking is endemic, where economic issues relating to agricultural production and the import and export of tobacco products are intertwined with heath concerns.

Smoking is both a personal lifestyle and a product of social, economic, and political forces, and its control must involve a broad strategy directed at individuals (e.g., education and information) and society at large (e.g., tax measures and bylaws limiting sales and use). Indeed, the whole field of population health can be encompassed by the issues raised in smoking and health, from establishing the burden of illness, to assessing risks and causality, to planning and evaluating interventions.

A custom loathsome to the eye, hateful to the nose, harmful to the brain, dangerous to the lungs, and in the black, stinking fume thereof, nearest resembling the horrible Stygian smoke of the pit that is bottomless.

King James I of England, *Counterblast to Tobacco*, 1604

Case Study 6.4.   Tracking Heart Disease Among World War II Airmen

Cohort studies of cardiovascular disease are the backbone of epidemiological research in the second half of the twentieth century. While Framingham is the best known, there is a host of others from around the world. A Canadian study known as the University of Manitoba Follow-Up Study (UMFUS), began in 1948 by enrolling 3,983 Royal Canadian Air Force pilots who survived the war (mean age, 31 years).[43]

A baseline medical examination included anthropometry, blood pressure, and resting electrocardiography (ECG). Periodic reexaminations (initially at five-year and later at three-year intervals) were performed by study participants' personal physicians. Annual contact with the study investigators was maintained by a return postcard, but more extensive questionnaires were mailed in later years to collect additional information such as smoking habits, family history, physical activity, occupation, and perceived stress level during the war.

By mid-1993, the study passed the 45-year mark. The study is still ongoing, and a variety of reports have been published. The vital status of 89% of the original cohort was known. Here are some facts to illustrate the scope of a cohort study of this size:

- 153,000 person-years of observations
- 69,000 ECGs received and coded
- 92,000 blood pressure readings on file
- 1,678 deaths have occurred
- 2,305 men were still alive, with a mean age of 74 years.

When funding of the research was exhausted, the study participants offered to pay for its continuance!

This study provides useful data on the risk factors, natural history, and prognosis of a variety of cardiovascular conditions. For example, it confirms the important role of risk factors such as obesity and hypertension in ischemic heart disease. It demonstrates the significance of many ECG abnormalities in the absence of clinically manifest cardiac disease. Thus atrial fibrillation is associated with a relative risk of 2.1 for stroke, 3.0 for congestive heart failure, 1.4 for cardiovascular mortality, and 1.3 for all-cause mortality, independent of preexisting cardiac disease, hypertension, smoking, and obesity. First-degree heart block, on the other hand, is found to be a relatively benign condition with little impact on ischemic heart disease morbidity or mortality.

The study shows that post-stroke survival is related to the pre-stroke blood pressure status: the higher the last recorded pre-stroke systolic blood pressure (SBP), the worse the survival experience;

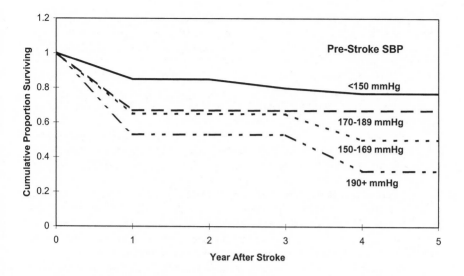

survival is also worse with a greater increase in SBP during the five-year pre-stroke period.

The prospective design is particularly suitable for tracking variables such as blood pressure. *Tracking* refers to the phenomenon whereby an individual maintains his ranking relative to others as he ages. The UMFUS measures tracking by computing the likelihood that a man whose blood pressure is in the top or bottom quintile will remain at these extremes five and more years later. Someone who was in the top quintile at age 40, when measured at age 45, was 1.9 times more likely than men his age to remain in the top quintile. (The "relative likelihood" is 1.0 if there is no tracking and if subsequent SBP is completely a random event unrelated to earlier SBP values). The relative likelihood is highest during the middle ages, from 45–55, and tracking tends to weaken with increasing intervals between measurements. The demonstration of tracking has implications for prevention—individuals at highest risk of hypertension can be identified at early adulthood.

Notes

1. Stroup and Teutsch (1998) provide a primer on quantitative analyses in public health. Woodward (1999) and Selvin (1996) are advanced epidemiology texts with extensive coverage of statistical analyses. Morse and Field (1995) offer a succinct handbook on analysis of qualitative data.

2. The politics of collecting public health data is discussed more fully in Krieger (1992).

3. The four basic levels (nominal, ordinal, interval, and ratio) can be attributed to the psychologist S. S. Stevens (1946), and they have remained in use in statistics and a variety of quantitative sciences. Note that *polytomous*, and not *polychotomous*,

corresponds with *dichotomous*. The Greek roots of dichotomous are not "di-" and "-chotomous" but "dicho-" (meaning "in two") and "-tomous" (meaning "to cut").

4. For a methodological discussion of ecological studies, see Morgenstern (1995), Greenland and Robins (1994), and Greenland (2001). For attempts to "rehabilitate" them, see Schwartz (1994) and Poole (1994). Krieger (1994) even warned of an "individual fallacy"! Diez-Roux (1998) argues for the need for multilevel analyses. An actual example, on cardiovascular risk factors and the neighborhood environment, can be found in Sundquist et al. (1999).

5. Every textbook of epidemiology has a somewhat different classification. See Kramer and Boivin (1987) for a cogent discussion and attempt to clear the confusion. Their ideas were further developed in Chapter 4 of Kramer's text (1988: 37–46).

6. There are excellent texts of RCTs (e.g., Friedman et al., 1996). Jadad (1998) is a useful primer presented in a question-and-answer format. Buck and Donner (1982) pointed out the differences in experimental design when evaluating non-therapeutic interventions such as prevention. A standard text on quasi-experiments long used by social scientists is the one by Cook and Campbell (1979).

7. Handbooks of survey research (e.g., Rossi et al., 1983; Frankfort-Nachmias and Nachmias, 1996) can be consulted for technical details on survey design, administration, and analysis. Frerichs and Shaheen (2001) discussed small community-based surveys in public health research. Etter and Perneger (2000) assessed the efficiency of snowball sampling in a survey of smokers.

8. In addition to coverage in standard epidemiology texts, there are several monographs on the case-control study; for example, Schlesselman (1982) and Breslow and Day (1980). A special issue of *Epidemiologic Reviews* (1994;16:1) is devoted exclusively to the case-control study. For the issues involved in the selection of controls, see Lasky and Stolley (1994) and the series of papers by Wacholder et al. (1992).

9. Cornfield's (1951) paper is a cornerstone of modern epidemiology. Miettinen (1976) showed that the "rare disease" assumption is not necessary. The relationship between the prevalence odds ratio and prevalence rate ratio is a function of the prevalence of D and the prevalence of E. For a discussion of their relative merits in cross-sectional studies, see Zocchetti et al. (1997).

10. See the reviews by Comstock (1994), Selby (1994), and Weiss (1994). The historical development of the case-control method is discussed in Lilienfeld and Lilienfeld (1979) and Susser (1985).

11. For a historical review of the cohort study, see Liddell (1988). A comprehensive monograph dealing exclusively with the cohort study is Breslow and Day (1987). Advanced texts in epidemiology such as Selvin (1996) and Kelsey et al. (1996) also contain substantial discussion of the cohort study.

12. See Feinstein and Horwitz (1982) and Feinstein (1988) on the RCT as gold standard. Arguments against the use of placebos can be found in Freedman et al. (1996).

13. For a more detailed description of the various types of validity, see Chapter 10 of Streiner and Norman (1995).

14. This is the Nurses Health Study, a large cohort study of over 120,000 women aged 30–55 years who were given a detailed questionnaire in 1976 and followed up for the development of cardiovascular and other chronic diseases. This study does not show an elevated risk of myocardial infarction or stroke associated with oral contraceptive use (Stampfer et al., 1988).

15. Greenland (1996) provides a quantitative approach to analyzing the potential impact of biases on study validity.

16. More detailed discussion of confounding can be found in advanced texts of epidemiology, such as Kleinbaum et al. (1982), Kelsey et al. (1996), and Rothman and Greenland (1998). See also the review by Greenland and Morgenstern (2001).

17. Explanations, examples, and citations for these biases can be found in Sackett's classic paper (1979).

18. Mantel and Haenszel's paper (1959) is a modern classic. It is reprinted in Greenland's collection of methodological papers (1987:111–41). More advanced students should consult the text by Fleiss (1981).

19. These techniques are discussed in detail in most advanced statistics texts (e.g., Kleinbaum et al., 1987; and Selvin, 1996). A self-learning text on logistic regression is also available (Kleinbaum, 1994). The easy availability of statistical software programs for personal computers has led to widespread abuse of these powerful statistical tools. For a thoughtful review of the appropriate use of multivariate techniques, see Hanley (1983).

20. Rothman's introductory text (2002) presents an extreme vision of epidemiology that is strongly methodological but divorced from social context or population health. The editorial lament is by Michels (2001).

21. Vainio and Boffetta (1994) reviewed various studies on the joint effects of asbestos and smoking on lung cancer. They postulated a biological mechanism of the interaction and suggested that a complex carcinogen may affect more than one stage of carcinogenesis. There is a variable pattern with examples of both the additive and multiplicative models. The multiplicative model tends to characterize insulation workers with high asbestos exposure.

22. For further discussion of interaction, see Kleinbaum et al. (1982:403–18); and Kahn and Sempos (1989:108–23).

23. The quotation is from Pope and Mays (1995), who published, in collaboration with other social scientists, a series of articles on qualitative research in health care in the *British Medical Journal*, which is subsequently collected in book form (Mays and Pope, 2000). The treatise on grounded theory was first published by Glaser and Strauss (1967). For an update, see Strauss and Corbin (1998).

24. The quotation is from Borman et al. (1986). For a discussion of the qualitative-quantitative divide in public health research, see Baum (1995).

25. Quoted in Denzin and Lincoln (1994:ix), one of the standard works on qualitative research methods. While authoritative, it is also densely theoretical.

26. Quoted from McKinlay (1993), who advocated the concept of *appropriate methodology*, which parallels that of *appropriate technology*, long accepted in international health programs.

27. This analytical framework, proposed by Browner et al. (1988), provides insight into underlying assumptions and logic that generate the structure, organization, and function of the medical systems being compared.

28. Observational methods are discussed further in Mays and Pope (2000). An example of the lack of correlation between self-report and direct observation is the study from Dhaka in Bangladesh on knowledge, attitude, and practices related to sanitation (Stanton et al., 1987).

29. For additional discussion of interviews, see Britten (1995).

30. See Kitzinger (1995) for further details and examples.

31. A useful introduction to the subject of research ethics as applied to epidemiology is the proceedings of the CIOMS conference (Bankowski et al., 1991),

which also reproduces the *International Guidelines*. The IEA's guidelines can be found in Last (1990). See also reviews by Soskolne (1989) and Coughlin and Beauchamp (1996). Callahan and Jennings (2002) discussed ethics and the broader discipline of public health.

32. See Lawlor and Stone (2001) on the implications of European and U.S. data protection legislations on public health practice and research.

33. See the Code of Ethics of the American Anthropological Association, approved in June 1998 (available on its web site, www.aaanet.org/committees/ethics/ethcode.htm).

34. See the review by Macaulay et al. (1999). The definition is from Green et al. (1995). A useful handbook on participatory research is Minkler and Wallerstein (2003).

35. The data are from Millar and Last (1988). The term *accident* is abhorred by injury prevention specialists since it connotes an event decided by fate and obscures the existence of preventable causes. They prefer "unintentional injuries" and use "crashes" for MVAs. Frost was appointed professor of epidemiology at Johns Hopkins University in Baltimore in 1921, the first one in the United States. For a discussion on statistical modelling in cohort analyses, see Holford (1991). Susser (2001) provides a historical perspective on cohort analysis.

36. Data for this case study are derived from Durkheim (1951 trans). See Berkman and Kawachi (2000:138–39) for an evaluation of his contributions to social epidemiology.

37. Crosby (1972) coined the term *Columbian exchange* to describe the import/export of flora, fauna, and microbes between the Old and New Worlds. From Europe, Native Americans received the horse, smallpox, and dandelion, among others. In the other direction went tobacco, corn, potato, and perhaps syphilis. A succinct history of tobacco can be found in the IARC monograph (1986), one of a series on carcinogenic agents. See Proctor (1997) on the Nazi war on tobacco and its political and historical context.

38. Mortality data from 1940–1960 are from Grove and Hetzel (1968), and for subsequent years, from various annual reports of *Health, United States*. Cancer of the respiratory system was the rubric used, rather than lung cancer specifically. All rates are directly standardized to the 1940 U.S. population. Cigarette consumption data originate from the U.S. Department of Agriculture.

39. Wynder and Graham (1950) and Levin et al. (1950) were published in the same issue of *JAMA*. According to the historical review by Susser (1985), the editors of *JAMA* were reluctant to publish the two papers because of the novelty of the findings.

40. Doll and Hill (1950) reported on the case-control study. The cohort study after 10 years of follow up was reported by Doll and Hill (1964). Subsequent reports appeared after 20 years (Doll and Peto, 1976) and 40 years of follow-up (Doll et al., 1994).

41. The Surgeon General's report on tobacco and health became an annual affair, keeping track of the burgeoning literature. Some reports have special themes, such as passive smoking, cardiovascular diseases, nicotine addiction, and ochronic obstructive lung diseases. The 1989 report commemorated the twenty-fifth anniversary of the first report.

42. The smoking and cancer literature is still growing. Vineis and Caporaso (1995) summarized the laboratory and experimental studies. Samet (1993) reviewed the epidemiological evidence, and Hennekens and Buring (1994) the strategies for control.

43. The UMFUS has spawned a large literature. Specific reports cited in this case study include Krahn et al. (1995) on atrial fibrillation, Mymin et al. (1986) on first-degree heart block, Rabkin et al. (1978) on blood pressure and stroke prognosis, and Tate et al. (1995) on blood pressure tracking.

EXERCISE 6.1.   Mantel-Haenszel Stratified Analysis

In a case-control study to evaluate the effectiveness of the Bacille-Calmette-Guérin (BCG) vaccine, cases of tuberculosis (TB) among Canadian Indian children under 15 years of age were selected from a provincial TB registry. Controls were randomly selected from the same communities from where the cases originated. The overall results can be presented in a 2 × 2 table:

	Cases	Controls
BCG	35	163
Non-BCG	36	50
Total	71	213

(a) Calculate the crude odds ratio to express the risk of vaccinated children in contracting TB.

The cases and controls can be stratified according to age:

	Stratum 1: Born 1965–1974			Stratum 2: Born 1975–1983	
	Cases	Controls		Cases	Controls
BCG	23	60	BCG	12	103
Non-BCG	29	33	Non-BCG	7	17

(b) Calculate the Mantel-Haenszel summary odds ratio combining data from the two strata.

Source: Young and Hershfield (1986)

EXERCISE 6.2.   Interaction of Smoking and Asbestos in Lung Cancer

The age-adjusted mortality rates for lung cancer (per 100,000 person-years) from two cohort studies in the United States and Canada are combined and arranged according to smoking and asbestos exposure status as follows.

	No asbestos	Asbestos
No smoking	11.3	58.4
Smoking	122.6	601.6

(a) Assigning the mortality rate of lung cancer among those exposed to neither asbestos nor smoking a value of 1.0, calculate the relative risk of lung cancer death among those exposed to asbestos but not smoking (RR_A), those exposed to smoking but not asbestos (RR_S), and those exposed to both risk factors (RR_{AS}).

(b) What is the relative risk of lung cancer from exposure to asbestos among smokers?

(c) Is there interaction based on an additive model? Is this indicative of synergism or antagonism?

(d) Do the data fit a multiplicative model?

Source: Saracci (1987)

EXERCISE 6.3.   Spot the Confounder!

Examine the following hypothetical studies and determine if the alleged confounder is indeed likely to be a confounder.

(a) A study found that people who use mouthwash are more likely to develop oral cancer. Can smoking be a confounder?

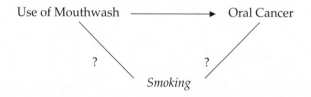

(b) Smoking causes lung cancer. Smokers also have yellow teeth. People with yellow teeth are also more likely to get lung cancer. Can yellow staining of teeth be the confounder?

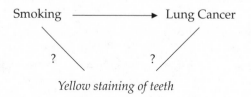

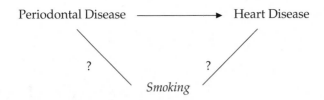

(c) Dental researchers have found that periodontal disease is a risk factor of heart disease. Since smoking is known to cause both heart disease and periodontal disease, can smoking be a confounder in the association between periodontal disease and heart disease?

7

Planning Population Health Interventions

Promoting Health, Preventing Disease

In Chapter 1, four tasks of population health were identified. Three of these were covered in the previous chapters—describing health, explaining causes, and predicting risks. This and the next chapter are concerned with the final task, that of controlling health problems.

Improving the health of the world's population was once thought to be a relatively simple matter: increase health services, build more hospitals, train more doctors, and so on. In the 1970s, the World Health Organization developed the concept of *primary health care* (PHC), which can qualify as a "paradigm shift" (see Chapter 1). In the landmark international conference in Alma Ata, USSR, in 1978, PHC was defined as:

> essential health care based on practical, scientifically sound and socially acceptable methods and technology made universally accessible to individuals and families in the community through their full participation and at a cost that the community and country can afford to maintain at every stage of their development in the spirit of self-reliance and self-determination.[1]

PHC was seen as the key instrument by which WHO's ambitious target of "Health for All by the Year 2000" (or HFA2000) would be achieved. In the years following, a debate arose within international development circles over the alternatives of *selective* vs. *comprehensive* PHC. Proponents of selective PHC argued that limited resources would prevent many health ministries from providing comprehensive PHC. Instead, resources should be concentrated on a limited number of strategies to achieve the most gains in health status for the least cost. Organizations such as UNICEF, for example, have promoted breast feeding, immunizations, and oral rehydration fluids—all inexpensive technologies—with spectacular reductions in childhood mortality in developing countries. Critics of this approach objected to its "biomedical" orientation and inadequate attention to redressing socioe-conomic inequities, improving basic infrastructure, and promoting commu-nity participation in health care that comprehensive PHC implies.[2]

PHC and HFA2000 are not designed only for developing countries. They are equally applicable to the industrialized countries, with adapta-tion to the much higher level of health care resources available, the differ-ent pattern of health and disease, and the existing mode of health services delivery. In the United States, the Surgeon General's landmark report *Healthy People*, released in 1979, identified five primary goals to enhance the health of Americans in five major life stages (infants, children, adoles-cents and young adults, adults, and older adults). Thus began the *Healthy People* process, which saw the publication in 1980 of detailed targets for measurable health objectives for the nation over the next decade, followed by *Healthy People 2000* (released in 1990) and *Healthy People 2010* (released in 2000). *Healthy People 2010* has two overarching goals: (1) increase qual-ity and years of healthy life, and (2) eliminate health disparities (with re-spect to gender, race/ethnicity, income/education, disability, geographic location, and sexual orientation). These two goals are essentially the same as those for *HP2000*. However, one goal in *HP2000*—that of achieving ac-cess to preventive services for all—was left out of *HP2010*.

To monitor the progress in achieving these goals, a variety of priority areas in health promotion, health protection, preventive services, and sur-veillance and data systems are identified. These objectives are all quantifi-able in terms of gains in health status (usually through reduction of disease), reduction in risk, and use of services. Brief descriptions of the 10 leading indicators used by *HP2010* can be found in Box 3.1 in Chapter 3.[3]

In 2000, the Institute of Medicine's Committee on Capitalizing on Social Science and Behavioral Research to Improve the Public's Health summa-rized the existing knowledge on promising and effective health promotion strategies.[4] Such interventions should:

1. Focus on generic social and behavioral determinants of disease, in-jury and disability;
2. Use multiple approaches and address multiple levels (from individ-uals to nations) of influence simultaneously;
3. Take account of special needs of target groups (based on age, sex, ethnicity, socioeconomic position);
4. Take long view of health outcomes, which may take years to become established;
5. Involve different sectors of society not traditionally associated with "health."

"Promoting health" and "preventing disease" are usually spoken in the same breath. Clearly both are needed to improve health of the population. Curiously, in some public health circles, the former is regarded as superior to the latter, because of its "positive" and "psychosocial" orientation. The emergence of new public health threats and resurgence of old foes in the early years of the twenty-first century is a strong reminder that disease prevention is still very much needed. Indeed, from a global perspective, the quality of life of millions of people will be immeasurably improved if we only "do" disease prevention, and leave health promotion for later, when more resources become available.

Population Health and the Health Care System

Up to this point, this book has not emphasized the health care system at all. Achievement of improved population health does involve the health care system, although neither exclusively nor predominantly. In most countries, whether developed or developing, the health care system serves several functions, of which improving the health of the population is one aspect. Others that come to mind include achieving equity, assuring quality, and creating employment.

Discussions of equity in health often confuse equity in health status with equity in health services. It should be clear that the latter is a secondary goal, subservient to the former. Services that are inequitably distributed should be redressed only if they have been shown to be effective, necessary, and beneficial. No one would argue for an equitable distribution of cigarettes, complete with price subsidy for disadvantaged populations! Similarly with quality of care—this cannot be the end in itself. We pursue quality only insofar that it will contribute to improved health. The best-run hospital has no patients, only administrators.

Components of the health care system that can potentially contribute to improved population health include public health and primary care. One attempt to combine primary care with public health is the concept of *community-oriented primary care* (COPC). As defined by its proponents, it refers to the complementary use of epidemiological and primary-care skills to address systematically the health care needs of a defined population.[5] COPC is not simply health services as traditionally provided by family physicians in their offices, but has the following features:

- Primary care is accessible, comprehensive, coordinated, continuous, and accountable;
- It is delivered within a defined community, which does not refer just to the users of a single physician practice; in fact, it aims to reorient the focus of services from "patients" ("numerator") to "the community" (denominator);
- It addresses major health problems by (1) defining and characterizing the population; (2) identifying community health problems; (3) modifying health care program to address priority health needs; and (4) monitoring the effectiveness of program modification.

While COPC has the potential to improve the health of a population by integrating curative and preventive health services, it is still the exception rather than the rule in the North American setting.

The remainder of this chapter focuses on the basic principles of disease prevention and health promotion, rather than on the organization, administration, and delivery of health services in general.

Types and Levels of Interventions

A health intervention can be defined as an action that reduces the frequency, duration, or severity of disease and promotes the health and well-being of the individual, family or community. Although such terms as *primary*, *secondary*, and *tertiary* prevention are often used in the public health literature, their inconsistent usage has led to some confusion, and they are best avoided, with the exception of primary prevention. Instead, five major types of interventions are recognized, based on various points in the natural history of disease where they act (Box 7.1). These are primary prevention, early detection, clinical treatment, rehabilitation, and palliation.

Primary prevention is often regarded as prevention in the true sense of the word; i.e., intervention occurring before the onset of disease. While the individual may be well, he or she may already be exposed to various behavioral and environmental risk factors whose presence promotes the development of disease. Primary prevention then reduces the level of risk factors in a population. There may also be situations where such exposure has not yet occurred; primary prevention then acts to prevent the exposure to risk factors in the first place (some authors emphasize the distinction by calling this *primordial* prevention).

There are three basic strategies for primary prevention:

1. Promoting healthy behavior, or *health promotion*: individuals are advised, cajoled, threatened to alter their behaviors relating to diet, personal and household hygiene, sexual activity, physical activity, tobacco and drug use, and safety practices at home, in the workplace, or during transportation.
2. Controlling environmental hazards: to ensure a safe and healthful indoor and outdoor environment by improving water supply, waste disposal, food hygiene, housing standards, air quality, occupational health, and the design of vehicles and corridors of transportation. This is often referred to as *health protection*.
3. Increasing host resistance, or reducing the susceptibility to disease, through improving nutritional status, immunizations, and chemoprophylaxis (i.e., the use of antibiotics after exposure to infection to abort the development of full-blown disease, or reduce its severity or contagiousness). Many of these activities are delivered within the context of personal health services.

BOX 7.1.   Natural History of Disease and Levels of Intervention

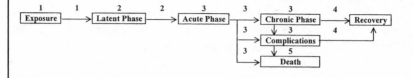

Impact on Measures of Health Status

	Incidence	Prevalence	Mortality	Case-Fatality	Quality of Life
1 Primary prevention	↓	↓	↓	–	–
2 Early detection	↑	↑	↓	↓	↑
3 Clinical treatment	–	↑	↓	↓	↑
4 Rehabilitation	–	–	–	–	↑
5 Palliation	–	–	–	–	↑

A comprehensive list of such interventions and the health conditions at which they are directed is given in Box 7.2. Primary prevention can be either active or passive. The former requires an individual to have the motivation to initiate a specific action, such as putting on a seatbelt, eating the right foods, brushing teeth, or stopping smoking. To prevent the same health problems by passive means—which do not require individual action—would involve airbags in cars that are activated upon impact, marketing of "lean" meats, fluoridation of community water supplies, and enacting municipal bylaws against smoking in public. It is not a matter of either-or, but of choosing the best mix of active and passive measures to achieve a stated health objective.

While primary prevention can be provided by all types of health care providers, it need not even be an exclusive responsibility of the health care system. As the list indicates, other sectors of society must also be involved if some of the strategies are to be implemented.

Early detection, also called *screening* when it is applied cheaply, rapidly, and on a large scale, takes place at the early stages of the disease process, usually before the onset of signs and symptoms. Sometimes these are presented as "packages" aimed at specific target groups at regular intervals—the periodic health examination (PHE). Screening is discussed in more detail below.

Clinical treatment can be offered to an individual when signs and symptoms of disease prompt the individual to seek help from a health professional. In the primary care setting, the treatment of minor illnesses

BOX 7.2.   Primary Prevention Strategies and Their Targeted Health Conditions

Strategy[6]	Health Conditions
Promoting Healthy Personal Behavior	
Nutrition and diet	Low birth weight, childhood infections, nutrient deficiencies, obesity, diabetes, cancer, hypertension, ischemic heart disease, dental caries
Personal/domestic hygiene	Diarrheal diseases, intestinal parasites, skin infections
Sexual behavior	Sexually transmitted diseases, unplanned pregnancy
Physical activity	Obesity, heart disease, diabetes, musculoskeletal problems
Tobacco use	Cancer, heart disease, chronic lung disease
Safety practices (vehicles, machinery)	Unintentional injuries
Alcohol and drug use	Addiction, dependence, abuse; unintentional injuries and violence; cirrhosis (alcohol), certain infections (intravenous drugs)
Contraceptive practices	Unplanned pregnancy
Knowledge of first aid	Injuries
Control of Environmental Hazards	
Water supply	Diarrheal diseases, intestinal parasites, skin infections
Waste disposal	Diarrheal diseases, intestinal parasites
Food hygiene	Diarrheal diseases, intestinal parasites
Air quality	Respiratory disease, toxic exposures
Housing quality	Respiratory disease, injuries, mental stress
Transportation safety	Unintentional injuries

(continued)

Occupational safety	Unintentional injuries, toxic exposures
Increasing Host Resistance/Reducing Susceptibility	
Immunizations	Selected infectious diseases
Chemoprophylaxis	Selected infectious diseases
Breast feeding	Childhood infections
Water fluoridation	Dental caries

using a small list of essential drugs can be effectively and competently performed by non-physicians such as nurses and health auxiliaries.[7]

Rehabilitation aims to return an individual after an illness or injury to full or partial functional capacity, and usually involves one or more of the rehabilitation professions, the use of prosthetic devices and physical aids, and active participation by the individual and his or her family. Rehabilitation sometimes also requires environmental redesign, such as restructuring the home, public buildings, and transportation to facilitate access, mobility, and the performance of daily activities.

An often-neglected intervention is palliation, offered to individuals with incurable or terminal illness for which adequate pain relief as well as other procedures to enhance the quality of life and maintain life support are needed. Much palliation takes place in long-term-care institutions, and, in recent years, hospices that cater to the physical and psychological needs of the terminally ill. In some communities there may be a cultural preference for the terminally ill to die at home among familiar surroundings.

Box 7.1 also shows the impact of these interventions on various indicators of population health status. The incidence of a disease can only be reduced through primary prevention. By detecting early disease among asymptomatic individuals, screening can actually, at least initially, increase the incidence and prevalence of a disease. Screening, if effective, can reduce mortality and, if followed by efficacious treatment, improve the quality of life. By improving survival, treatment also increases prevalence.

This chapter is concerned primarily with the first two types of interventions, which are traditionally included under the rubric of prevention. Public health workers are firm believers in the adage that prevention is better than cure. It should be recognized, however, that prevention does entail resource costs and health risks. As with treatment, preventive strategies also need to be rigorously evaluated (see Chapter 8) if the objective of improving health status is to be achieved.[8]

The economic argument for prevention is actually fallacious. Prevention rarely reduces health expenditures, contrary to popular belief. While the mortality rate of the population in a given year may decrease, in reality

---

BOX 7.3.   Words and Origins

One of the earliest forms of health protection was quarantine, physical separation of the sick from the well. During the Black Death in medieval Europe, officials in Venice inspected all ships entering port. While the sick were barred from leaving the ship, even apparently well visitors were also detained for 40 days to see if disease would develop in the interval. "Quarante giorni" became *quarantine*. Quarantine works if the period of isolation exceeds the incubation period of the disease—the duration from infection to the appearance of signs and symptoms ("incubate"—to hatch, from the Latin *incubare*, to lie on). It is interesting to observe that in 2003, during the outbreak of the Severe Acute Respiratory Syndrome (SARS) in China, Hong Kong, Taiwan, Canada, and other countries, quarantine was used extensively, in the face of a new pathogen for which there was no effective treatment or vaccine.

Edward Jenner (1749–1823) pioneered vaccination in 1796 by injecting into the arm of a young boy materials from the pustule of a patient with cowpox (*vacca* being the Latin word for "cow"). It replaced an early, riskier practice of variolation, which used the pus from smallpox patients (smallpox: *Variola*, a name in use since the sixth century). The history of smallpox and its eradication is chronicled in Case Study 7.1. In 1881, Louis Pasteur (1822–1895), in honor of Jenner, generalized the use of the term *vaccination* to include the preventive inoculation of all kinds of infectious agents.

Prophylaxis [from the Greek *pro* (before) + *phulaxis* (guarding)] is sometimes used to mean prevention in general. In the control of infectious diseases, *chemoprophylaxis* refers to the use of drugs to prevent the development of disease after infection, as in prescribing isoniazid for those who have converted from negative to positive on tuberculin testing. In cancer control, the term *chemoprevention* is used, referring to the use of naturally occurring or synthetic substances (beta-carotene in certain foods, the drug tamoxifen, etc.) that inhibit carcinogenesis. For obscure reasons, the polysyllabic word *prophylactics* is widely used by the general public to mean condoms!

---

deaths are never prevented, only postponed. The more effective prevention is, the longer people live, and the higher the costs of social and health services for the elderly! According to British epidemiologist Geoffrey Rose, the only and sufficient argument for prevention is a humanitarian one—it is better to be healthy than ill or dead. The benefits of prevention may only be appreciated at the population level. Indeed, many preventive measures that brings large benefits to the community often offer little to each participating individual (the prevention paradox). Sometimes, individuals may actually suffer harm, as in complications from immunizations.

An important consideration in the implementation of a health intervention is its intended target. Should it be directed only at individuals who are at high risk, or should it be applied to the entire population? Rose contrasted the high risk strategy (HRS) with the population strategy (PS). HRS is familiar to clinicians—it is selective, individual-based, and avoids interference with those not at special risk. Its overall impact in terms of reduction of the disease burden in the population may be small, although individuals receiving the intervention tend to benefit the most. PS recognizes that the occurrence of diseases reflects the behavior and circumstances of society as a whole, which is more than a collection of individuals. Diseases and risk factors vary tremendously across populations. By shifting the entire distribution of a risk factor in a favorable direction, large benefits tend to accrue to the whole population. Data from large cohort studies and randomized trials suggest that a reduction of only 2 mmHg of a population's mean diastolic blood pressure (DBP) can decrease new stroke cases by as much as 14%, which is comparable to targeted medical treatment of all individuals with DBP $\geq$ 95 mmHg. A population strategy involving public education and regulatory changes is far less costly than screening high-risk individuals and administering antihypertensive drugs. The lowering of fat consumption by the entire population is believed to be more effective in reducing heart disease incidence than prescribing cholesterol-lowering drugs for individuals with very high plasma cholesterol values. Fluoridating a community's water supply protects everybody from dental caries, whether they brush their teeth or not. The HRS puts the focus on relative risk, while the PS emphasizes the population attributable risk (see Chapter 5) in determining what is important for interventions.[9]

Criteria for Screening

Screening is intrinsically attractive—one would want to detect disease before it is too late for effective treatment to succeed. In the 1920s the American Medical Association was recommending the annual physical examination for healthy persons. It is hardly surprising that the physician's perfunctory listening for heart murmurs, palpating for a large spleen, and tapping the knee to elicit the reflex, among other ministrations that constitute the "routine" physical, are unlikely to be of much use in detecting nasty diseases lurking in the body. Screening has evolved towards the execution of specific maneuvers directed at specific diseases and target groups such as children, elderly men, pregnant women, and so on.

A definition of *screening* was offered by the Commission on Chronic Illness, a national voluntary agency in the United States formed in the 1950s to study means to control the emergent chronic diseases:

the presumptive identification of unrecognized disease or defect by the application of tests, examinations, or other procedures which can be applied rapidly. [They] sort out apparently well persons who probably have a disease from those who probably do not.[10]

Wilson and Jungner, in a 1968 WHO monograph, enumerated 10 criteria upon which the decision to conduct screening should be based:

1. The condition sought should be an important health problem;
2. There should be an accepted treatment for patients with recognized disease;
3. Facilities for diagnosis and treatment should be available;
4. There should be a recognizable latent or early symptomatic stage;
5. There should be a suitable test or examination;
6. The test should be acceptable to the population;
7. The natural history of the condition, including development from latent to declared disease, should be adequately understood;
8. There should be an agreed policy on whom to treat as patients;
9. The cost of case-finding should be economically balanced in relation to possible expenditure on medical care as a whole;
10. Case-finding should be a continuing process and not a "once and for all" project.

Other authors have proposed similar guidelines. Some add conditions that a test should have been shown to be effective by randomized controlled trials and that those who have been screened positive and recommended treatment are likely to comply with it.[11]

In the 1970s the Canadian Task Force on the Periodic Health Examinations spearheaded the critical review of the literature for evidence of effectiveness and published guidelines for physicians. This was followed by the U.S. Preventive Services Task Force in 1984. The two organizations collaborate closely, and their guidelines are largely comparable. These reports are not concerned exclusively with screening or early detection, but also evaluate other preventive services such as counseling, immunizations, dietary supplementation, etc.[12] The quality of the evidence that the intervention is effective is central to the whole enterprise. Both task forces rank studies on the basis of research design, with randomized controlled trials at the top (category I); followed by non-randomized trials (II-1); cohort or case-control studies (II-2); multiple time series, uncontrolled experiments (II-3); and lastly, expert opinions, clinical experience, and descriptive studies (III).

As the examples in Box 7.4 illustrate, not all "A" procedures are supported by Category I evidence. There are many situations where an RCT is not feasible, unethical, or too costly. Some interventions cannot be randomized or blinded. Some outcomes may be too rare and would require a large sample and long followup.[13]

Enthusiasts for screening are often fooled by biases that produce apparent benefits when none in fact exists. *Lead-time bias* occurs when

BOX 7.4.   To Screen or Not to Screen?

The following are examples of screening maneuvers considered by the Canadian and U.S. Task Forces, with their associated ratings in terms of strength of recommendation and quality of evidence of effectiveness.[14]

Screening maneuver	Disease/ health condition	Age-sex group	Highest level of evidence
A. Good evidence to support inclusion			
phenylalanine level	phenylketonuria	newborn	II-3
thyroxine/thyroid stimulating hormone level	congenital hypothyroidism	newborn	II-3
hip examination	congenital dislocation of hip	infants	II-2
mammography ± clinical examination	breast cancer	F, 50-69	I
Papanicolaou smear	cervical cancer	sexually active F	II-2
blood pressure measurement	hypertension	≥21	I
hepatitis B surface antigen	hepatitis B	pregnant F	I
D(Rh) antibodies	D(Rh) incompatibility	pregnant F	I
urine culture	bacteriuria	pregnant F	I
B. Fair evidence to support inclusion			
height and weight measurement	obesity	all ages	I
growth monitoring	short stature (endocrine)	infants	II-2
vision examination	amblyopia, strabismus	preschoolers	II-1
rubella antibodies	congenital rubella syndrome	F, childbearing age	II-2
serum total cholesterol	coronary heart disease	M, 35–65; F, 45–65	I
fecal occult blood ± sigmoidoscopy	colorectal cancer	≥50	I
hemoglobin/ hematocrit	anemia	pregnant F	II-1
maternal serum multiple-marker	Down's syndrome	pregnant F	II-2
maternal α-fetoprotein	neural tube defects	pregnant F	II-2
fetal ultrasonography during 2nd trimester	perinatal mortality/ morbidity	pregnant F	I

(continued)

Screening maneuver	Disease/ health condition	Age-sex group	Highest level of evidence
C. Poor evidence to support inclusion			
hemoglobin	anemia	infants	I
hearing test	hearing impairment	children > 3	II-2
back examination	scoliosis	adolescents	II-2
electrocardiography	coronary heart disease	middle age, elderly	II-2
mammography	breast cancer	F, 40–49	I
glucose challenge test	diabetes	adults	II-2
D. Fair evidence to support exclusion			
Denver developmental scale	developmental problems	preschoolers	I
General Health Questionnaire	depression	adults	I
chest X-ray/sputum cytology	lung cancer	adults	I
prostate specific antigen/digital rectal exam	prostate cancer	M, adults	II-2
E. Good evidence to support exclusion			
urine dipstick	urinary infection	children	I
Mantoux skin test	tuberculosis	all ages	II-2

screening advances the time of diagnosis among those screened, apparently increasing survival time. (Think of the Book of Life: suppose, on page 10, cancer develops insidiously inside your body; on page 20, clinical signs and symptoms appear, which lead to detection; and on page 30, you die. There are thus 10 pages between detection and death. If screening results in detection occurring earlier, say, on page 15, but you still die on page 30, it gives the impression of prolonging life by five pages. It is only if screening results in death occurring beyond page 30, say page 35, that it can be considered effective in prolonging life.)

Another bias, called *length bias*, occurs when screening preferentially detects slow-growing disease and misses aggressive and rapidly progressive cases that are present in the population only briefly. The group that is screened thus appears to have a better survival because of the higher proportion of low-grade lesions and non–life-threatening disease.

Screening need not be directed only at detecting the presence of disease. Often it is done in the context of establishing the risk profile of an individual

BOX 7.5. What Works in Community Prevention?

The U.S. and Canadian preventive services task forces mentioned earlier are directed mainly at personal health services, especially those under the supervision of physicians and the primary care system. In 1996 the Task Force on Community Preventive Services, under the leadership of the CDC, was convened to conduct and publish systematic reviews on community-based interventions to prevent disease and promote health.[15] Such interventions are graded into: (1) recommended—strong evidence; (2) recommended—sufficient evidence; (3) insufficient evidence to determine effectiveness; and (4) recommended against. Among interventions that have been graded as "recommended based on strong evidence" are:

Topic	Intervention
I. Changing health-risk behaviors	
Reducing exposure to environmental smoke	—Smoking bans and restrictions
Reducing initiation/increasing cessation of smoking	—Increasing unit price of tobacco products; mass media campaign
Increasing physical activity	—Community-wide campaigns
	—School-based physical education; individually-adapted behavior change programs; social support in community settings
	—Enhanced access to facilities + information outreach
II. Reducing specific health conditions	
Dental caries	—Community water fluoridation; school-based dental sealant delivery programs
Diabetes	—Case management
Motor vehicle occupant injury	—Blood alcohol concentration laws; maintaining legal drinking age at 21; sobriety checkpoints
	—Child safety seat laws; distribution and education programs
	—Enactment and enforcement of safety belt laws

(continued)

Topic	Intervention
Vaccine-preventable diseases	—Expanding access to vaccination services in medical offices or public health clinics; reducing out-of-pocket costs —Client reminder/recall systems —Provider reminder/recall systems; assessment and feedback for providers
III. Addressing environmental challenges	
Promote healthy social environments	—Early childhood development programs

for certain diseases. For example, cholesterol screening is not done to detect the presence of heart disease, but the level of risk for future heart disease. While most physiological variables are continuously distributed, cutoff points that followup action is based on are arbitrary, dichotomizing individuals into "positive" and "negative" (see Chapter 3). Invitations for screening have a tendency to emphasize the benefits of participation, while underplaying the possible harms and uncertainties. Categorizing an individual as being "at risk"—called "labeling"—has been shown to be associated with adverse psychological effects. Some authorities—for example, the National Screening Committee in the United Kingdom—advocate a shift from the traditional public health approach to screening to one based on individual, informed choice. Although the participation rate may be affected, it is believed that individuals participating in screening after having made an informed choice to do so are more likely to have realistic expectations and a stronger motivation to change their behavior.[16]

Behavioral Models for Health Promotion

Because the health conditions it targets comprise the most important contemporary causes of morbidity and mortality, health promotion has become the major strategy in primary prevention.[17] The key element in this strategy is changing behavior, which may be health-directed or health-related. Health-directed behavior is conscious behavior with the goal to improve health (e.g., eating low-fat foods), whereas health-related behavior is unconscious, pursued for non-health purposes but with health consequences (e.g., losing weight to improve one's physical appearance, living in a house with flush toilets). Traditional health education is directed at voluntary changes in behavior by individuals. It is now subsumed under health promotion, which is broadened to include also environmental

PRECEDE

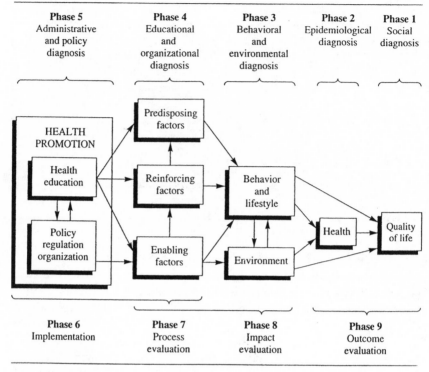

Figure 7.1. The PRECEDE/PROCEED model of health promotion planning. Reprinted from: Green LW, Kreuter MW. *Health Promotion Planning: An Educational and Environmental Approach*, 2nd ed., with kind permission from Mayfield Publishing Company.

supports (policy, regulatory, and organizational) for both individual actions and social conditions that are conducive to health. Promoters of health promotion attempt to deflect much criticism aimed at health education for being preoccupied with causation and intervention at the individual level by showing their awareness of social responsibility for health and their willingness to seek broader institutional and social change.

Lawrence Green and associates have developed a framework for planning, implementing, and evaluating health promotion, called PRECEDE-PROCEED (Figure 7.1). PRECEDE is an acronym of "predisposing, reinforcing, enabling constructs in educational and environmental diagnosis and evaluation" while PROCEED stands for "policy, regulatory, organizational constructs in educational and environmental development." Predisposing factors are characteristics of a person that motivate behavior prior to the occurrence of the behavior, and include knowledge, attitudes, beliefs, values, and perceptions. Enabling factors are characteristics of the environment that facilitate action and any skill or resource required to attain a specific behavior. Reinforcing factors represent either rewards or punishments that follow or are anticipated as a consequence of a behavior, serving to strengthen the motivation for the behavior after it occurs. As an example, a person who takes up jogging knows about and believes in the health benefits of physical exercise. A safe, tree-lined neighborhood provides an ideal environment for jogging, and having an executive job gives her maximum flexibility to pursue the activity during working hours. Evidence of some weight loss and a perception that her job appears less stressful as a result of the jogging encourage her to persist in her daily routine.

In planning specific health promotion activities, it is necessary to understand why people behave as they do when dealing with health and disease. Health promotion planners have drawn on the work of social scientists and adapted some of their models of human behavior to health.[18] The *health belief model* (HBM) was developed in the 1950s when psychologists at the U.S. Public Health Service attempted to understand the widespread failure of people to accept disease prevention and screening. The model contends that individuals behave in a particular way based on their perception of (1) how susceptible they are to the disease, (2) how serious the disease is, (3) what benefits they will derive from taking preventive/curative action, and (4) what it will cost them. Thus a smoker may know full well the serious health consequences, but does not think anything will happen to him. After weighing the benefit of quitting against the disadvantages (irritability, weight gain) he decides to continue smoking. In the words of Irwin Rosenstock, one of the model's early proponents, "the combined levels of susceptibility and severity provides the energy or force to act, and the perception of benefits (less barriers) provides a preferred path of action." The decision-making process is triggered by some stimulus (or cue to action) which can be internal (a symptom) or external (mass media, advice from others, illness of a family member). Perceptions of susceptibility and severity are also modified by demographic and psychosocial variables.

Complementary to the HBM is *social cognitive theory*, developed by Albert Bandura, which "embraces an interactional model of causation in which environmental events, personal factors, and behavior all operate as interacting determinants of each other." The theory emphasizes the social origin of human thought and the role of thought in human motivation and action; i.e., cognitive control. An individual learns by direct experience and, more frequently, by observing other's behaviors and consequences. In the process of such "modeling," the person acquires rules for generating and regulating behavior, without the need for trial and error. Behavior is strongly influenced by self-regulation, evaluating one's action in terms of personal standards; and self-reflection, analyzing experience to alter thinking. Confidence in one's own ability to perform a task, which affects whether a thought is translated into action, is called *self-efficacy*.

In their *theory of reasoned action*, Icek Ajzen and Martin Fishbein contend that behavior is governed by intentions, which in turn are determined by personal and societal attitudes towards the behavior. *Attitude* is formed by a person's belief that a particular behavior will lead to certain outcomes and his own evaluation of these outcomes. The opinion of influential individuals or groups ("referents") in the community provide the social norm that motivates the individual to decide to comply or not. Thus a new mother's breastfeeding behavior is determined by her intentions about breastfeeding before and during pregnancy. Such intentions are formed by her personal beliefs that breastfeeding is beneficial on one hand, and the favorable opinions of spouses, parents, and community leaders on the other.

These overlapping psychosocial theories and models are often implicitly incorporated in the design and implementation of community-based health promotion programs, such as the North Karelia (see Case Study 7.3), the Stanford Five Cities, and the Minnesota Heart Health projects.

Cross-Cultural Considerations

In the 1950s, Benjamin Paul, one of the pioneers of integrating the social sciences into international health and development work, warned against cultural misunderstanding when planning and implementing interventions. Public health workers from Western countries (or for that matter, local workers trained in the Western scientific tradition) tend to think of the targets of their interventions as "captives of blind customs," whereas they themselves are rational beings free of cultural peculiarities. They think that their ways are more advanced and that the local people need to "catch up" to their level. They also fail to recognize the linkages between different customs and beliefs within a cultural complex, and that introduction of a health intervention may have unexpected dislocations in other aspects of community life. An example is building latrines in rural areas of developing countries so people would not have to defecate in the bush and contaminate the water supply. Yet many such sanitation programs are poorly accepted or used. In some villages, women take time off from their grinding domestic chores and go to the river banks as a group, not only to perform toiletry and bathing, but to socialize. Understandably, they are not prepared to give up this important custom. Steven Polgar, a medical anthropologist, enumerated four common fallacies in cross-cultural health interventions:

1. Fallacy of the empty vessel—there are no established health customs, only a void waiting for whatever program is being introduced;
2. Fallacy of the separate capsule—health beliefs and practices are separate compartments from the larger culture;

3. Fallacy of the single pyramid—society is monolithic, hierarchically organized, and all one needs to do is to convince the leaders and the rest will follow suit;
4. Fallacy of the interchangeable faces—all natives are alike![19]

Ellen Corin, another medical anthropologist, offers the following general principles for health intervention programs:[20]

- Programs have to be culturally and socially acceptable and appropriate.
- They have to build on and reinforce a community's strengths and insights and not contribute to a collective sense of inadequacy or fragility by well-intentioned actions.
- Before trying to modify attitudes and behaviors it is important to understand their cultural origins and significance, their present function, and their place within community life.
- It is important to assess local perceptions of the relative importance and the degrees of tolerance or intolerance of various problems in a given community.
- The concept of "at-risk group" should be complemented by that of "target conditions," which arise out of a complex web of social and cultural determinants in a given environment.

A Broader View of Prevention

In discussing strategies to improve the health of populations, all too frequently attention is focused on specific interventions, such as those evaluated by the U.S. Preventive Services Task Force and the Canadian Task Force on the Periodic Health Examination. While such groups have made a major contribution by emphasizing the need for rigorous scientific standards in determining effectiveness, their focus is primarily clinical prevention—preventive activities such as screening, counseling, and immunizations, which are performed by physicians in their practices. Sometimes the bigger picture becomes lost. In fact, the improvement of health ultimately requires moving out of the health sector altogether. John McKinlay, among others, advocated moving "upstream" from individual-based treatment (downstream), through primary prevention and screening (midstream), towards a social policy approach.[21] Upstream interventions include efforts to change government policies, organizational practices, and provider behaviors, which affect the entire population and its social norms and macroeconomic structure. It is thus not so much fine-tuning public health policy, but developing a *healthy public policy*, that will have the most impact on health.

Individual behavior changes cannot occur if they are persistently thwarted by the environment and social norms. On the other hand,

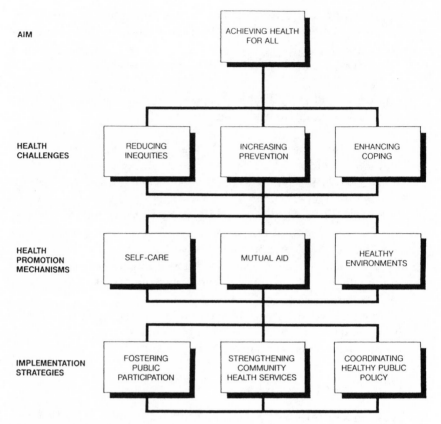

Figure 7.2. A conceptual framework for population health. Reprinted from *Achieving Health for All: A Framework for Health Promotion.* Ottawa: Health and Welfare Canada, 1986.

governments and legislatures are reluctant to initiate policy changes or enact regulations if there is no widespread social consensus that such changes are desirable. Clearly, there is no single formula for improving the health of populations. All possible avenues must be explored, from the "macro" to the "micro."

Figure 7.2 presents one vision of a strategy to improve population health that incorporates individual and community action, and health services and public policy.

The definition of primary health care at the beginning of this chapter recognizes the linkage between health and community development. Community development has many interpretations and understandings. A useful definition, taken from a standard text on applied anthropology, is as follows:

> Community development is a process of social action in which the people of a community organize themselves for planning and action; define their

---

BOX 7.6.   Upstream and Downstream in Diabetes Prevention

There is an epidemic of diabetes in many populations around the world. Among the risk factors found to be associated with the emergence of diabetes are genetic susceptibility, age, sex, ethnicity, socioeconomic status, obesity, body fat distribution, physical activity, diet, and stress. These operate at a variety of levels, from the molecular to the population. Traditionally, diabetes is managed in the clinical setting, the preserve of physicians, nutritionists, and diabetes educators. There is an increasing recognition that diabetes should be viewed as a public health problem. John McKinlay and Lisa Marceau conceived of a balanced strategy to prevent and control diabetes that involve upstream (healthy public policy), midstream (prevention), and downstream (treatment) measures.[22]

Upstream measures:	National health insurance (in those countries that don't have them)
	Tax incentives for private-sector screening
	Environmental programs to facilitate exercise
Midstream measures:	Community-based primary prevention (directed at diet and physical activity)
	Physician-provider education
	Work site risk reduction
Downstream measures:	Local community screening
	Individual counseling to modify lifestyles
	Tight glycemic control

---

common and individual needs and problems, make group and individual plans to meet their needs and solve their problems; execute the plans with a maximum reliance on community resources; and supplement these resources where necessary with services and materials from . . . agencies outside the community.[23]

Community development must permeate health planning at all stages. While recognizing the difficulties of translating rhetoric into practical actions, health planners must constantly evaluate their proposals in terms of whether they enhance or inhibit community development.

Broadening the definition of health and recognizing the importance of addressing the determinants does not mean that the health care system must take on responsibilities in all areas that have an impact on health. That education, employment, and housing have an overwhelming impact on health status does not mean that the health care system should be teaching children arithmetic, conducting adult literacy and job training

classes, or building safe and affordable homes. At the political level, decisions can certainly be made that resources allocated to conventional
health services may well be diverted to non–health care but health-
enhancing programs such as improving housing. Within the arena of the
health care system, the scope of health care services must be limited for
them to be manageable and effective. The health care system cannot do
everything, but for the things that it does do, it must do well. In the next
chapter, the basic concepts and techniques of health program evaluation
are discussed.

Summary

This chapter introduces the strategies directed at improving the health of
populations, from comprehensive, community-oriented primary care to
specific interventions that correspond to different stages in the natural
history of disease: primary prevention, early detection, treatment, rehabilitation, and palliation. Primary prevention reduces exposure to risk factors prior to the development of disease and can be achieved through
promoting healthy personal behaviors, controlling environmental hazards, and increasing host resistance and reducing susceptibility to disease.
A combination of active and passive measures should be attempted for
any health objective. The largest health benefit, however, is more likely to
result from a population strategy than a high-risk strategy, by shifting the
entire distribution of a risk factor in the population in a favorable direction. Screening—early detection applied cheaply, rapidly, and on a mass
scale—should be implemented only if certain conditions are met, especially the existence of good-quality evidence of its effectiveness. Lead-
time and length biases can produce apparent improvement in survival.
The planning of health promotion requires understanding of behavioral
change, of which several theoretical models have been developed. Health
intervention in the cross-cultural setting must avoid certain pitfalls and
fallacies. Ultimately, the goal of improving the health of populations cannot be achieved by the health sector alone. Health programs must move
upstream towards healthy public policy and community development.

Case Study 7.1.   The Global Eradication of Smallpox

The eradication of smallpox from the face of the earth counts as one
of the most important achievements of the human species in the
twentieth century. Smallpox is an acute viral disease characterized
by pustular eruptions on the skin and associated with severe debility and often death.[24] It is spread primarily through the respiratory
route. There is no effective treatment other than supportive care.
Survivors are disfigured by pockmarks but are conferred lifelong
immunity. The smallpox virus (variola) is a member of the orthopox

viruses, which also include cowpox, monkeypox, and others. It is a uniquely human disease with no known animal reservoir.

The disease is of great antiquity—the scars still visible on the skin of some Egyptian mummies are suggestive of smallpox. Ancient Chinese and Indian medical texts provide clinical descriptions of the disease. By the tenth century it was already endemic throughout the populated centers of the known world, spread by trade, wars, exploration, and migration. The arrival of Europeans in the Americas triggered devastating epidemics that decimated entire tribes of Native Americans. By the end of the eighteenth century, smallpox was truly a global disease. It was no respecter of class or wealth, afflicting royalty, bishops, and peasants alike.

Efforts to prevent smallpox in the form of variolation were developed in China and India by the tenth century. Small quantities of pustular fluid or powdered dried scabs from a patient containing live virus were introduced to a healthy person by the intranasal route in China and subcutaneous route in India. The subcutaneous method was introduced to Europe via the Ottoman Empire. Lady Mary Wortley Montagu (1689–1742), whose husband was the British ambassador to Constantinople and who was severely pockmarked herself, was credited with the introduction of variolation to Britain, where it was widely practiced in all strata of society. The practice was effective, but also dangerous. The inoculated could die from smallpox, while family and community contacts could become infected.

Edward Jenner (1749–1823), an English country doctor, noted that variolation failed to "take" in individuals who had contracted cowpox before. It was widely believed in Europe at the time that milkmaids, who frequently contracted cowpox from cows, appeared not to be susceptible to smallpox. Jenner believed that cowpox somehow conferred protection against smallpox, and he tested his idea in 1796 when he inoculated a boy with cowpox matter taken from the hand of a milkmaid. Several weeks later he inoculated the boy with smallpox, but it did not take. Jenner published his observations in a book in 1798. He was prophetic when he predicted in his book that with vaccination, smallpox would one day be eradicated. Despite some opposition, the practice was soon widely disseminated. By the middle of the nineteenth century, smallpox vaccination was made legally compulsory in most European countries.

Certain virological and epidemiological characteristics of smallpox favor its eradication. It is a serious disease that is easily recognized without the need for sophisticated clinical training or laboratory facilities. There is no asymptomatic long-term carrier state; i.e., all infected persons can be identified, allowing contacts to be vaccinated, the main control strategy. For the virus to be maintained in a population, the chain of transmission from person to person must be

maintained. There is no animal reservoir to replenish the virus supply after it has died out in the human population, and insect vectors
are not involved in transmission. The period of infectivity is relatively short (two to three weeks), making it easy for patient isolation
to prevent spread.

The smallpox vaccine is highly effective—the vaccinated maintains 100% immunity for about three years, which then slowly
wanes over 10 years. It leaves a telltale scar, an important feature in
regions where there is little record keeping. It can be cheaply produced, and the freeze-dried form is heat-stable and can withstand
the tropical heat without spoiling.

The efficacy of smallpox vaccination was never demonstrated by
a randomized controlled trial. Yet wherever it was introduced the
practice had such a dramatic effect on incidence and mortality that
few could challenge its efficacy.

The graph below compares mortality rate in two German states in
the nineteenth century, where a law of compulsory vaccination at
age two and revaccination at age 12 was introduced in 1874; and
Austria, where there was no such law.

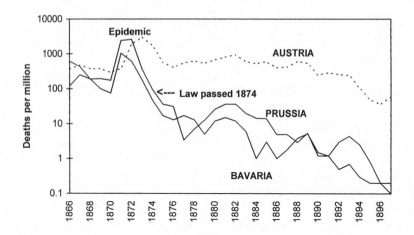

One type of evidence of efficacy is the comparison of secondary attack rates in the course of an outbreak investigation. Various studies
in India and Pakistan during the 1960s indicated that contacts who
had been vaccinated were much less likely to develop smallpox than
those who had not been vaccinated (with relative risks ranging from
0.03 to 0.09, which translates into protective efficacy of at least 90%).

By the 1940s most industrialized countries were already free of endemic smallpox, although they were still subject to importations and
hence maintained vaccination programs for the general population,
especially travelers to endemic countries. In the developing countries,

smallpox continued to rage. In 1959, the Twelfth World Health Assembly (WHA) first resolved to eradicate smallpox globally, but there was no special program with a dedicated budget, and little progress was made. In 1966, at the Nineteenth WHA, an intensified program with specially designated funds was launched.

The program consisted of a special unit at WHO headquarters in Geneva and also in regional offices located in endemic areas. Since quality vaccine was critical to the success of the program, international centers for quality control were set up in Toronto and Bilthoven, Netherlands. While special epidemiological and administrative assistance was provided to member states, it was individual national programs that carried out the task of surveillance, case detection, and outbreak containment. This strategy, when carried out promptly and vigorously, was more cost-effective than mass vaccination of the entire national population. As cases dwindled, the net was cast far and wide to identify outbreaks and vaccinate contacts. A "rumor registry" was even set up. Specimens from suspicious cases were sent to sophisticated virological diagnostic centers at Atlanta and Moscow to rule out or confirm smallpox. There were "pockmark surveys" to detect afflicted children who had been born after the last survey.

A country was declared free of smallpox when two years had elapsed after the last known case. Several countries had setbacks after initially declaring eradication. Slowly but surely, the number of countries still reporting cases declined. The progress continued despite international wars, civil strife, and natural disasters. The very last naturally occurring case was discovered in October 1977 in Somalia.

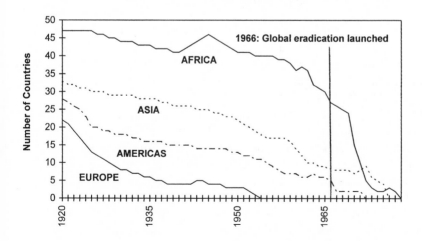

In September 1978 two cases occurred in Birmingham, England, in a laboratory outbreak. No further cases, natural or laboratory-acquired, occurred after 1978. In May 1980, the Thirty-third World

Health Assembly finally declared that "the world and all its peoples have won freedom from smallpox." By 1985, routine vaccination programs were discontinued in all countries of the world, and travelers were no longer required to obtain a smallpox vaccination certificate. WHO did recommend stockpiling 200 million doses of vaccine as a precaution against any unanticipated outbreak in the future.

As natural smallpox no longer exists and the proportion of the population still immune is rapidly dwindling, laboratory accidents, sabotage, terrorism, and biological warfare involving smallpox pose a real threat to world health. The WHO requested that laboratories around the world destroy or voluntarily transfer remaining stocks to four designated laboratories in the United States, U.S.S.R., England, and South Africa. By the mid 1980s, only two maximum-security laboratories, at the CDC in Atlanta and the Research Institute of Viral Preparations in Moscow, continued to maintain stocks of smallpox virus. In the 1990s there was renewed debate regarding whether these stocks should be destroyed so that the world would be truly free of smallpox. It is unclear who else, other than these two sites, possesses the virus. It is this uncertainty that led to the renewed concerns about bioterrorism, especially after the events of September 11, 2001. In December 2002, the President of the United States announced a plan to protect the American people against the threat of smallpox attacks by hostile groups or governments, whereby health care workers, first responders, military, and other critical personnel are offered smallpox vaccination.

Case Study 7.2.   Is Mammography Good for Women?

Cancer of the breast is the most important cancer among women in the developed countries.[25] As shown in the graph on the next page, based on data on Canadian women, the age-standardized incidence rate has been steadily rising, while mortality has remained stable. It is estimated that the lifetime probability of developing breast cancer is 11%, while that of dying from the disease is 4%. The disease is associated with considerable psychosocial distress. The treatment may be disfiguring and severely compromises the quality of life among survivors.

The effectiveness of mammography screening in reducing breast cancer mortality among women over the age of 50 has been firmly established. One of the earliest randomized controlled trials of mammography is the Health Insurance Plan (HIP) Study in New York conducted in the early 1960s. To date seven RCTs have been reported around the world. For women between ages of 40 and 49, among whom the incidence is low and the ability of mammography to detect tumors in the relatively dense breasts is reduced, the benefits are not as strong or consistent. One of the largest RCTs, the Canadian

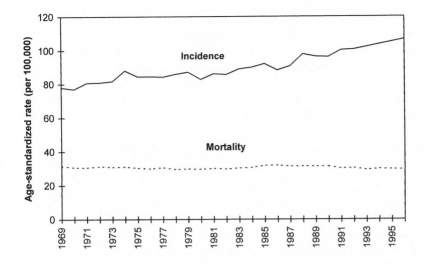

National Breast Screening Study (NBSS), was launched in the early 1980s with the specific objective of assessing effectiveness among women in the 40–49 age group. The negative results of this study were hotly contested, especially by radiologists. Data pertaining to the 40–49 age group from the seven trials are summarized below.

Study	Years of follow-up	Sample size	Relative risk (95% confidence interval)
HIP, United States (1963–1970)	18	29,133	0.8 (0.53–1.11)
Malmö, Sweden (1976–1990)	10–16	25,770	0.6 (0.45–0.89)
Two County, Sweden (1977–1985)	13	35,448	0.9 (0.54–1.41)
Edinburgh, United Kingdom (1979–1988)	10–14	21,774	0.8 (0.51–1.32)
Stockholm, Sweden (1981–1985)	11	21,950	1.1 (0.54–2.17)
Gothenburg, Sweden (1982–1992)	10	25,941	0.6 (0.31–0.96)
NBSS, Canada (1980–1988)	11	49,430	1.1 (0.83–1.56)

Between 1995 and 2000, six meta-analyses (a statistical procedure to combine results from different studies) were published. The combined RR ranged from 0.82 to 1.04. The one with the longest followup period showed the best protective effect (RR = 0.82, 95% CI 0.71–0.95). Most of the others showed overall no statistically significant differences between screened and non-screened participants.

The same scientific data, however, led to divergent recommendations by different expert groups. Breast cancer screening has moved beyond the weighing of scientific evidence, to the public arena, where politicians, the mass media, and special interest groups join in the increasingly emotional and acrimonious debate. It is an excellent example of the conflict between scientific evidence and strongly held beliefs, vested professional and financial interests, and established practice.

In 1993 the U.S. National Cancer Institute (NCI) reversed its stance based on the conclusion of an international workshop that there was insufficient evidence that screening was effective in reducing mortality in the 40–49 age group. This only served to increase the intensity of the debate (and confusion among the public). In the hope of resolving the issue, the National Institutes of Health (NIH) convened a consensus development conference in 1997. The panel concluded that "the data currently available do not warrant a universal recommendation for mammography for all women in their forties." The expert panel was roundly condemned by those who favored screening. The director of the NCI, a molecular biologist, publicly criticized the report. The NCI then convened its own National Cancer Advisory Board to review the report and came to the opposite conclusion, that women aged 40–49 should be screened every one to two years, hence reversing its position once again. The NIH consensus panel's chair was summoned to a special hearing of a Senate subcommittee on health services appropriations where various politicians challenged the scientific competence and integrity of the panel. The Senate then voted unanimously in favor of a nonbinding resolution supporting mammography for women in their 40s. Some sensational media reports even labeled the panel as anti-women.

The Canadian Task Force on the Periodic Health Examination (later changed to Preventive Health Care) concluded in 2001 updated its recommendation that "current evidence does not suggest the inclusion in, or its exclusion from, the periodic health examination of women aged 40–49 years," which represents a change from the previous recommendation that there was fair evidence to exclude it altogether.

Even though there is no controversy surrounding screening in older women, surveys indicate that among American women aged 50–64, only 65% had received a mammogram in the past year, and for women 65 and above, 54%. Those with more education are more likely to have been screened. Thus those who would definitely benefit from screening do not participate, while those for whom the benefit of screening is uncertain are being urged to participate.

Case Study 7.3.   Community-Based Heart Disease Prevention in North Karelia

Beginning in the 1940s, ischemic heart disease (IHD) became increasingly the most important cause of death in the industrialized countries. Mortality rates, however, varied substantially between countries, with

Finland claiming the dubious distinction of having one of the world's highest mortality rates of IHD. Within the country, certain counties in the east, including North Karelia near the Russian border, had the highest rates. In 1971, a delegation of politicians and citizens from North Karelia petitioned the national government for urgent action to control the IHD epidemic. As a result, a heart disease prevention project was launched, a collaboration between the local and national governments, the health and education ministries, the Finnish Heart Association, health professionals, and academics.

North Karelia is a predominantly rural county (population in 1970: 185,000), its main economic activities being dairy farming and forestry. Compared to the rest of Finland, it had a lower SES with high prevalence of smoking, hypertension, and hypercholesterolemia. The North Karelia Project began in 1972 with a baseline risk-factor survey.[26] The project had the long-term objective of reducing the incidence and mortality of IHD, and shorter-term objectives of reduction in risk-factor levels, targeting smoking, hypertension, and serum cholesterol levels. The neighboring county of Kuopio was chosen as the non-intervention site.

The project was designed as a community-based one, with public education on heart disease and its risk factors the main strategy. Mass media were used extensively, and a variety of health education materials were produced. Existing health care infrastructure was utilized, but with reorganization of services to accommodate the new emphasis on education. Community opinion leaders were identified and given special training. Finally, personal services were complemented by environmental changes such as the restriction of smoking in public areas, reduction of animal fat in local dairy produce and sausages, promotion of vegetable gardening, and marketing of nutritious foods in local stores.

Repeat risk factor surveys were done at 5, 10, 15, and 20 years after the baseline one in 1972. Surveillance of IHD incidence and mortality was also instituted. Changes in the prevalence of smoking, hypertension (diastolic blood pressure ≥95 mmHg), and high total serum cholesterol (≥6.5 mmol/L) are shown in the graphs on the next page.

During the first five years, total cholesterol and blood pressure (both mean values and proportion with high levels) declined more steeply in North Karelia than in Kuopio, but subsequent changes have been about the same in both areas. The decline leveled off (or even worsened) between the 1982 and 1987 surveys. This resulted in new nationwide preventive activities, which appear to have an impact in the last five years, when major declines in cholesterol and blood pressure were observed. Smoking in men declined more in North Karelia than in Kuopio during the first 10 years, with North Karelia maintaining a lower prevalence as both continued to decline

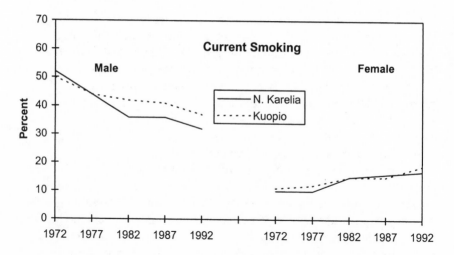

less steeply in the last 10 years. Among women, both areas showed an increase. During this period, IHD incidence also declined in both areas. Regression analyses indicate that the proportion of decline in incidence attributable to changes in the three risk factors was substantially larger in North Karelia than in Kuopio. Interestingly, the decline in smoking among men seems to have affected the incidence of lung cancer as well.

The North Karelia Project demonstrates that multifaceted, community-based health promotion programs can have a measurable impact on risk-factor prevalence and disease incidence. That the benefit has not been as great relative to a non-program region suggests the diffusion of program awareness and behavioral change. Indeed,

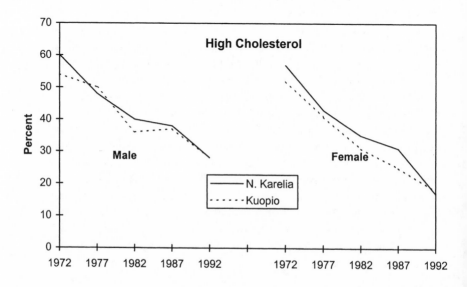

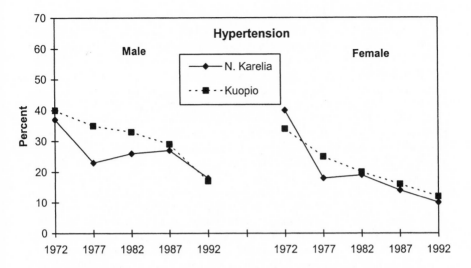

the North Karelia Project was soon replicated on a nationwide basis in Finland, although North Karelia continues to be a population "laboratory" in testing innovative health promotion strategies.

Notes

1. The full text of the Alma-Ata Declaration can be found in WHO's archives, available from its web site: www.who.int/hpr/backgroundhp/almaata.htm
2. An explanation of selective primary health care was provided by Walsh and Warren (1979). For critiques, see Rifkin and Walt (1986) and Briscoe (1984).
3. See the documents *Healthy People 2000 Final Review* and *Healthy People 2010: Understanding and Improving Health,* available from the Healthy People web site (www.healthypeople.gov)
4. See Smedley and Syme (2000).
5. The definition was cited by Nutting et al. (1985) from Kark's 1981 monograph. The APHA has also published a "how-to" manual (Rhyne et al., 1998).
6. This table is modified from that provided in the World Bank handbook by Jamison et al. (1993).
7. Health auxiliaries are employed extensively in many developing countries, and a substantial literature has been accumulated (see, for example, Fendall, 1972; and Storms, 1979). In developed countries, they are usually employed in remote, underserviced areas. See Case Study 8.1 on a randomized controlled trial to evaluate the effectiveness of nurse-practitioners in an urban family practice setting.
8. See the provocatively titled monograph *Is Prevention Better Than Cure?* by Russell (1986). It should also be pointed out that clinicians often demand rigorous proof of effectiveness from preventive strategies, yet much of clinical practice consists of therapies that have never been evaluated. "Evidence-based medicine," much in vogue now, is long overdue.
9. Rose presented his ideas on prevention in his classic paper on sick individuals and sick populations (1985), later expanded into a monograph (1992). His classic paper was reprinted in 2001 in the *International Journal of Epidemiology* (30:427–32) with commentaries. Data on blood pressure reduction are from Cook et al. (1995).

10. The Commission on Chronic Illness (1957:45) was founded by the American Hospital, Medical, Public Health, and Public Welfare Associations in recognition of the emergent disease burden due to chronic diseases and the need for new strategies to control them. For a comprehensive review of screening in chronic diseases, see Morrison (1992).

11. See Wilson and Jungner (1968) for elaboration on the 10 principles. Cadman et al. (1984) provide a slightly different approach.

12. The Canadian Task Force on the Periodic Health Examination published its first report in 1979, with periodic updates since then. A comprehensive handbook was published in 1994. The U.S. Preventive Services Task Force published its first report in 1989 and a second edition in 1996.

13. See Susser (1995) on the place of RCTs in community health. Smith et al. (1997) demonstrated that RCTs are underused in community health interventions even when they are recommended and feasible; the few that are published in community health journals generally lack methodological rigor.

14. Where the two reports differ in their rating, the maneuver is placed in the higher category. Only recommendations for various age-sex groups in the general North American population are included here, although the reports also make references to specific high-risk groups where screening is appropriate.

15. For an overview and rationale of the *Guide to Community Preventive Services*, see Truman et al. (2000). The regularly updated database of reviews is available from the Guide's web site: www.thecommunityguide.org.

16. See Marteau and Kinmonth (2002) on individual informed choice in screening. For a review of the behavioral and psychological consequences of labeling in hypertension, see Macdonald et al. (1984).

17. Much of this section is based on the text on health promotion planning by Green and Kreuter (1991).

18. See Rosenstock's paper in the monograph on the health belief model, edited by Becker (1974). Social cognitive theory (Bandura, 1986) is also called social learning theory. Ajzen and Fishbein (1980) updated their earlier versions of the theory of reasoned action. Fincham (1992) reviewed the theoretical bases of community health promotion programs as applied to heart disease.

19. See Paul (1958), who focuses on sanitation programs. See also his 1955 book for more case studies of community reactions to health interventions. Polgar's four fallacies are cited by Landy (1977:233) in the introduction to Paul's paper reprinted in his selections of readings in medical anthropology.

20. See Corin (1994:129). The recommendation regarding at-risk groups echoes that of Rose (1992) discussed earlier. Rubel and Garro (1992) point out the importance of understanding the health culture of patients in tuberculosis control programs.

21. See McKinlay (1993). Schmid et al. (1995) used cardiovascular disease prevention as an example where environmental and policy approaches should complement individual health education.

22. See McKinlay and Marceau (2000). A review of the global burden of diabetes can be found in King et al. (1998). See Vinicor (1998) for an explanation of the public health approach to diabetes.

23. The definition is from Van Willigen (1993:92).

24. Anything anyone could possibly want to know about smallpox can be found in the massive, 1,460-page tome published by the WHO to document and celebrate the eradication program (Fenner et al., 1988). The data used in the

graphs are from pp. 171 and 273. Visit the WHO and CDC web sites for current developments in smallpox preparedness.

25. Information on various cancers can be obtained from NCI's CancerInfo web site (www.nci.nih.gov/cancerinfo). The NIH Consensus Development Conference Statement No. 103 is reprinted in *Journal of the National Cancer Institute* 1997; 89:1015–26. See Hendrick et al. (1997) for a meta-analysis of the seven RCTs, and Gotzsche and Olsen (2000) for the two "unbiased" trials. References to individual studies used in the meta-analyses can be found in these sources. A reporter for *Science* (Taubes, 1997) referred to the dispute over the mammography recommendations as a "brawl." See Ringash et al. (2001) for the Canadian Task Force on Preventive Health Care report.

26. The North Karelia Project has produced much literature. For details of the background and design of the project, see the project monograph (National Public Health Laboratory of Finland, 1981). Vartiainen et al. (1994) summarized the risk-factor changes during the 20-year period. The impact of risk-factor change on the incidence of ischemic heart disease was analyzed by Salonen et al. (1989) and on lung cancer incidence by Luostarinen et al. (1995). For a systematic review of RCTs of multiple risk-factor interventions in preventing coronary heart disease, see Ebrahim and Smith (1997).

EXERCISE 7.1.   Designing a Hypertension Control Program

Design an intervention program to control hypertension in your community. In your proposal, address the following issues:

(a)   Is hypertension a significant health problem in your community? What data are already available to allow you to assess the burden of illness? What additional data need to be collected?

(b)   What is the significance of hypertension in population terms? Why should anything be done to control it?

(c)   How can hypertension be prevented or controlled? What is the quality of the evidence that these strategies are effective?

(d)   Given the population characteristics of your community, what is the best approach to take? What are the relative merits of primary prevention, early detection and screening, treatment, and rehabilitation? Should you focus on active or passive measures, individuals at high risk or the total population?

(e)   What socioeconomic, cultural, and political barriers can be expected in implementing your proposed program?

Consult the American Public Health Association's manual on chronic disease control (Brownson et al., 1998). If you don't like hypertension, pick another health problem—tuberculosis, diabetes, Alzheimer's disease, etc.

8

Evaluating Health Programs for Populations

A Framework for Evaluation

The last chapter was concerned with planning and implementing interventions to improve the health of populations. In order to determine if such programs are performing as planned and have achieved their goals and objectives, they need to be evaluated. According to a WHO guidebook, evaluation is a "systematic way of learning from experience and using the lessons learned to improve current activities and promote better planning by careful selection of alternatives for future action." The purpose of health program evaluation is to "improve health programs and the health infrastructure for delivering them and to guide the allocation of resources in current and future programs.[1]"

Evaluation is thus an integral part of the managerial process and plays a key role in decision-making. Evaluation may be *formative*, when it is primarily concerned with improving and fine-tuning the ongoing operation of a program, or *summative*, when it is done after the end of a program and aims to benefit similar programs in the future. Evaluation should be planned at the outset of a program and should not be regarded as a freestanding activity, as its results are important in the planning and implementation phases as well. A more appropriate view of evaluation is that of a "loop," rather than linear. Figure 8.1 introduces the concept of the measurement iterative loop. Iteration is a mathematical procedure whereby an operation is repeated, each time coming closer to the desired results. It is envisioned that, even for proven effective interventions, repeated cycles of the loop are needed to achieve the desired health outcome.

Before launching an evaluation, we should make a preliminary assessment of the "evaluability" of the program; i.e., determine if evaluation is even feasible. Whether the program's objectives are realistic and well-defined, its assumptions are plausible, the intended users of the evaluation are identified, and the time and resources to conduct the evaluation

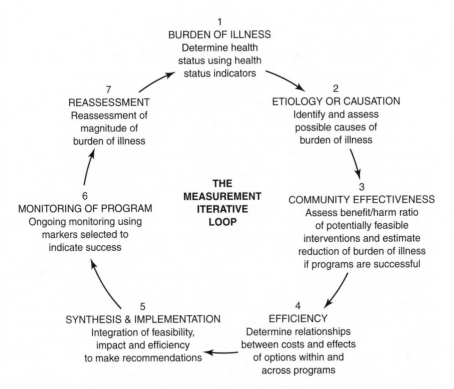

Figure 8.1. The measurement iterative loop. Reprinted from: Tugwell P, Bennett KJ, Sackett DL, Haynes RB. The measurement interative loop: A framework for the critical appraisal of need, benefits, and costs of health interventions. *J Chron Dis* 1985; 38:339–51, with kind permission from Elsevier Science, Inc.

are available, are questions that need to be addressed at the outset. The evaluator should also be aware of the political context of the evaluation. An externally imposed evaluation, if perceived to be providing the justification for discontinuing a program, is likely to devastate staff morale and engender opposition and non-cooperation. The link to the target audience, or users of the evaluation, especially decision-makers or policy makers, is particularly important. Their responsibilities and expertise will affect the type of questions asked and the evaluation design chosen.

A useful framework for classifying types of evaluation was proposed by nutritionist Jean-Pierre Habicht and his colleagues, with particular relevance to health and nutrition interventions but applicable to other areas as well.[2] This framework has two axes. One axis refers to the type of indicators used, which may be concerned with performance and/or impact, and addresses the question "What does one want to measure?" The other axis refers to the type of inference needed—adequacy, plausibility and probability—which addresses the question "How sure does one want to be" that the observed effects are due to the program?

Performance refers to the provision, utilization, and coverage of the program. Are services available and accessible to the target population? Are they of good quality? Are they acceptable (politically, socially, culturally)? Once provided, are the services being used? Finally, what proportion of the target population was reached by the program? *Impact* refers to the overall effect of the program on the health status of the population, or in an even broader sense, on equity, social justice, and economic development. In a performance evaluation, data on program activities are collected from those implementing the program and recipients of the services. In impact evaluation, health and behavioral indicators are measured in either program recipients or the target population.

In assessing *adequacy*, comparison is made with predetermined criteria—has the program met its original objectives? For adequacy of performance, program activities are monitored to determine if they are performed as planned in the initial implementation schedule, in terms of the milestones achieved. There is adequacy of impact if the observed changes in health status or behavioral indicators are in the expected direction and magnitude.

In assessing *plausibility*, one would like to determine if the program appears to have an effect above and beyond those of non-program influences. To arrive at such an inference, comparison needs to be made between a group that received the intervention and one that did not. These groups can be selected from program recipients "before" and "after" the intervention. They can also be assembled opportunistically—for example, between geographical areas where the implementation has been staggered, resulting in some areas' receiving it sooner than others; or some areas' not receiving it altogether for administrative or political reasons. The intervention group should have better performance or impact indicators than the non-intervention group.

The most stringent inference is *probability*, whereby an effect of the program can be demonstrated and attributed to the program with a measurable level of statistical probability, which requires randomization in the creation of intervention and "control" groups.

There are several key concepts in evaluation, which are often mixed up in everyday usage. These are *efficacy*, *effectiveness*, and *efficiency*. Their use was standardized by Archibald Cochrane (1909–1988) in his influential book *Effectiveness and Efficiency*, published in 1972. An important legacy of "Archie" Cochrane was the development of the Cochrane Collaboration (see Box 8.3), named in his honor. Efficacy is the extent to which a specific intervention produces a beneficial result under ideal conditions. Cochrane and a generation of clinical epidemiologists following him would insist that efficacy should preferably be established by a randomized controlled trial. While an intervention known to be non-efficacious should never have been adopted in the first place, in the real world, many interventions with untested efficacy are introduced and widely used—examples abound in both clinical medicine and public health. Effectiveness measures the extent to which a specific intervention, when deployed in the field in routine circumstances, does what it is intended to do. Whereas efficacy determines if something *can* work, effectiveness tells us if it *does* work. Efficacy is demonstrated in the controlled environment of a laboratory or a hospital ward, effectiveness is assessed under conditions of the "real world." Thus an oral contraceptive can be shown to be efficacious in the laboratory (suppresses ovulation in mice) and in a clinical trial conducted by highly motivated and skilled personnel in a highly selected group of fully compliant, paid volunteers. When it is offered to the general community as a family planning program, the effectiveness may be compromised by such factors as spoilage, incorrect advice given by staff, poor acceptance due to cultural barriers, political and religious opposition, etc.

Efficiency is an economic concept that relates the human, financial, and other resources expended in the program to the results obtained (more discussion below). It usually implies obtaining the desired results at minimal cost. Clearly, effectiveness has to be established first—an ineffective program should never be contemplated, no matter how little it will cost.

Of the several components of performance evaluation mentioned earlier, quality of care has traditionally been emphasized in characterizing the health care provided by an institution, program, or individual providers. Since the 1960s, Avedis Donabedian has contributed much to the study of quality and its measurement.[3] In Donabedian's scheme, quality is conceived of as having three dimensions: structure, process and outcome. Originally applied mainly in the medical care setting (hospital and physician offices), the concept is equally applicable to population health programs. *Structure* refers to the attributes of the setting in which care occurs: the material (facilities, equipment, finances), human resources (number and qualifications of staff), and organizational structure of the program or institution. *Process* is what the program actually does—the items of services that it delivers. *Outcome* comprises the effects on the health status of the population served. Health care planners and administrators traditionally tend to focus more on structure and process (e.g., hospital accreditation surveys) than on outcome. It can be seen that outcome evaluation covers much the same ground as impact evaluation, as discussed earlier.

Technology Assessment, Diffusion, and Transfer

Technology assessment can be considered a special case of program evaluation, when the focus is on products, processes, and practices. *Technology* is defined by economist John Kenneth Galbraith (b. 1908) in his book *The New Industrial State* as "the systematic application of scientific or other organized knowledge to practical tasks." In the health care context, technology usually refers to drugs, vaccines, medical devices (such as cardiac pacemakers), and therapeutic and diagnostic procedures (e.g., angiography).[4]

The International Network of Agencies for Health Technology Assessment (INAHTA) defines *health technology assessment* (HTA) as "a multidisciplinary field of policy analysis. It studies the medical, social, ethical, and economic implications of development, diffusion, and use of health technology." It is a burgeoning field, and many countries have established offices/agencies dedicated to HTA. INAHTA has 40 member organizations from around the world. The U.S. Congress established the Office of Technology Assessment in 1972, which introduced a health program in 1975, but closed it down in 1995. HTA is now part of the mandate of the Agency for Health Care Research and Quality. In Canada, the Canadian Coordinating Office for Health Technology Assessment has been in existence since 1989, supported by various federal and provincial health ministries.[5]

HTA is not just more research. There are four distinguishing features[6]:

1. Policy orientation
2. Interdisciplinary content and process
3. Multiple methods
4. Dissemination and communication

HTA thus bridges research and policy-making. The two spheres of activities, however, do need to remain separate. Health policy-making must be informed by, but not limited to, scientific evidence. Health policy is also influenced by contextual factors: the political and social climate in which decisions are made. Research needs to be sensitive to the policy-making process, but cannot be dictated to by policy-makers in posing the research questions, implementing the research, and interpreting the results.

A technology can be considered to have a lifecycle of its own, usually represented by: *innovation → early diffusion → incorporation → wide utilization → abandonment*. Generally, far more technologies are introduced than abandoned. These stages highlight the difference between efficacy and effectiveness. In the innovation stage, the efficacy of a technology is established, based on studies of a limited number of subjects within a narrow range of values of the relevant indicator of the health condition (blood pressure, alcohol consumption, etc.). During early diffusion, the technology is applied to a broader range of subjects, where the efficacy is lower, with the result that the overall effectiveness becomes reduced considerably. Effectiveness is further compromised during the wide utilization phase.

It has been the experience in most developed countries that a technology will be used if it is available, even when effectiveness has not been demonstrated. Indeed, for most medical technologies, efficacy or effectiveness is seldom established prior to their widespread diffusion. Often they are promoted merely on the basis of case reports or case series. John McKinlay elaborated seven stages to characterize the typical "career" of a medical technology: (1) promising report; (2) professional/organizational adoption; (3) public acceptance; (4) standard procedure and observational reports; (5) randomized controlled trial; (6) professional denunciation; and (7) erosion and discreditation. It can be seen that the sequence is entirely illogical, but unfortunately it does describe how most medical technologies are diffused, a process that is wasteful of scarce resources. It is much better to establish and demonstrate effectiveness first, preferably through the use of RCTs, prior to adoption, acceptance, and proliferation as a standard procedure.[7]

Technologies are often transferred from developed to developing countries, as foreign aid or market expansion (the two are often indistinguishable). Often a finished product is simply transferred without transmitting

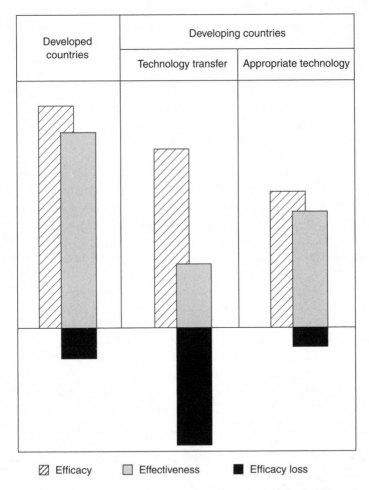

Figure 8.2. Effect of local conditions on the effectiveness of a health technology. Reprinted from: Panerai RB, Mohr JP. *Health Technology Assessment: Methodologies for Developing Countries.* Washington, DC: Pan American Health Organization, 1989, with kind permission from the publisher.

the knowledge that developed the technology or the skills to operate the technology. There are many obstacles to effective technology transfer. The recipient country is usually severely limited in health resources and scientific and technical capacity to fully utilize the new technology. The disease pattern is usually vastly different, sometimes negating the need for the technology itself. There may be cultural barriers to effective implementation, and the technology itself may even be harmful to local culture. The political climate may be too unstable to sustain the operation and maintenance of the technology.

A certain amount of efficacy loss is to be expected when a technology is widely diffused. Such efficacy loss can be even greater in technology transfer to developing countries (Figure 8.2). The use of appropriate technology (AT) is one way to minimize efficacy loss even if the efficacy of the locally designed alternative technology is less than the preferred standard used in developed countries.

Evaluation Methods

All the types of research designs discussed in Chapter 6 can be used in evaluation, especially to determine effectiveness. "Exposure," instead of being a causal agent for a disease, can be an intervention, procedure, service, or program. Chapter 7 refers to a hierarchy of research designs with respect to the quality of the evidence for effectiveness in screening programs. The randomized controlled trial (RCT) is generally considered to offer the highest level of evidence (Case Study 8.1 illustrates the use of the RCT to evaluate the effectiveness of a cadre of health professionals). *Trend analysis*, the graphical presentation of the occurrence of a target condition before and after the initiation of an intervention, is an example of a descriptive study that can sometimes demonstrate the dramatic effects of an intervention (see the graph in Case Study 7.1 on the effect of compulsory vaccination on the smallpox mortality trend in the nineteenth century).

Often an RCT evaluating a particular intervention shows a positive effect, but is judged statistically insignificant due to the small sample size. By combining the results of several independent studies on the same topic, using a procedure known as meta-analysis, it is possible to demonstrate a significant effect. This is an improvement over the traditional narrative literature review. A numerical summary such as an odds ratio or effect size can be computed. Case Study 8.4 provides an example of a meta-analysis of adolescent smoking prevention studies. Meta-analyses are based on published data and may not even require the participation or cooperation of the original studies' authors. An elaboration involves actual pooling of individual-level datasets obtained directly from the authors and performing reanalysis of the pooled dataset.[8] One should be

---

BOX 8.1.   Measuring the Protective Effectiveness of Vaccines

As indicated in Chapter 7, many diseases can be effectively prevented by immunizations. It is common to evaluate the efficacy of a vaccine during its developmental and pre-licensure phase, usually by a randomised controlled trial in a highly selected population.[9] Once the vaccine has been deployed in the field, its effectiveness can be evaluated by a variety of methods, including RCTs, cohort studies, and case-control studies. Often these are done in the midst of an epidemic outbreak of the disease to determine if the vaccine has failed.

Vaccine effectiveness (VE) or protective effect (PE) can be expressed as a percentage and computed from:

$$VE = (ARU - ARV)/ARU \times 100\%$$

where ARU is the attack rate (i.e., cumulative incidence) of disease among the unvaccinated and ARV the rate among the vaccinated. Since ARV/ARU is the relative risk (RR) of disease, the formula can be rewritten as $(1 - RR) \times 100\%$. If a vaccine is protective, $ARU > ARV$ and $RR < 1$. If a case-control study is done, the OR can be used in place of RR.

VE is also related to the extent of coverage of the vaccine (PPV— proportion of population vaccinated) and the proportion of cases vaccinated (PCV). Unless VE is 100%, there will always be some cases occurring among those who have been vaccinated, and thus represent vaccine failures. The relationship is as follows:

$$PCV = [PPV - (PPV \times VE)] / [1 - (PPV \times VE)]$$

As vaccine coverage improves, PCV will also increase, giving the impression of widespread vaccine failure. For example, if a highly effective vaccine with VE of 90% and 90% of the population has been vaccinated, in an outbreak, 47% of the cases that occurred would be among individuals who had been vaccinated. If the same vaccine covers only 10% of the population, PCV will only be 1%. A high PCV does not necessarily indicate that the vaccine is no longer effective.

---

aware of publication bias, as studies showing an effect are more likely than negative ones to be published. The meta-analyst also has no control over the quality of data collection in the individual studies.

Note that evaluation need not even be thought of as "research," with the goal of contributing to the pool of universal knowledge and perhaps even with an eye to posterity. It may be primarily location-specific, and its

BOX 8.2.   Evaluating Interventions to Reduce Health Inequalities

As Chapter 4 showed, considerable research has been conducted into the existence and explanation of socioeconomic inequalities in health. Clearly, the reduction of inequalities within the population is an important and worthwhile goal, even if overall, the entire population's health has not improved as a result of the intervention. Many interventions are amenable to the experimental design—the randomized controlled trial if individuals are involved, and the community intervention trial if groups of people (such as entire communities) are involved. Johan Mackenbach and Louise Gunning-Schepers present a useful schema that summarizes the basic designs and analytical approaches to conducting such studies.[10]

SES	Event rate BEFORE	Intervention	Event rate AFTER
High	$H_0 \longrightarrow$	Yes $\longrightarrow$	H_1
	$h_0 \longrightarrow$	No $\longrightarrow$	h_1
Low	$L_0 \longrightarrow$	Yes $\longrightarrow$	L_1
	$l_0 \longrightarrow$	No $\longrightarrow$	l_1

High SES group is represented by (H/h) and low SES by (L/l). The experimental group (which received the intervention) is represented by capital letters, and the control group (no interventions) by lowercase letters. The subscript 0 refers to the event rate (mortality rate of a disease) before, and 1 to the event rate after the interventions.
    A variety of designs is available:

Design	Hypothesis to be tested		Assumptions
A	$[(L_1 - H_1) - (L_0 - H_0)]$	$< \ [(l_1 - h_1) - (l_0 - h_0)]$	nil
B_1	$(L_1 - L_0)$	$< \ (l_1 - l_0)$	$(H_0 - H_1) = (h_0 - h_1)$
B_2	L_1	$< \ l_1$	$(H_0 - H_1) = (h_0 - h_1);$ $L_0 - l_0$
C_1	$(L_1 - H_1)$	$< \ (L_0 - H_0)$	$(l_1 - h_1) = (l_0 - h_0)$
C_2	L_1	$< \ L_0$	$(l_1 - h_1) = (l_0 - h_0);$ $H_1 = H_0$
D_1	$(L_1 - H_1)$	$< \ (l_1 - h_1)$	$(L_0 - H_0) = (l_0 - h_0)$
D_2	L_1	$< \ l_1$	$(L_0 - H_0) = (l_0 - h_0);$ $H_1 = H_1$

    (A) is the "full" model, which requires the most data collection points. The others require less complex measurement but more assumptions have to be made.

BOX 8.3.   The Cochrane Collaboration and Systematic Reviews

The Cochrane Collaboration is an international nonprofit and independent organization, dedicated to making up-to-date, accurate information about the effects of health care readily available worldwide.[11] Founded in 1993, it produces and disseminates systematic reviews of health care interventions and promotes the search for evidence in the form of clinical trials and other studies. Reviews are published electronically in the *Cochrane Database of Systematic Reviews* and included in the Cochrane Library. Preparation and maintenance of Cochrane reviews is the responsibility of international collaborative review groups, composed primarily of health care professionals and researchers. The Collaboration also operates the Cochrane Central Register of Controlled Trials (CENTRAL), an international effort to search the world's journals and other sources of information and create an unbiased source of data for systematic reviews. Cochrane Centres have been established in many countries; these are not directly involved in the reviews, but exist to help establish and support the review groups.

The Collaboration envisions a systematic review as comprising the following steps:

1. State objectives of the review, and outline eligibility criteria.
2. Search for studies that seem to meet eligibility criteria.
3. Tabulate characteristics of each study identified and assess its methodological quality.
4. Apply eligibility criteria, and justify any exclusions.
5. Assemble the most complete dataset feasible, with involvement of investigators, if possible.
6. Analyze results of eligible studies, and use statistical synthesis of data (meta-analysis), if appropriate and possible.
7. Perform sensitivity analysis and subgroup analysis, if appropriate and possible.
8. Prepare a structured report of the review, stating aims, describing materials and methods, and reporting results.

Although the reviews that have been published are predominantly clinical (e.g., drug therapies for various diseases), there are also prevention-oriented studies; for example, on vaccines for pneumonoccal infections, screening for oral cancer, prevention of falls among the elderly, and the impact of tobacco advertising on promoting adolescent smoking behavior, among others.

lessons may or may not be generalizable or relevant to other settings. The vast majority of program evaluations are never published in the scientific literature accessible to the general public.

Qualitative methods (also discussed in Chapter 6) are often used in evaluation, particularly in the context of a case study of a particular program. This may involve structured interviews of key informants, focus groups, content analysis of program documents, and participant observation.

Expert opinions are often relied upon, especially in the absence of "hard" data. There are formal methods to obtain the opinions of experts in aid of evaluation and decision-making, one of which is the *Delphi method*, originally developed by the RAND Corporation. (Students with a classical bent may have heard of the Delphic oracle: At a temple in Delphi in ancient Greece, priestesses with special prophetic powers served as intermediaries between the god Apollo and earthly mortals.) A questionnaire is presented to a panel of respondents, usually recognized experts in the field. Based on their pooled responses, a summary report is fed back to the respondents, followed by a new questionnaire. After several rounds of questions and responses, the range of opinions is progressively refined and narrowed, until either consensus is reached or there is saturation, when no further gain in consensus can be expected. The process is anonymous, and no single respondent dominates the process. The results can also be quantified; for example, summing and ranking the scores derived from the responses to the questions.

Another formal method of gathering expert opinions is the *consensus development conference*, developed by the NIH. A panel of experts is convened, and with the assistance of staff researchers, they prepare a detailed literature review that forms the basis of the panel's deliberation. A report is then prepared and presented at a conference, with public participation. The NIH has published many such consensus statements, the products of the consensus development conferences. Sometimes they are very controversial, such as the one on mammography screening for women under age 50 (see Case Study 7.2). While consensus is great when it occurs, one is often reminded of a quotation from former Israeli diplomat Abba Eban (1905–2002), who said: "Consensus means that lots of people say collectively what nobody believes individually!"[12]

Economic Appraisal

Demonstrating the effectiveness of a program or intervention is only part of the evaluation. Because health systems operate in an environment of scarce resources, the program needs to be justified in economic terms; i.e., demonstrate its efficiency. Health economists have developed an array of methods, subsumed under the term *economic appraisal* or *evaluation*. A textbook defines it as "comparative analysis of alternative courses of action in terms of both their costs and consequences." *Costs* refers to the economic

---

BOX 8.4.   Ten Basic Notions of Health Economics

Health economists Michael Drummond, Gregory Stoddart, and their colleagues introduced 10 "basic notions of health economics" in a primer directed at clinicians (who are generally unsophisticated in economics, like the rest of humanity), in an attempt to clear away some common misconceptions and identify implicit assumptions:[13]

1. Human wants are unlimited but resources are finite.
2. Economics is as much about benefits as it is about costs.
3. The costs of health programs are not restricted to health care facilities, or even to the health sector.
4. Choices in health care and health planning inescapably involve value judgements.
5. Many of the simple rules of market operation do not apply in the case of health care.
6. Consideration of costs is not necessarily unethical.
7. Most choices in health care relate to changes in the level or extent of a given activity; the relevant evaluation concerns these marginal changes, not the total activity.
8. The provision of health care is but one way of improving the health of the population.
9. As a community we prefer to postpone costs and to bring forward benefits.
10. Equity in health care may be desirable, but reducing inequalities usually comes at a price.

---

resources consumed or expended by the program (inputs) and *consequences* to the health effects, outcomes, or outputs.[14]

A community desires and expects to get certain health services or programs, usually without knowing their costs—this is referred to as its *want*. It is to be distinguished from *need*, which is supposedly "objectively" defined, usually by experts, based on an analysis of the health status of the population. It is their perspective on what ought to be provided and is sometimes further specified as "professionally defined need." When costs are known to the consumers, wants will be modified and translated into *demand* for services, which is the willingness or ability to seek, use and pay for services. However, when need is not perceived by consumers, it may not be expressed as either a want or demand. Need is sometimes also equated with "potential demand." Ordinarily a service will be supplied by the health care system in response to the expressed demand. *Use* is a measure of demand that is satisfied or met. Often supply itself drives demand, resulting in inappropriate use. In an ideal health system, want = need = demand = supply = use.

Costs are usually expressed in units of currency. In international comparative studies, there is a tendency to use U.S. dollars as the "universal" currency.

There are three types of consequences, which distinguish the three basic types of economic appraisals:

1. *Cost-effectiveness analysis* (CEA): costs are compared to health effects, in units of mortality, morbidity or some health status measure. For example, it costs $x to prevent one death from influenza by vaccination among the elderly institutionalized population.
2. *Cost-benefit analysis* (CBA): here the consequences are expressed as economic benefits, in units of currency that can then be directly compared to the costs. For example, for every dollar spent on the obligatory installation of airbags in cars, there are $x in benefits through reduced health-care costs of crash victims.
3. *Cost-utility analysis* (CUA): as in CEA, the consequences are also expressed in health terms, but in utilities rather than some natural units of health status. In economics, *utility* is the preference for, or desirability of, a specific outcome. In the health context, it is the value or worth assigned to a level of health by an individual or a community (would you rather be dead or alive? healthy or sick? endure a long, lingering death from cancer or suffer a heart attack?). Preference scales can be devised, some of which involve "willingness to pay" (an individual may express the preference of paying, hypothetically of course, $5 to avoid the common cold, $500 for a fracture of the ankle, and $5 million for paraplegia). Such utility values can then be incorporated into quality adjusted life-years (QALYs were first discussed in Chapter 3).

Because both costs and benefits are in the same unit, CBA can be used to compare totally different fields of activity; for example, paving roads vs. hiring doctors. CEA and CUA tend to be used to evaluate different strategies within the same sector; for example, oral rehydration fluids vs. piped water supply to reduce diarrheal disease.

Simply describing the cost of a program, or whether it saves lives or not, is strictly speaking not economic evaluation. Even when both are investigated concurrently but if no alternatives are examined, it is considered only a partial evaluation. Full economic evaluation, as the definition above indicates, requires both costs and consequences, and alternatives. There are situations, however, when an alternative may not be explicitly stated, as when "no action" or the status quo is the implied alternative. When there are several alternatives, but only their costs but not the consequences are assessed, it is referred to as "cost analysis," which is another type of partial evaluation. Cost analyses are useful in cases where the effectiveness of the various alternatives has already been firmly established and where costs alone will be the deciding factor.

While economic appraisal is a powerful tool for decision-making in health care, there are important limitations. Every step along the way in the analyses, there are assumptions and approximations. Costs are not easily determined. CEA, CBA, and CUA by themselves only assess effectiveness relative to costs; they do not actually establish that the program or intervention is effective. Such information is derived from the literature or determined in an earlier, separate study. An important limitation is that such methods do not take into account the distribution of costs and effects. The promotion of social equity or political advantage by a program is usually not part of the economic appraisal, but nevertheless forms part, perhaps even the major part, of the decision-making process. There is another assumption in that the achievement of cost savings will free up resources for other worthwhile projects.

The critical aspect of all economic appraisals is the estimation of costs. While the identification of direct costs is relatively straightforward, deciding how far one should cast the net in counting indirect costs is far more complex. In population health, the societal perspective is usually taken—the costs and benefits to society as a whole rather than to an institution or even the health care system. A narrow institution or agency perspective tends not to worry about transferring costs to other payers. Operating costs need to be distinguished from capital costs—the former is recurrent whereas the latter represents a one-time investment which depreciates over time. Equipment, land, and buildings are rarely used for only one program, and apportioning costs to different programs is, again, not a simple matter. Assigning a dollar figure to materials, supplies, salaries, and travel is generally not controversial, but not so non-market items such as volunteer time. Costs spread over a period of years need to take inflation into account, hence the need to express costs in constant dollars or current dollars. Costs and benefits also need to be discounted because of time preference, a case of "payment now and gratification later." Most people would rather have money now than later, but money not used now can be invested and is worth more in the future. Spending now is thus costlier; conversely, future benefits are less valued than current ones. The "discount rate" is usually measured by the common borrowing costs over and above inflation. In North America, public investments are often discounted at 5% because it is the rate over inflation at which governments typically borrow funds.

Costs can be fixed or variable. Fixed costs do not vary according to the quantity of output. Thus a hospital building has to be heated, whether there are only ten patients or a hundred. The cost of gasoline used by a vaccination outreach team varies according to the number of kilometers traveled. The average cost of a program is its total cost divided by the quantity of output. It should be distinguished from the marginal cost, which is the additional cost of producing an extra unit of output. For example, the average cost per village in a malaria control team's territory of 10 villages may be, say, $100. Adding an extra village to the 10, however, will probably incur only an additional $20—the marginal cost, which may be substantially less than the average cost.

Decision-Making in Health Care

The techniques of economic evaluation described above serve a more general purpose than determining the worth of a particular program. Economic evaluation provides information for health policy-makers to make rational decisions in the allocation of scarce resources. While decision-making can be entirely arbitrary, whimsical, and based on nothing more than political expediency, it can also be made formal, logical, and explicit using a modeling technique known as decision analysis. It is a process of making choices in the face of uncertainty, and has its origin in the theory of games developed by mathematician John von Neumann (1903–1957) and economist Oskar Morgenstern (1902–1977).[15]

A decision analysis consists of five steps:

1. Define all alternative choices.
2. Estimate the probability of each chance outcome;
3. Assign a relative value or utility to each potential outcome;
4. Calculate the best alternative; and
5. Perform sensitivity analyses (see below).

Box 8.5 provides an example of a decision tree, a graphical presentation of decision analysis.

BOX 8.5.   A Decision Tree for Prenatal Screening Policies to Detect Down's Syndrome

A decision analysis was conducted by the Oxfordshire Health Authority in England to compare different options for prenatal screening for Down's syndrome. Individuals who screened positive on the blood test were offered amniocentesis, and, if Down's syndrome was confirmed, termination of pregnancy. The different options were compared in terms of unaffected births, cases of Down's syndrome born alive, miscarriages with Down's syndrome, amniocentesis performed, miscarriages resulting from amniocentesis, costs of screening, and number of women offered screening. The resulting decision tree looks like this:

(continued)

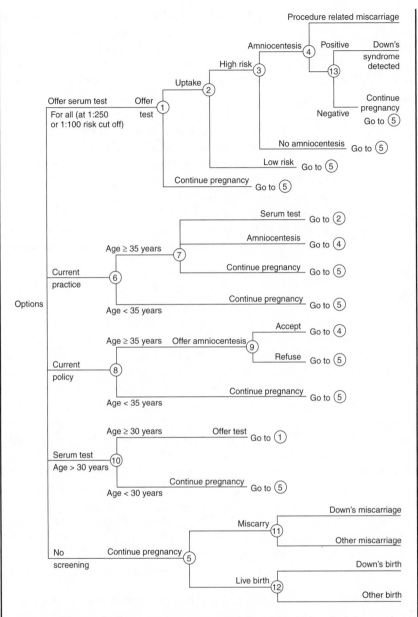

Reprinted from: Fletcher J, Hicks NR, Kay JDS, Boyd PA. Using decision analysis to compare policies for antenatal screening for Down's syndrome. *British Medical Journal* 1995; 311:351–56, with kind permission from the British Medical Association, London.

Sensitivity analysis is the procedure whereby the assumptions, values of variables, or method of data collection are changed, either singly or in combination, to determine if the overall conclusions are affected. A study is deemed to be *robust* if it arrives at more or less the same general conclusion under a variety of scenarios. There are several types of sensitivity analysis:

1. Simple sensitivity analysis—one or more parameters is varied across a plausible range (one-way or multi-way);
2. Threshold analysis—identifying a critical value of parameters above or below which the conclusion of a study will change;
3. Analysis of extremes—pessimistic (high cost/low effectiveness) vs. optimistic (low cost/high effectiveness);
4. Probabilistic sensitivity analysis—incorporate likelihood of various scenarios; assign ranges and distributions to uncertain variables.

Summary

Evaluation allows the population health practitioner to learn from experience, improve current activities, and allocate resources rationally. Efficacious strategies tested under ideal conditions may not be fully effective when deployed in the field. Efficacy loss is especially marked when technology is transferred from developed to developing countries. Because health systems operate in an environment of scarce resources, effective programs still need to be justified in terms of economic efficiency, which can be demonstrated by means of cost-effectiveness, cost-benefit, and cost-utility analyses. These types of economic evaluations all relate costs to consequences, but differ in how consequences are measured: as health effects, in monetary units, or in quality-adjusted life years, respectively. To aid the decision-maker in the face of uncertainty, a modeling technique known as "decision analysis" can be used, which makes explicit the alternate choices, their probability of occurrence, and the value associated with each potential outcome.

Case Study 8.1.   Nurse-Practitioners in Primary Care

In many countries and regions, physicians are perceived to be in short supply, or at least poorly distributed. In the 1960s and 1970s, various types of alternative health care providers or physician substitutes who are less costly to produce and support were tried in a variety of settings, in both developed and developing countries. Evaluations of such projects had mostly focused on the process rather than the outcome of care, and used an observational rather than experimental designs.

In the early 1970s a randomized controlled trial was conducted in a primary care clinic in the southwestern Ontario city of Burlington.[16] Families who had made contact with the two-physician practice over an 18-month period were randomly allocated to two groups: (1) a "usual care" group, with 1,058 families (2,796 members) who continued to receive their care from the two family physicians (FP); and (2) an "intervention" group, with 540 families (1,529 members) who were assigned to two nurse-practitioners (NP) for their first-contact health care needs. The 2 : 1 FP : NP ratio was based on the assumption that the optimal patient load for NPs was half that of FPs. Patients were contacted and explained the purpose and plan of the study. Those allocated to the intervention group were asked to make an appointment with a NP the next time they needed to use the clinic's services.

There were very few refusals to participate (0.2% of the families in the FP group and 0.9% in the NP group). Over the one-year period of study, the attrition rate was 0.9% in the FP and 0.7% in the NP group. While NPs were designated as first-contact providers in the intervention group, about one-third of cases required referrals to a physician for further care. This study was therefore not a strict comparison of FP vs. NP, but two systems of care, one using FPs exclusively, the other using NPs primarily but with physician support.

Both process and outcome measures were used in the evaluation. The process of medical care was evaluated by the use of "tracers," in this case, the appropriateness of the management of 10 health conditions and the prescription of 13 common drugs was rated according to predetermined criteria. The FPs and NPs participating in the study were not aware of which conditions or drugs had been selected for rating. Of 392 episodes of care involving the indicator conditions, FPs were rated adequate in 66% and NPs in 69%. For the 510 prescriptions written, 75% of those by FPs and 71% of those by NPs were rated appropriate. None of these differences was statistically significant.

There was also no significant difference in terms of the following outcome (i.e., health status) measures: physical function index, activity of daily living, days free from bed disability, emotional function index, social function index, crude mortality rate, and level of satisfaction.

This project demonstrates that the use of NPs in a FP practice is both safe and effective. In terms of cost to society, NPs represent substantial savings, hence it is also efficient. However, such an innovation was not adopted widely in North America because participating physicians would suffer financial loss. NP services are generally not reimbursable by public and private third-party payers. For the innovation to be adopted and disseminated, structural change in the health care system, especially the financing of health services, provider attitudes, and interprofessional rivalry, needs to occur. A decade after this RCT was published, the principal investigator of the study, Walter Spitzer, lamented the "slow death of a good idea" in an editorial. Milton Roemer, a researcher of international health systems, observed that in developed countries, "physician extenders" such as NPs were used almost exclusively among the urban and rural poor. He contended that such social inequity stemmed from the developed countries' failure to require primary care physicians to serve in places of need.

Case Study 8.2.   Fluoridation of Community Water Supply to Prevent Dental Caries

The decay of teeth, or dental caries, is present in almost all human populations. It involves the destruction of the hard structures of the teeth, a process initiated by certain bacteria in a susceptible host and promoted by a sugar-rich environment within the oral cavity. One of the most successful preventive strategies is fluoridation of the community water supply, an example of primary and passive prevention, directed at the entire population rather than only at high-risk groups (see Chapter 7).[17] Fluoride, when incorporated into the enamel, increases the resistance of teeth to the cariogenic action of bacteria. Fluoride also occurs naturally in widely varying concentrations depending on the locality.

The caries experience of an individual can be measured by the *DMFT* index, the number of decayed, missing, and filled permanent teeth. For deciduous teeth, the corresponding index is indicated by lowercase letters *dmft*.

In 1901, an observant dentist working in Colorado Springs, Frederick McKay, noticed a high number of children with stained teeth, or mottling of the enamel. Over the next several years he continued his investigations. He further noted that despite the damage to the enamel, children with mottled teeth were not more susceptible to caries. It was not until 1930 that the cause of mottling was traced to the fluoride content of drinking water. At high concentrations, fluoride causes fluorosis, but at low concentrations, it protects against caries. In the 1940s, the U.S. Public Health Service assigned a young dental officer, Trendley Dean (1893–1962), to begin a research program into the association between fluoride in water and dental caries.

In an ecological study (see Chapter 6), Dean and coworkers correlated the mean fluoride content of the public water supply in 21 cities in four states with the mean DMFT indices of over 7,000 white children aged 12–14 living in these localities:

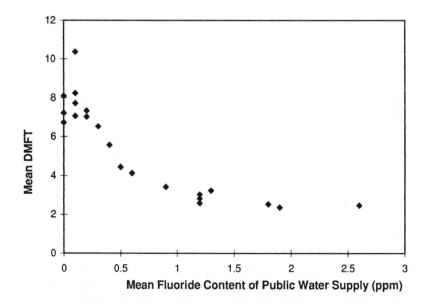

Each dot in the graph represents one of the 21 cities. It can be seen that the mean DMFT index of children living in a locality decreases as the mean fluoride concentration of the water supply increases.

Beginning in 1945, community trials of artificially adding fluoride to the public water systems began in four communities in the United States and Canada (Grand Rapids, MI; Newburgh, NY; Evanston, IL; and Brantford, ON), each paired with a control community without the intervention (Muskegon, MI; Kingston, NY; Oak Park, IL; and Sarnia, ON). These studies established the effectiveness and safety of fluoridation. Results from the Newburgh/Kingston, NY, study after 10 years are shown below. At each of the age groups the fluoridated community had much a lower DMFT index, with a dramatic reduction of around 50%.

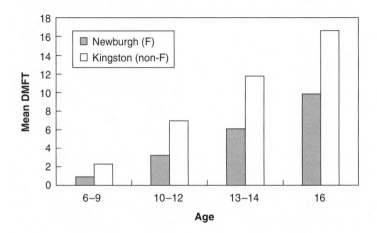

By the 1990s, 113 studies had been conducted in 23 countries. The most frequently reported effect (the *mode*) is 40%–49% reduction in dmft and 50%–59% in DMFT. In communities that had discontinued fluoridation, a reversal in the caries prevalence was reported within a few years. The magnitude of the reduction in caries prevalence tends to be smaller in more recent studies compared to the earlier trials. This is the result of the widespread availability of fluoride toothpastes and prophylactic treatment with topical fluorides, offering protection even in communities with a fluoride-deficient water supply.

A study in England, comparing the dental health of five-year-olds in fluoridated with non-fluoridated communities, found that the regression line showing the association between mean dmft and the Townsend score, an index of socioeconomic deprivation, is significantly steeper for non-fluoridated communities, suggesting that community water fluoridation reduces inequalities in dental health.

Fluoridation has been shown to be cost-effective. In the United States, it has been estimated that it costs only about 50 cents per person per year. The cost of one dental filling is equivalent to the cost of providing fluoridated public water to an individual for a lifetime. While there are alternatives that are active preventive measures requiring individual action (brushing with fluoride toothpaste) or professional intervention (topical fluoride), fluoridation of community water supplies still occupies a central place in preventive dental health care because of its equity, high compliance, and cost-effectiveness.

In 1993, 135 million Americans lived in communities with water systems where the fluoride level was artificially adjusted. Another 10 million lived in areas with an adequate fluoride level from natural sources. Thus about 56% of the total population of the United States, or 62% of the U.S. population on public water systems, are provided with adequate fluoride. The *Healthy People 2000* objective set the target of 75% of the population, which was not achieved, and the target remains unchanged for *HP 2010*. While engineering and administrative expertise is needed to maintain optimal levels, the major obstacle to the wider dissemination of a cost-effective intervention is mainly political. The deliberate "contamination" of drinking water with a chemical substance is objected to by some environmentalist groups, which have promoted claims of cancer and other detrimental effects. In many communities, such groups have been successful in reversing long-standing policies of fluoridation. The debate sometimes pits scientific evidence (or the interpretation of it) against the perception of professional power and corporate interests. Fluoridation offers another good example of risk assessment and risk management, discussed earlier in Chapter 5.

Case Study 8.3.   Economic Evaluation of Neonatal Intensive Care

The availability of neonatal intensive care units has resulted in improved chance of survival of premature and low-birth-weight infants who would otherwise have died. However, operating such units requires expensive equipment and highly skilled medical personnel. In the 1970s, a regional perinatal program was introduced in Hamilton-Wentworth County, a predominantly urban and industrialized region in southern Ontario, Canada.[18] The program consisted of three tiers of increasingly sophisticated and costly perinatal services, with level 3 offering neonatal intensive care for high-risk infants at a university hospital.

An economic evaluation of the regional perinatal program was conducted. It was a population-based study that adopted the societal perspective, rather than that of an institution or even that of the health care system. The following types of data were collected:

Health outcomes: (1) mortality, and (2) life-years adjusted for quality using utility values (preference) assigned by a sample of parents to various health states constructed from measures of physical function, role function, social/emotional function, and health problems.

Costs (expressed in constant 1978 Canadian dollars): direct cost of intensive care, share of costs of support services and overhead, physician charges, convalescent care, ambulance transport; cost of followup care (health care, special services, appliances, schooling, etc.). The anticipated lifetime earnings of survivors were subtracted from costs to yield a net economic cost. Information on current services used by survivors was obtained by interviewing parents of survivors; data on future costs and outcomes were estimated by two developmental pediatricians based on the medical history of each child, specifying a probability distribution for various outcomes

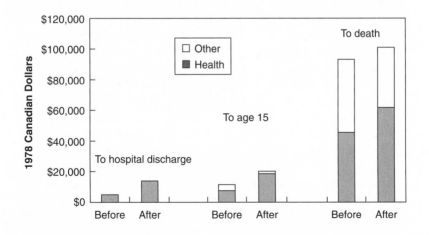

forecast. All costs were considered, regardless of who was responsible for payment (individual, government, insurance company, etc.).

With future costs, earnings, and benefits undiscounted, the following results were obtained: Among infants with birth weight (BW) 1,000–1,499 gms, 62% survived in the pre-program eras (1964–1969), compared to 77% after the regional program was in operation (1973–1977). The life-years per live birth and the QALY per live birth projected to age 15 and to death all increased by 23%–31% in the post-program period.

The cost of medical care of each live birth weighing 1,000–1,499 grams up to the time of hospital discharge was $14,200, 2.6 times the cost in the pre–intensive care era. The total (health and other) cost up to age 15 was $20,700, a 1.7-fold increase. Projected to death, the lifetime cost was $100,100, an increase of only 8%.

Thus health has improved, but so have costs. In terms of economic efficiency, the data can be used in CEA, CUA, and CBA:

		Birth weight 1,000–1,499 g	Birth weight 500–999 g
Cost-effectiveness analysis:			
Cost/additional survivor	at discharge	$59,500	$102,500
Cost/life-year gained	at age 15	$4,100	$9,400
	at death	$900	$5,100
Cost-utility analysis:			
Cost/QALY gained	at age 15	$5,100	$30,900
	at death	$900	$9,100
Cost-benefit analysis:			
Net economic benefit/live birth	at death	$24,700	−$3,700

Thus it can be seen that by every measure of economic evaluation, the impact of neonatal intensive care was more favorable among infants with BW between 1,000 and 1,499 grams than those weighing 500–999 grams. Sensitivity analysis was also performed. As the discount rate was increased from 0 to 10%, all measures became less favorable—higher costs were associated with the same level of effect or benefit. For those with BW 1,000–1,499 grams, the net economic benefit became negative when the discount rate increased beyond 3.5%. At 5%, the usual rate used in most economic evaluations, the net economic loss per live birth was $2,600 for BW 1,000–1,499 grams and $16,100 for BW 500–999 grams. The various measures did not vary much when the life expectancy was altered, or when assumptions of those lost to followup changed from "all damaged" to "all well." Variation in utility values affected those in the 500 to 999-gram group and less so the 1,000 to 1,499-gram group. Moreover, at each scenario, the direction of the difference between the two BW groups was unaffected by changes in the factor.

Case Study 8.4.   A Meta-Analysis of Adolescent Smoking Programs

A variety of approaches has been used in intervention programs to prevent adolescents from smoking.[19] These can be categorized into the following:

1. "Rational": providing factual information about smoking and its health consequences;
2. "Social reinforcement": increasing self-esteem, decreasing alienation and developing decision-making skills, with little specific focus on smoking per se;
3. "Social norm": providing alternatives to smoking such as participation in community improvement projects, vocational training, and recreational activities;
4. "Developmental": developing skills to recognize and resist social pressures to smoke.

A review of 94 school-based programs classified them into these four orientations and also scored for methodological rigor. Results of the meta-analysis based on the 48 methodologically stronger studies were presented separately. Three outcomes were measured: effect on knowledge, attitude, and behavior. An effect size was computed for the post-test and first follow-up, based on the formula $(X_e - X_c)/SD_c$, where X is the mean score and SD its standard deviation; the subscript e refers to the experimental group and c the control group.

The following graph shows the overall behavioral effect sizes according to program orientation, measured at the post-test, first, and second followup.

It can be seen that programs with a social reinforcement and social norms orientation reported positive and significant effect sizes consistently; for developmental orientation, the effects were initially positive but became negative by the second followup; programs using the rational approach had only minimal effect. In terms of impact on knowledge, programs of all four types had strong and positive effects, ranging from 0.22 to 0.95, with little or no decline between the post-test and first follow-up. With regard to attitude, only

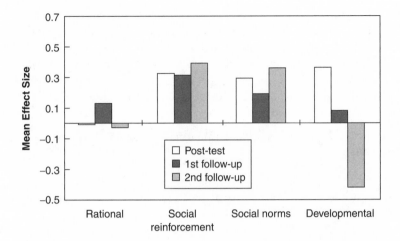

programs with the social reinforcement orientation had any significant impact, with a effect size of 0.59.

It can be concluded that school-based smoking prevention programs that rely on providing information on the harmful effects of smoking tend to improve knowledge but do not affect attitude or change behaviors. Programs that are not specifically directed at smoking but focus on increasing self-esteem and reducing alienation, and those offering activities as alternatives to smoking, are most likely to result in behavioral change.

Notes

1. These *Guiding Principles* (WHO, 1981) were published as part of the Health for All Series, which aimed to make key concepts understandable and accessible. Standard texts on health program evaluation (e.g., Veney and Kaluzny, 1998) should be consulted. Valente (2002) focuses specifically on evaluating health promotion programs.

2. See Habicht et al. (1999).

3. For a short summary of his contribution to the quality of care literature, see Donabedian (1988).

4. See the monographs by the Institute of Medicine (1985) and the Pan-American Health Organization (Panerai and Mohr, 1989). The quotation from Galbraith is cited by Panerai and Mohr (1989:1).

5. The Agency for Health Care Research and Quality replaces the Agency for Health Care Policy and Research (AHCPR) in 1999 (www.ahrq.gov). The International Network of Agencies for Health Technology Assessment web site (www.inahta.org) provides links to all the national agencies, including CCOHTA (www. ccohta.ca). Current projects and many publications are available.

6. See the commentary by Battista and Hodge (1999).

7. See McKinlay (1981).

8. Meta-analyses are discussed fully in the text by Petitti (2000). See also Blettner et al. (1999) for a comparison of traditional reviews, meta-analyses, and pooled analyses in observational studies.

9. See Orenstein et al. (1988) for a comprehensive review of the methodological issues in vaccine evaluations.

10. Modified from Mackenbach and Gunning-Schepers (1997).

11. Visit the Cochrane Collaboration's web site, www.cochrane.org, for further information.

12. For a review and critique of consensus methods, see Lomas (1991), where the quotation attributed to Abba Eban can be found.

13. Cited from Drummond et al. (1987).

14. An excellent introductory text on economic evaluation is that by Drummond et al. (1997) from which the definition is quoted (8–9). See Doubilet et al. (1986) on the varied use and misuse of the term "cost-effective." Haddix et al. (1996) discuss economic evaluation in public health programs.

15. See the general review by McNeil and Pauker (1984) on decision analysis and Briggs et al. (1994) on sensitivity analysis. General texts by Haddix et al. (1996) and Petitti (2000) also discuss decision analysis.

16. Data for this case study are obtained from Spitzer et al. (1974). See also the editorial by Spitzer (1984) and article by Roemer (1977) for further discussion of NPs and other physician extenders/substitutes.

17. For a comprehensive review of the prevention of oral disease, including fluorides, see the monograph by Murray (1996). Data for the graphs are from Dean et al. (1942) and Ast and Schlesinger (1956). An example of the reversal of caries prevalence after discontinuation of fluoridation was reported by Attwood and Blinkhorn (1991) in Scotland. The study of the impact of fluoridation on dental health inequalities is from Riley et al. (1999). A sociological and political analysis of the public controversy over fluoridation can be found in Martin (1991).

18. Data for this case study are based on Boyle et al. (1983).

19. Data on the meta-analysis are obtained from Bruvold (1993). The typology of prevention programs is based on work on drug abuse by Battjes (1985).

EXERCISE 8.1.   Evaluation Case Studies

From the abstracts provided, determine what type of economic evaluation has been conducted.

(a) Toxoplasmosis, a disease caused by the protozoan *Toxoplasma gondii*, is a zoonosis affecting cats (the final host), although many mammals, including human beings, can become infected (intermediate hosts). In healthy adults it is a relatively mild disease, but in a pregnant woman, the parasite can be transmitted to the fetus and cause severe damage to the brain and the eyes. Prevention is therefore important to relieve individual suffering and avoid costs to society. A study in Norway compares two strategies to prevent congenital toxoplasmosis: (1) health education of pregnant women on avoidance of infection; and (2) serological surveillance in pregnancy, prenatal diagnosis and antibiotic therapy.

The cost per woman is 20 Norwegian kroner (NOK) for strategy (1) and 215 NOK for strategy (2). The benefits are influenced by many uncertain factors such as the discount rate, the incidence of infection, the intrauterine transmission rate, the outcome of the pregnancy, the prognosis of the offspring, the sensitivity of the screening tests, and the effectiveness of the program. In one analysis, the ratio of benefit to cost is 9.0 for strategy (1) and 1.13 for strategy (2).

(b) Diabetes is associated with many serious complications, one of which is disease of the small retinal blood vessels (retinopathy) which may lead to blindness if undetected and untreated. A study demonstrates that, in the United States, screening and treatment of eye disease in patients with diabetes costs $1,757 per person-year of sight saved and $3,190 per quality-adjusted life-year saved. The cost/QALY is considerably lower than for many commonly accepted medical interventions reported in the literature.

(c) The treatment of renal failure involves removing toxic waste products in the blood by dialysis, of which there are two basic approaches—hemodialysis and peritoneal dialysis. A study in one Canadian pediatric hospital shows that the total annual cost of home-based continuous peritoneal dialysis for a typical uncomplicated case is CDN$47,569, about 63% of the total annual cost of ambulatory, hospital-based hemodialysis. For the range of complication probabilities considered, expected total costs are always lower with peritoneal dialysis than with hemodialysis.

(d) Hepatitis B is a serious infection that may lead to the chronic carrier state, cirrhosis, and liver cancer. Universal vaccination is recommended by many jurisdictions to eliminate the transmission of the virus, although the age at which it occurs varies. In British Columbia, Canada, public health nurses have administered the vaccine to sixth-grade students in schools since the early 1990s. An economic evaluation found that vaccinating each child cost $44, evenly split between the cost of the vaccine and the cost of administering it. Considering direct costs only, vaccination resulted in incremental costs of $161 and $2,135 for each acute and chronic infection prevented, respectively, and $2,145 for each additional life year gained. The analysis was insensitive to changing various epidemiological and economic variables (such as the probability of chronic infection following acute infection, the cost of vaccination).

(e) Tuberculosis (TB) is a major health problem globally. Efficacious drug therapy exists, which cures the individuals with the disease and interrupts transmission of the infection. The World Health Organization recommends the use of DOTS (directly observed treatment, short course). WHO developed a mathematical model that made use of routinely collected data and applied it to the world's largest TB control program involving over 500 million people in 12 provinces of China. Over a period of seven years since the early 1990s, it was found that counties that had been enrolled in the program had prevented at least 46% of the TB deaths that would otherwise have occurred.

Source: The data used in this exercise have been obtained from (a) Stray-Pedersen and Jenum (1992); (b) Javitt and Aiello (1996); (c) Coyte et al. (1996); (d) Krahn et al. (1998); and (e) Dye et al. (2000).

9

Improving the Health
of Populations

This Final Chapter Shall Be Written by You!

The writing of this chapter can be done as a small-group project or submitted as a term paper by individual students. The intent is to apply everything you have learned from this book to a specific, defined population. You should demonstrate your ability to seek out information from the scientific literature and statistical databases, critically appraise its worth, integrate and organize your thoughts and ideas, and, finally, produce a chapter that is coherent, comprehensible, and concise.

Select any population—for example:

- Infants/children/adolescents
- Ethnic minorities
- Disabled
- Adults/elderly
- Indigenous/aboriginal peoples
- Industrial workers
- Men/women
- Migrants/refugees
- Farmers/fishermen

Determine the scope of your coverage: global, national, regional, or local. For the population you have selected, organize your paper as follows:

1. *The demographic situation:* What is the estimated size of this population? What are the characteristics of this population? As an example, Figure 9.1 shows the size of the elderly population in the United States.
2. *Significant health problems:* What is the health status of this population? What are its major health problems? Cite statistical data in support, critique the quality of the data, and identify data gaps. As

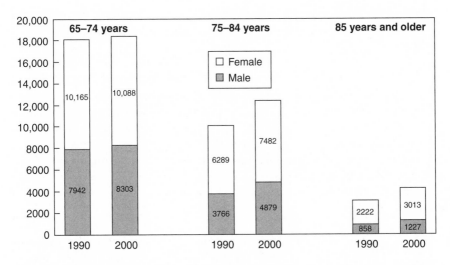

Figure 9.1. Growth in U.S. population aged 65 years and above, 1990 to 2000. Source: Hetzel and Smith (2001).

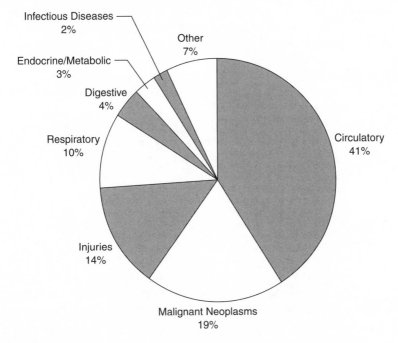

Figure 9.2. Percent distribution of causes of death among farm workers in 24 U.S. states, 1984–1993. Source: Colt et al. (2001).

an example, Figure 9.2 shows the distribution of deaths by cause among farm workers in 24 states.

3. *Determinants of health:* What are the factors that produce the health problems in this population? Is there evidence that these factors are

---

BOX 9.1.   Improving the Health of Hispanic/Latino Americans

The overall health profile of Hispanics/Latinos presents a striking so-cioeconomic disparity when compared with the health status of the rest of the American population. Nevertheless, much can be done to improve the health of this population by implementing health promotion and disease prevention (HPDP) interventions. The challenge is to develop and implement efficacious HPDP strategies for improving the health of Hispanics/Latinos across the country. HPDP interventions targeted to Hispanics/Latinos are essential for achieving the Hispanic/Latino-specific health care objectives for the nation by the year 2000.

Summary of key strategies

1. Encourage and endorse authorizing legislation at the federal level to direct federal funds for the development and evaluation of HPDP programs directed toward Hispanic/Latino groups.
2. Integrate paraprofessionals, informal community leaders, ethnic/folk healers, "prometoras de salud," and other community health workers in HPDP programming for the Hispanic/Latino community, and provide appropriate recognition and incentives for their participation.
3. Use appropriate media resources and community networks at local, state, and federal levels to educate Hispanic/Latino communities regarding HPDP issues.
4. Establish guidelines for Hispanic/Latino national and community-based organizations for accepting corporate contributions; corporations' products and services must be compatible with HPDP goals.
5. Make HPDP issues (including environmental issues) critical elements in the regulations and implementation of the North American Free Trade Agreement (NAFTA).
6. Develop a mass media marketing plan that informs the public on how to gain access to and properly utilize health and related services. This plan should target Spanish-speaking and bilingual Hispanics, especially in areas where little or no information is available (state and local).

Source: *The Surgeon General's T-O-D-O-S Report* (www.omhrc.gov/haa/HAA2pg/PlansReports1.htm)

---

responsible? Are there competing theories or perspectives on the causes of health problems in this population? As an example, Figure 9.3 shows the socioeconomic disparities between the aboriginal and non-aboriginal women of Canada.

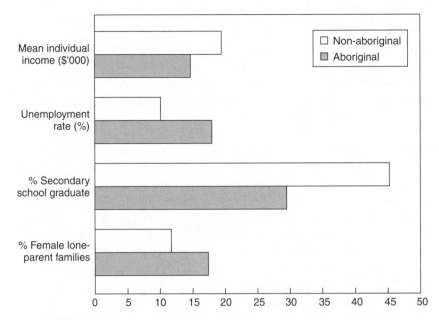

Figure 9.3. Selected socioeconomic indicators of aboriginal and non-aboriginal women in Canada, 1996. Source: Indian and Northern Affairs Canada (2001).

4. *Potential interventions:* What can be done to improve the health of this population? What is the evidence that the interventions work? Are there alternatives? Box 9.1 reproduces sections of the Surgeon General's TODOS Report, part of the Hispanic Agenda for Action of the U.S. Department of Health and Human Services.

Guide to Resources

To help you get started, and to supplement any MEDLINE search that you may have done, here are some recent background monographs and reviews. The web sites of national and international health agencies should be consulted, especially for access to documents and statistical databases (e.g., the Census Bureau for the latest demographic data of specific populations).

The literature on the health of children is vast. Pless (1994) provides a useful review of the epidemiology of childhood disorders. For a global perspective, see UNICEF's annual *State of the World's Children* report, available from its web site (www.unicef.org). Clement (2002) focuses on vulnerable children, such as the homeless, migrants, and inner city residents. There are actually few works that deal with adults (other than women) as a specific population with unique health needs, an example being Feachem et al. (1992), which focuses on developing countries.

The health of women is a rapidly developing field with a burgeoning literature. While gynecology texts have been around for centuries, a new breed of women's health text began to appear in the 1990s; for example, Ness and Kuller (1998) and Waller and McPherson (2003). Kuh and Hardy (2002) used the life-course approach. Dan (1994) offered an overview of the various theoretical perspectives. Reviews of women's health in developing countries include Santow (1995), with a focus on social disadvantages, and a World Bank discussion paper (Tinker et al., 1994). Krieger (2003) explained the difference between sex and gender and their connections to health.

The elderly is another demographic group on which a substantial literature exists. To start off, you may wish to consult a text on geriatrics/gerontology (e.g., Tallis et al., 1998). Epidemiological reviews of common health problems can be found in Wallace and Woolson (1992), and Ebrahim and Kalache (1996). For a brief global overview, see Butler (1997).

The *Report of the Secretary's Task Force on Black and Minority Health* (DHHS, 1985) is a landmark study of the health needs of disadvantaged ethnic minorities in the United States. Visit the web site of the Office of Minority Health (www.omhrc.gov). Health issues in the Black and Latino communities were examined by Braithwaite and Taylor (2001) and Aguirre-Molina and others (2001), respectively. The CDC prepared a demographic and health summary of the U.S. Hispanic/Latino population for the 2002 National Hispanic Health Leadership Summit (www.cdc.gov/nchs/data/hpdata2010/chcsummit.pdf)

The health of indigenous/aboriginal populations in Canada and the United States was reviewed by Young (1994) and Waldram et al. (1995). The August 1, 2003, issue of *Morbidity and Mortality Weekly Report* was devoted to health disparities experienced by American Indians and Alaska Natives. A World Bank study investigated poverty among indigenous peoples in Latin America (Psacharopoulos and Patrinos, 1994). The advocacy group Cultural Survival reported on the state of indigenous peoples globally (Miller, 1993).

A special issue of the journal *International Migration* contained articles on various aspects of the health of migrants (Siem and Bollini, 1992). The perilous state of the world's refugees is evident from the annual report of the United Nations High Commissioner for Refugees, available from its web site (www.unhcr.ch). Muecke (1992) contrasted the different paradigms in which the issue of refugee health can be discussed. The health problems associated with forced movements of populations (as refugees and victims of coerced resettlement or environmental catastrophes) in tropical Africa were reviewed by Prothero (1994).

For those unfamiliar with the substantial literature on the health of workers, a standard text on occupational health/epidemiology (e.g., Levy and Wegman, 2000) provides an introduction. Kraut (1994) demonstrated how the burden of illness can be estimated and what sources of data are available. Gottlieb et al. (1992) discussed the health risks experienced by blue-collar workers. A collection of papers on agricultural health and safety was edited by McDuffie et al. (1995). The *American Journal of Industrial Medicine* devoted a special issue to migrant and seasonal farm workers (Zahm and Blair, 2001). See also the review by Villarejo (2003). Visit the web sites of the National Institute of Occupational Safety and Health (www.cdc.gov/niosh/homepage.html) and the Occupational Safety and Health Administration of the Department of Labor (www.osha.gov).

Basic demographic and socioeconomic data on disabled Americans can be found in a Census Bureau report (McNeil, 1993). Consult the report of a National Academy of Sciences panel on disabilities and their prevention (Pope and Tarlov, 1991). The definitions and determinants of handicaps are reviewed by Shaar and McCarthy (1994). Barnes (2003) discusses disability from a sociological perspective. Priestley (2003) uses a life-course approach.

Bibliography

Abramson JH, Abramson ZH. *Making Sense of Data: A Self-Instruction Manual on the Interpretation of Epidemiological Data.* 3rd ed. New York: Oxford University Press, 2001.

Aguirre-Molina M, Molina C, Zambrana RE. *Health Issues in the Latino Community.* San Francisco: Jossey-Bass, 2001.

Ahmad OB, Boschi-Pinto C, Lopez AD, Murray CJL, Lozano R, Inoue M. *Age Standardization of Rates: A New WHO Standard.* GPE Discussion Paper Series No. 31. EIP/GPE/EBD. Geneva: World Health Organization (n.d., circa 2001).

Ajzen I, Fishbein M. *Understanding Attitudes and Predicting Social Behavior.* Englewood Cliffs, NJ: Prentice-Hall, 1980.

Albrecht GL, Fitzpatrick R, Scrimshaw SC (eds.), *The Handbook of Social Studies in Health and Medicine.* London: Sage, 2000.

Alland A. *Adaptation in Cultural Evolution: An Approach to Medical Anthropology.* New York: Columbia University Press, 1970.

Allison AC. Protection afforded by sickle cell trait against subtertian malarial infection. *Br Med J* 1954; i:290–94.

American Psychiatric Association. *Diagnostic and Statistical Manual of Mental Disorders. DSM-IV-Text Revision.* Washington, DC: APA, 2000.

Anderson RM. Populations, infectious disease and immunity: A very nonlinear world. *Phil Trans Roy Soc Lond B* 1994; 346:457–505.

Andrieu N, Goldstein AM. Epidemiologic and genetic approaches in the study of gene-environment interaction: An overview of available methods. *Epidemiol Rev* 1998; 20:137–47.

Anonymous. Population health looking upstream. *Lancet* 1994; 343:429–30.

Aral SO. Sexually transmitted diseases: Magnitude, determinants and consequences. *Int J STD AIDS* 2001; 12:211–15.

Albrecht GL, Fitzpatrick R, Scrimshaw SC (eds.), *The Handbook of Social Studies in Health and Medicine.* London: Sage Publications, 2000.

Armstrong BG. Comparing standardized mortality ratios. *Ann Epidemiol* 1995; 5:60–64.

Armstrong D. *Political Anatomy of the Body: Medical Knowledge in Britain in the Twentieth Century.* Cambridge: Cambridge University Press, 1983.

Armstrong D. The invention of infant mortality. *Soc Health Illness* 1986; 8:211–32.

Armstrong D. *Outline of Sociology as Applied to Medicine*. 4th ed. Oxford: Butterworth-Heinemann, 1994.

Armstrong D. The rise of surveillance medicine. *Soc Health Illness* 1995; 17:393–404.

Arnesen T, Nord E. The value of DALY life: Problems with ethics and validity of disability adjusted life years. *Br Med J* 1999; 319:1423–25.

Ast DB, Schlesinger ER. The conclusion of a ten-year study of water fluoridation. *Am J Public Health* 1956; 46:265–71.

Attwood D, Blinkhorn AS. Dental health in school children five years after water fluoridation ceased in south-west Scotland. *Int Dent J* 1991; 41:43–48.

Baird PA, Anderson TW, Newcombe HB, Lowry RB. Genetic disorders in children and young adults: A population study. *Am J Hum Genet* 1988; 42:672–93.

Bandura A. *Social Foundations of Thought and Action: A Social Cognitive Theory*. Englewood Cliffs, NJ: Prentice-Hall, 1986.

Bankowski Z, Bryant JH, Last JM (eds.), *Ethics and Epidemiology: International Guidelines*. Geneva: CIOMS, 1991.

Bard D, Verger P, Hubert P. Chernobyl, 10 years after: Health consequences. *Epidemiol Rev* 1997; 19: 187–204.

Barker DJP. *Mothers, Babies and Health in Later Life*. Edinburgh: Churchill Livingstone, 1998.

Barker DJP, Eriksson JG, Forsén T, Osmond C. Fetal origins of adult disease: Strength of effects and biological basis. *Int J Epidemiol* 2002; 31: 1235–39.

Barnes C. *Disability*. Cambridge: Cambridge University Press, 2003.

Barss P, Smith G, Baker S, Mohan D. *Injury Prevention: An International Perspective*. New York: Oxford University Press, 1998.

Bashir SA, Estève J. Analysing the difference due to risk and demographic factors for incidence or mortality. *Int J Epidemiol* 2000; 29:878–84.

Battista RN, Hodge MJ. The evolving paradigm of health technology assessment: Reflections for the millennium. *Can Med Assoc J* 1999; 160:1464–67.

Battjes RJ. Prevention of adolescent drug abuse. *Int J Addict* 1985; 20:1113–34.

Baum F. Researching public health: Behind the qualitative-quantitative methodological debate. *Soc Sci Med* 1995; 40:459–68.

Beaglehole R, Magnus P. The search for new risk factors for coronary heart disease: Occupational therapy for epidemiologists? *Int J Epidemiol* 2002; 31:1117–22.

Beck U. *Risk Society: Towards a New Modernity*. London: Sage, 1992.

Becker MH (ed.), *The Health Belief Model and Personal Health Behavior*. Thorofare, NJ: Charles B. Slack, Inc. 1974. [Reprint of winter 1974 issue of *Health Education Monographs*.]

Bellamy R. Susceptibility to mycobacterial infections: The importance of host genetics. *Genes Immun* 2003; 4:4–11.

Benfante R. Studies of cardiovascular disease and cause-specific mortality trends in Japanese-American men living in Hawaii and risk factor comparisons with other Japanese populations in the Pacific region: A review. *Hum Biol* 1992; 64:791–805.

Bennett P, Calman K (eds.), *Risk Communication and Public Health*. New York: Oxford University Press, 1999.

Ben-Shlomo Y, Kuh D. A life course approach to chronic disease epidemiology: Conceptual models, empirical challenges and interdisciplinary perspectives. *Int J Epidemiol* 2002; 31:285–93.

Bentham G, Aase A. Incidence of malignant melanoma of the skin in Norway, 1955–1989: Associations with solar ultraviolet radiation, income and holidays abroad. *Int J Epidemiol* 1996; 25:1132–38.

Berger PL, Luckmann T. *The Social Construction of Reality: A Treatise in the Sociology of Knowledge*. Garden City, NY: Doubleday, 1966.

Berkman LF. Assessing the physical health effects of social networks and social support. *Annu Rev Public Health* 1984; 5:413–32.

Berkman LF, Kawachi I (eds.), *Social Epidemiology*. New York: Oxford University Press, 2000.

Bernstein PL. *Against the Gods: The Remarkable Story of Risk*. New York: John Wiley, 1996.

Bhopal R. Paradigms in epidemiology textbooks: In the footsteps of Thomas Kuhn. *Am J Public Health* 1999; 89:1162–65.

Björntorp P, Brodoff BN (eds.), *Obesity*. Philadelphia: J.B. Lippincott, 1992.

Blackburn S, ed. *The Oxford Dictionary of Philosophy*. Oxford: Oxford University Press, 1994.

Blaser MJ. The bacteria behind ulcers. *Sci Am* 1996; 274(2):104–7.

Blettner M, Sauerbrei W, Schlehofer B, Scheuchenpflug T, Friedenreich C. Traditional reviews, meta-analyses and pooled analyses in epidemiology. *Int J Epidemiol* 1999; 28:1–9.

Blum D, Feachem RG. Measuring the impact of water supply and sanitation investments on diarrheal diseases: problems of methodology. *Int J Epidemiol* 1983; 12:357–65.

Borman KM, LeCompt MD, Goetz JP. Ethnographic and qualitative research design and why it doesn't work. *Am Behavioral Scientist* 1986; 30:42–57.

Bouchard C. Current understanding of the etiology of obesity: Genetic and non-genetic factors. *Am J Clin Nutr* 1991; 53:1561S–65S.

Boyle M, Torrance G, Sinclair J, Horwood S. Economic evaluation of neonatal intensive care of very-low-birth-weight infants. *N Engl J Med* 1983; 308:1330–37.

Braithwaite RL, Taylor SE (eds.), *Health Issues in the Black Community*. 2nd ed. San Francisco: Jossey-Bass, 2001.

Brennan TA, Carter RF. Legal and scientific probability of causation of cancer and other environmental disease in individuals. *Health Polit Policy Law* 1985; 10:33–80.

Breslow L. A quantitative approach to the World Health Organization definition of health: Physical, mental and social well being. *Int J Epidemiol* 1972; 1:347–50.

Breslow NE, Day NE (eds.), *Statistical Methods in Cancer Research: Vol. I—The*

Analysis of Case-Control Studies. Lyon: International Agency for Research on Cancer, 1980.

Breslow NE, Day NE (eds.), *Statistical Methods in Cancer Research: Vol. II—The Design and Analysis of Cohort Studies.* Lyon: International Agency for Research on Cancer, 1987.

Briggs A, Sculpher M, Buxton M. Uncertainty in the economic evaluation of health care technologies: The role of sensitivity analysis. *Health Econ* 1994; 3:95–104.

Bright RA, Avorn J, Everitt DE. Medicaid data as a resource for epidemiologic studies: Strengths and limitations. *J Clin Epidemiol* 1989; 42:937–45.

Briscoe J. Water supply and health in developing countries: selective primary health care revisited. *Am J Public Health* 1984; 74: 1009–13.

Britten N. Qualitative interviews in medical research. *Br Med J* 1995; 311: 251–53.

Browner CH, Ortiz de Montellano BR, Rubel AJ. A methodology for cross-cultural ethnomedical research. *Curr Anthropol* 1988; 29:681–702.

Brownson RC, Remington PL, Davis JR (eds.), *Chronic Disease Epidemiology and Control.* 2nd ed. Washington, DC: American Public Health Association, 1998.

Brunner E, Marmot M. Social organization, stress and health. In: Marmot M, Wilkinson RG (eds.), *Social Determinants of Health.* Oxford: Oxford University Press, 1999:17–43.

Bruvold WH. A meta-analysis of adolescent smoking prevention programs. *Am J Public Health* 1993; 83:872–80.

Buck C. Popper's philosophy for epidemiologists. *Int J Epidemiol* 1975; 4:159–68.

Buck C, Donner A. The design of controlled experiments in the evaluation of non-therapeutic interventions. *J Chron Dis* 1982; 35:531–38.

Buck C, Llopis A, Nájera E, Terris M (eds.), *The Challenge of Epidemiology: Issues and Selected Readings.* Washington, DC: Pan American Health Organization, 1988.

Buehler JW, Smith LF, Wallace EM, Heath CW, Kusiak R, Herndon JL. Unexplained deaths in a children's hospital: An epidemiologic assessment. *N Engl J Med* 1985; 313:211–16.

Bunker JP, Frazier HS, Mosteller F. Improving health: Measuring effects of medical care. *Milbank Q* 1994; 72:225–58.

Butler RN. Population aging and health. *Br Med J* 1997; 315:1082–84.

Cadman D, Chambers L, Feldman W, Sackett D. Assessing the effectiveness of community screening programs. *JAMA* 1984; 251:1580–85.

Cairncross S, Carruthers I, Curtis D, et al., *Evaluation of Village Water Supply Planning.* New York: John Wiley and Sons, 1980.

Callahan D, Jennings B. Ethics and public health: Forging a strong relationship. *Am J Public Health* 2002; 92:169–76.

Canadian Task Force on the Periodic Health Examination. *The Canadian Guide to Clinical Preventive Health Care.* Ottawa: Health Canada, 1994.

Carriere KC, Roos LL. Comparing standardized rates of events. *Am J Epidemiol* 1994; 140:472–82.

Carrington M, Hoelzel AR (eds.), *Molecular Epidemiology: A Practical Approach.* Oxford: Oxford University Press, 2001.

Carter KC. The germ theory, beriberi, and the deficiency theory of disease. *Med Hist* 1977; 21:119–36.

Carter KC. Koch's postulates in relation to the work of Jacob Henle and Edwin Klebs. *Med Hist* 1985; 29:353–74.

Cassel J. The contribution of the social environment to host resistance. *Am J Epidemiol* 1976; 104:107–23.

Cassell EJ. *The Healer's Art: A New Approach to the Doctor-Patient Relationship.* Philadelphia: Lippincott, 1976.

Cavalli-Sforza LL, Menozzi P, Piazza A. *The History and Geography of Human Genes.* Princeton: Princeton University Press, 1994.

Centerwall BS. Homicide and the prevalence of handguns: Canada and the United States, 1976 to 1980. *Am J Epidemiol* 1991; 134:1245–60.

Chandramohan D, Maude GH, Rodrigues LC, Hays RJ. Verbal autopsies for adult deaths: Issues in their development and validation. *Int J Epidemiol* 1994; 23:213–22.

Chandramohan D, Setel P, Quigley M. Effect of misclassification of causes of death in verbal autopsy: Can it be adjusted? *Int J Epidemiol* 2001; 30: 509–14.

Chesnais J-C. *The Demographic Transition: Stages, Patterns, and Economic Implications. A Longitudinal Study of Sixty-Seven Countries Covering the Period 1720–1984.* Kreager E, Kreager P (trans.). Oxford: Clarendon Press, 1992.

Chiang CL. Competing risks in mortality analysis. *Annu Rev Public Health* 1991; 12:281–307.

Clement MS. *Children at Health Risk.* Malden, MA: Blackwell Science, 2003.

Cliff AD, Haggett P. *Atlas of Disease Distributions: Analytic Approaches to Epidemiological Data.* Oxford: Blackwell, 1988.

Coburn D, Denny K, Mykhalovskiy E, McDonough P, Robertson A, Love R. Population health in Canada: A brief critique. *Am J Public Health* 2003; 93:392–96.

Cockerham WC. *Medical Sociology.* 7th ed. Englewood Cliffs, NJ: Prentice-Hall, 1997.

Cohen MM, Young TK, Hammerstrand K. Ethnic variation in surgical rates and outcomes: Cholecystectomy in Manitoba, 1972–1984. *Am J Public Health* 1989; 79:751–55.

Colgrove J. The McKeown thesis: A historical controversy and its enduring influence. *Am J Public Health* 2002; 92:725–29.

Collishaw NE, Tostowaryk W, Wigle DT. Mortality attributable to tobacco use in Canada. *Can J Public Health* 1988; 79:166–69.

Colt JS, Stallones L, Cameron LL, Dosemeci M, Zahm SH. Proportionate mortality among U.S. migrant and seasonal farmworkers in twenty-four states. *Am J Ind Med* 2001; 40:604–611.

Commission on Chronic Illness. *Chronic Illness in the United States.* Vol. I. *Prevention of Chronic Illness.* Cambridge: Harvard University Press, 1957.

Comstock GW. Evaluating vaccination effectiveness and vaccine efficacy by means of case-control studies. *Epidemiol Rev* 1994; 16:77–89.

Cook NR, Cohen J, Herbert PR, Taylor JO, Hennekens CH. Implications of small reductions in diastolic blood pressure for primary prevention. *Arch Intern Med* 1995; 155:701–9.

Cook TD, Campbell DT. *Quasi-Experimentation: Design and Analysis Issues for Field Settings*. Boston: Houghton Mifflin, 1979.

Cooke GS, Hill AVS. Genetics of susceptibility to human infectious disease. *Nat Rev Genet* 2001; 2:967–77.

Cooper RS. Race, genes, and health—new wine in old bottles? *Int J Epidemiol* 2003; 32:23–25.

Copi IM, Cohen C. *Introduction to Logic*. 8th ed. New York: Macmillan, 1990.

Coreil J, Levin JS, Jaco EG. Life style—an emergent concept in the sociomedical sciences. *Cult Med Psychiatry* 1985; 9:423–37.

Corin E. The social and cultural matrix of health and disease. In: Evans RG, Barer ML, Marmor TR (eds.), *Why Are Some People Healthy and Others Not? The Determinants of Health of Populations*. New York: Aldine de Gruyter, 1994:93–132.

Cornfield J. A method of estimating comparative rates from clinical data. Applications to cancer of the lung, breast, and cervix. *J Natl Cancer Inst* 1951; 11:1269–75.

Cornfield J. The estimation of the probability of developing a disease in the presence of competing risks. *Am J Public Health* 1957; 47:601–7.

Coughlin SS, Beauchamp TC (eds.), *Ethics and Epidemiology*. New York: Oxford University Press, 1996.

Coughlin SS, Benichou J, Weed DL. Attributable risk estimation in case-control studies. *Epidemiol Rev* 1994; 16:51–64.

Coulthart MB, Cashman NR. Variant Creutzfeldt-Jakob disease: A summary of current scientific knowledge in relation to public health. *Can Med Assoc J* 2001; 165:51–58.

Covello VT, Mumpower J. Risk analysis and risk management: An historical perspective. *Risk Anal* 1985; 5:103–20.

Covello VT, Sandman PM, Slovic P. Guidelines for communicating information about chemical risks effectively and responsibly. In: Mayo DG, Hollander RD (eds.), *Acceptable Evidence: Science and Values in Risk Management*. New York: Oxford University Press, 1991:66–90.

Cowan WM, Kopnisky KL, Hyman SE. The Human Genome Project and its impact on psychiatry. *Annu Rev Neurosci* 2002; 25:1–50.1

Coyte PC, Young LG, Tipper BL, Mitchell VM, Stoffman PR, Willumsen J, Geary DF. An economic evaluation of hospital based hemodialysis and home-based peritoneal dialysis for pediatric patients. *Am J Kid Dis* 1996; 27:557–65.

Crosby AW. *The Columbian Exchange: Biological and Cultural Consequences of 1492*. Westport, CT: Greenwood Press, 1972.

Dan AJ (ed.), *Reframing Women's Health: Multidisciplinary Research and Practice*. Thousand Oaks, CA: Sage, 1994.

Davey Smith G. The uses of "Uses of Epidemiology." *Int J Epidemiol* 2001; 30:1146–55.

Dawber TR. *The Framingham Study: The Epidemiology of Atherosclerotic Disease.* Cambridge, MA: Harvard University Press, 1980.

Day NE. Cumulative rate and cumulative risk. In: Parkin DM, Muir CS, Whelan SL, Gao YT, Ferlay J, Powell J (eds.), *Cancer Incidence in Five Continents. Volume VI.* Lyon: International Agency for Research on Cancer, 1992:862–64.

De Gruijl FR. Skin cancer and solar UV radiation. *Eur J Cancer* 1999; 35:2003–9.

Dean HT, Arnold FA, Elvove E. Domestic water and dental caries. *Public Health Rep* 1942; 57:1155–79.

Dean K (ed.), *Population Health Research: Linking Theory and Methods.* London: Sage, 1993.

Denzin NK, Lincoln YS. *Handbook of Qualitative Research.* Thousand Oaks, CA: Sage, 1994.

Department of Health and Human Services. *Report of the Secretary's Task Force on Black and Minority Health.* Vol. 1. Executive Summary. Washington, DC: Government Printing Office, 1985.

Department of Health and Human Services. *Reducing the Health Consequences of Smoking—25 Years of Progress: A Report of the Surgeon General.* Rockville, MD: DHHS/PHS/CDC, 1989.

Department of Health and Human Services. *Strategies to Control Tobacco Use in the United States: A Blueprint for Public Health Action in the 1990s.* Bethesda, MD: DHHS, 1991.

Department of Health and Human Services. *Physical Activity and Health: A Report of the Surgeon General.* Atlanta, GA: Centers for Disease Control and Prevention; and MacLean, VA: International Medical Publishing, 1996.

Department of Health and Human Services. *The Surgeon General's Call to Action to Prevent and Decrease Overweight and Obesity.* Rockville, MD: Office of the Surgeon General, 2001.

Department of Health, Education and Welfare. *Healthy People: The Surgeon General's Report on Health Promotion and Disease Prevention.* Washington, DC: DHEW/ Public Health Service, 1979.

Detels R, McEwen J, Beaglehole R, Tanaka H (eds.), *Oxford Textbook of Public Health* [3 vols]. New York: Oxford University Press, 2002.

Diez-Roux AV. Bringing context back into epidemiology: Variables and fallacies in multilevel analysis. *Am J Public Health* 1998; 88:216–22.

Dittman S, Wharton M, Vitek C, Ciotti M, Galazka A, Guichard S, Hardy I, et al. Successful control of epidemic diphtheria in the states of the former Union of Soviet Socialist Republics: Lessons learned. *J Infect Dis* 2000; 18(Suppl 1):S10–S22.

Dohrenwend BP, Levav I, Shrout PE. Socio-economic status and psychiatric disorders: The causation-selection issue. *Science* 1992; 255:946–52.

Doll R. Sir Austin Bradford Hill and the progress of medical science. *Br Med J* 1992; 305:1521–26.

Doll R, Hill AB. Smoking and carcinoma of the lung: Preliminary report. *Br Med J* 1950; ii:739–48.

Doll R, Hill AB. Mortality in relation to smoking: Ten years' observations of British doctors. *Br Med J* 1964; i:1399–1410, 1460–67.

Doll R, Peto R. Mortality in relation to smoking: 20 years' observations on male British doctors. *Br Med J* 1976; ii:1525–36.

Doll R, Peto R. *The Causes of Cancer*. New York: Oxford University Press, 1981.

Doll R, Peto R, Wheatley K, Gray R, Sutherland I. Mortality in relation to smoking: 40 years' observations on male British doctors. *Br Med J* 1994; 309: 901–11.

Donabedian A. The quality of care: How can it be assessed? *JAMA* 1988; 260:1743–48.

Donovan JL, Frankel SJ, Eyles JD. Assessing the need for health status measurement. *J Epidemiol Commun Health* 1993; 47:158–62.

Doubilet P, Weinstein M, McNeil B. Use and misuse of the term "cost-effective" in medicine. *N Engl J Med* 1986; 314:253–56.

Douglas M, Wildavsky A. *Risk and Culture: An Essay on the Selection of Technical and Environmental Dangers*. Berkeley, CA: University of California Press, 1982.

Drummond M, O'Brien B, Stoddart G, Torrance GW. *Methods for the Economic Evaluation of Health Care Programmes*. 2nd ed. Oxford: Oxford University Press, 1997.

Drummond M, Stoddart G, Labelle R, Cushman R. Health economics: An introduction for clinicians. *Ann Intern Med* 1987; 107:88–92.

Dubos R. *Man, Medicine and Environment*. New York: Praeger, 1968.

Dunn HL. Record linkage. *Am J Public Health* 1946; 36:1412–16.

Durkheim E. *Suicide: A Study in Sociology*. Glencoe, Il: The Free Press, 1951.

Dye C, Zhao F, Scheele S, Williams B. Evaluating the impact of tuberculosis control: Number of deaths prevented by short-course chemotherapy in China. *Int J Epidemiol* 2000; 29:558–64.

Eaton SB, Konner M. Paleolithic nutrition: A consideration of its nature and current implications. *N Engl J Med* 1985; 312:283–89.

Ebrahim S, Kalache A (eds.), *Epidemiology in Old Age*. London: BMJ Publishing Group, 1996.

Ebrahim S, Smith GD. Systematic review of randomized controlled trials of multiple risk factor interventions for preventing coronary heart disease. *Brit Med J* 1997; 314:1666–74.

Egeland GM, Perham-Hester KA, Hook EB. Use of capture-recapture analysis in fetal alcohol syndrome surveillance in Alaska. *Am J Epidemiol* 1995; 141:335–41.

Eichelberger MR, Gotshall CS, Feely HB, Harstad P, Bowman LM. Parental attitudes and knowledge of child safety. *Am J Dis Child* 1990; 144:714–20.

Eisenberg L. Disease and illness: Distinctions between professional and popular ideas of sickness. *Cult Med Psychiatry* 1977; 1:9–23.

Elandt-Johnson RC. Definition of rates: Some remarks on their use and misuse. *Am J Epidemiol* 1975; 102:267–71.

Elliott P, Wakefield J, Best N, Briggs D. *Spatial Epidemiology: Methods and Applications*. New York: Oxford University Press, 2001.

Epstein S. *Impure Science: AIDS, Activism and the Politics of Knowledge*. Berkeley: University of California Press, 1996.

Erickson P, Wilson R, Shannon I. Years of healthy life. *Health People Statistical*

Notes No. 7. Hyattsville, MD: National Center for Health Statistics, 1995.

Esrey SA, Habicht J-P. Epidemiologic evidence for health benefits from improved water and sanitation in developing countries. *Epidemiol Rev* 1986; 8:117–28.

Etter JF, Perneger TV. Snowball sampling by mail: Application to a survey of smokers in the general population. *Int J Epidemiol* 2000; 29:43–48.

Evans AS. Causation and disease: A chronological journey. *Am J Epidemiol* 1978; 108:249–58.

Evans GW, Kantrowitz E. Socioeconomic status and health: The potential role of environmental risk exposure. *Annu Rev Public Health* 2002; 23:303–31.

Evans R. A retrospective on the "New Perspectives." *J Health Polit Policy Law* 1982; 7:325–44.

Evans RG, Barer ML, Marmor TR (eds.), *Why Are Some People Healthy and Others Not? The Determinants of Health of Populations.* New York: Aldine de Gruyter, 1994.

Evans RG, Stoddart GL. Producing health, consuming health care. *Soc Sci Med* 1990; 31:1347–63.

Evans RG, Stoddart GL. Consuming research, producing policy? *Am J Public Health* 2003; 93:371–79.

Eyler JM. *Victorian Social Medicine: The Idea and Methods of William Farr.* Baltimore: Johns Hopkins University Press, 1979.

Ezzati M, Lopez AD, Rodgers A, Hoorn SV, Murray CJL, Comparative Risk Assessment Collaborating Group. Selected major risk factors and global and regional burden of disease. *Lancet* 2002; 360:1347–60.

Feachem RGA, Kjellstrom T, Murray CJL, Over M, Phillips MA (eds.), *The Health of Adults in the Developing World.* New York: Oxford University Press, 1992.

Feinstein AR. Scientific standards in epidemiologic studies of the menace of daily life. *Science* 1988; 242:1257–63.

Feinstein AR, Chan CK, Esdaile JM, Horwitz RI, McFarlane MJ, Wells CK. Mathematical models and scientific reality in occurrence rates for disease. *Am J Public Health* 1989; 79:1303–4.

Feinstein AR, Cicchetti DV. High agreement but low kappa: I. The problem of two paradoxes. *J Clin Epidemiol* 1990; 43:543–49.

Feinstein AR, Horwitz RI. Double standards, scientific methods, and epidemiologic research. *N Engl J Med* 1982; 307:1611–17.

Fendall NRE. *Auxiliaries in Health Care: Programmes in Developing Countries.* Baltimore: The John Hopkins University Press, 1972.

Fenner F, Henderson DA, Arita I, Jezek Z, Ladnyi ID. *Smallpox and Its Eradication.* Geneva: World Health Organization, 1988.

Field MJ, Gold MR (eds.), *Summarizing Population Health: Directions for the Development and Application of Population Metrics.* Committee on Summary Measures of Population Health, Institute of Medicine. Washington, DC: National Academy Press, 1998.

Fincham S. Community health promotion programs. *Soc Sci Med* 1992; 35: 239–49.

Fisher EB, Haire-Joshu D, Morgan GD, Rehberg H, Rost K. Smoking and smoking cessation. *Am Rev Resp Dis* 1990; 142:702–20.

Flanders WD, O'Brien TR. Inappropriate comparisons of incidence and prevalence in epidemiologic research. *Am J Public Health* 1989; 79:1301–3.

Fleiss JL. *Statistical Methods for Rates and Proportions*. 2nd ed. New York: Wiley, 1981.

Franco EL, Duarte-Franco E, Ferenczy A. Cervical cancer: Epidemiology, prevention and the role of human papillomavirus infection. *Can Med Assoc J* 2001; 164:1017–25.

Frank JW. Why "population health." *Can J Public Health* 1995; 86:162–64.

Frankfort-Nahmias C, Nahmias D. *Research Methods in the Social Sciences*. 5th ed. New York: St. Martin's Press, 1996.

Freedman B, Glass KC, Weijer C. Placebo orthodoxy in clinical research. II. Ethical, legal and regulatory myths. *J Law Med Ethics* 1996; 24:252–59.

Freedman B, Weijer C, Glass KC. Placebo orthodoxy in clinical research. I. Empirical and methodological myths. *J Law Med Ethics* 1996; 24:243–51.

Freeman J, Hutchison GB. Prevalence, incidence and duration. *Am J Epidemiol* 1980; 112:707–23.

Freirichs RR, Shaheen MA. Small community-bassed surveys. *Annu Rev Public Health* 2001; 22:231–47.

Friedman LM, Furberg CD, DeMets DL. *Fundamentals of Clinical Trials*. 3rd ed. St Louis: Mosby, 1996.

Fries JF. Aging, natural death, and the compression of morbidity. *N Engl J Med* 1980; 303:130–36.

Fries JF. Compression of morbidity in the elderly. *Vaccine* 2000; 18:1584–89.

Gail MH, Benichou J (eds.), *Encyclopedia of Epidemiologic Methods*. Chichester: Wiley, 2000.

Gajdusek DC. Unconventional viruses and the origin and disappearance of kuru. *Science* 1977; 197:943–60.

Gardner JW, Sanborn JS. Years of potential life lost (YPLL)—what does it measure? *Epidemiology* 1990; 1:322–29.

Garro L. Explaining high blood pressure: Variation in knowledge about illness. *Am Ethnologist* 1988; 15:98–119.

Gazmararian JA, Foxman B, Yen LT, Morgenstern H, Edington DW. Comparing the predictive accuracy of health risk appraisal: The Centers of Disease Control versus Carter Center Program. *Am J Public Health* 1991; 81:1296–301.

Gee EM. Misconceptions and misapprehensions about population aging. *Int J Epidemiol* 2002; 31:750–53.

Gibson RS. *Principles of Nutritional Assessment*. New York: Oxford University Press, 1990.

Giddens A. *Modernity and Self-Identity*. Cambridge: Polity, 1991.

Glaser BG, Strauss AL. *The Discovery of Grounded Theory: Strategies for Qualitative Research*. Chicago: Aldine, 1967.

Gold MR, Stevenson D, Fryback DG. HALYs and QALYs and DALYs, Oh My: Similarities and differences in summary measures of population health. *Annu Rev Public Health* 2002; 23:115–34.

Goldman L. Statistics and the science of society in early Victorian Britain: An intellectual context for the General Register Office. *Soc Hist Med* 1991; 4:415–34.

González MA, Artalejo FR, Calero JR. Relationship between socioeconomic status and ischemic heart disease in cohort and case-control studies, 1960–1993. *Int J Epidemiol* 1998; 27:350–58.

Goodman RA, Buehler JW, Koplan JP. The epidemiologic field investigation: Science and judgement in public health practice. *Am J Epidemiol* 1990; 132:9–16.

Gottlieb NH, Weinstein RP, Baun WB, Bernacki EJ. A profile of health risks among blue-collar workers. *J Occup Med* 1992; 34:61–68.

Gotzsche PC, Olsen O. Is screening for breast cancer with mammography justifiable? *Lancet* 2000; 355:129–34.

Green E, Short SD, Duarte-Davidson R, Levy LS. Public and professional perceptions of environmental and health risks. In: Bennett P, Calman K (eds.), *Risk Communication and Public Health*. New York: Oxford University Press, 1999:51–64.

Green LW, George MA, Daniel M, Frankish CJ, Herbert CJ, Bowie WR, O'Neill M. *Participatory Research in Health Promotion in Canada*. Ottawa: The Royal Society of Canada, 1995.

Green LW, Kreuter MW. *Health Promotion Planning: An Educational and Environmental Approach*. 2nd ed. Mountain View, CA: Mayfield, 1991.

Green LW, Ottoson JM. *Community and Population Health*. 8th ed. Boston: WCB/McGraw-Hill, 1999.

Greenland S, ed. *Evolution of Epidemiologic Ideas: Annotated Readings on Concepts and Methods*. Chestnut Hill, MA: Epidemiologic Resources Inc., 1987.

Greenland S. Interpretation and choice of effect measures in epidemiologic analyses. *Am J Epidemiol* 1987; 125:761–68.

Greenland S. Basic methods for sensitivity analysis of biases. *Int J Epidemiol* 1996; 25:1107–16.

Greenland S. Induction versus Popper: Substance versus semantics. *Int J Epidemiol* 1998; 27:543–48.

Greenland S. Relation of probability of causation to relative risk and doubling dose: A methodologic error that has become a social problem. *Am J Public Health* 1999; 89:1166–69.

Greenland S. Ecologic versus individual-level sources of bias in ecologic estimates of contextual health effects. *Int J Epidemiol* 2001; 30:1343–50.

Greenland S, Morgenstern H. Confounding in health research. *Annu Rev Public Health* 2001; 22:189–212.

Greenland S, Robins J. Conceptual problems in the definition and interpretation of attributable fractions. *Am J Epidemiol* 1988; 128:1185–97.

Greenland S, Robins J. Ecologic studies—biases, misconceptions and counterexamples. *Am J Epidemiol* 1994; 139:747–71.

Gregg MB (ed.), *Field Epidemiology*. 2nd ed. New York: Oxford University Press, 2002.

Gribble JN, Preston S (eds.), *The Epidemiological Transition: Policy and Planning*

Implications for Developing Countries. Washington, DC: National Academy Press, 1993.

Grove RD, Hetzel AM. *Vital Statistics Rates in the United States, 1940–1960.* Washington, DC: National Center for Health Statistics, 1968.

Grover SA, Coupal L, Hu XP. Identifying adults at increased risk of coronary heart disease: How well do the current cholesterol guidelines work? *JAMA* 1995; 274:801–6.

Habicht JP, Victora CG, Vaughan JP. Evaluation designs for adequacy, plausibility and probability of public health programme performance and impact. *Int J Epidemiol* 1999; 28:10–18.

Hacking I. *The Emergence of Probability: A Philosophical Study of Early Ideas about Probability, Induction, and Statistical Inference.* London: Cambridge University Press, 1975.

Haddix AC, Teutsch SM, Shaffer PA, Duñet DO (eds.), *Prevention Effectiveness: A Guide to Decision Analysis and Economic Evaluation.* New York: Oxford University Press, 1996.

Hahn RA. *Sickness and Healing: An Anthropological Perspective.* New Haven, CT: Yale University Press, 1995.

Hahn RA (ed.), *Anthropology in Public Health: Bridging Differences in Culture and Society.* New York: Oxford University Press, 1999.

Hamlin C. *Public Health and Social Justice in the Age of Chadwick.* Cambridge: Cambridge University Press, 1997.

Hanley JA. Appropriate use of multivariate analysis. *Annu Rev Public Health* 1983; 4:155–80.

Hansluwka HE. Measuring the health of populations: Indicators and interpretations. *Soc Sci Med* 1985; 20:1207–24.

Harding JE. The nutritional basis of the fetal origins of adult disease. *Int J Epidemiol* 2001; 30:15–23.

Hardman AE. Physical activity and health: current issues and research needs. *Int J Epidemiol* 2001; 30:1193–97.

Harlow SD, Linet MS. Agreement between questionnaire data and medical records: The evidence for accuracy of recall. *Am J Epidemiol* 1989; 129:233–48.

Hayes MV. On the epistemology of risk: Language, logic and social science. *Soc Sci Med* 1992; 35:401–7.

Health Canada. *Strategies for Population Health: Investing in the Health of Canadians.* Ottawa, 1994.

Health and Welfare Canada. *A New Perspectives on the Health of Canadians.* Ottawa: DNHW, 1974.

Health and Welfare Canada. *Achieving Health for All.* Ottawa: DNHW, 1986.

Helman CG. *Culture, Health and Illness.* 4th ed. Oxford: Butterworth-Heinemann, 2000.

Hendrick RE, Smith RA, Rutledge JH III, Smart CR. Benefit of screening mammography in women aged 40–49: A new meta-analysis of randomized controlled trials. *J Natl Cancer Inst Monogr* 1997; 22:87–92.

Hennekens CH, Buring JE. Contributions of observational evidence and clinical trials in cancer prevention. *Cancer* 1994; 74(Suppl 9):2625–29.

Hertz-Picciotto I. Epidemiology and quantitative risk assessment: A bridge from science to policy. *Am J Public Health* 1995; 85:491–93.

Hertzman C, Power C, Matthews S, Manor O. Using an interactive framework of society and lifecourse to explain self-rated health in early adulthood. *Soc Sci Med* 2001; 53:1575–85.

Hetzel L, Smith A. The 65 years and over population: 2000. *Census 2000 Brief*. Washington, DC: US Census Bureau, 2001 (C2KBR/01-10).

Higgins MW, Luepker RV (eds.), *Trends in Coronary Heart Disease Mortality: The Influence of Medical Care*. New York: Oxford University Press, 1988.

Hill AB. The environment and disease: association or causation? *Proc Roy Soc Med* 1965; 58:295–300.

Hill AB, Hill ID. *Bradford Hill's Principles of Medical Statistics*. 12th ed. Sevenoaks, Kent: Edward Arnold, 1991.

Holford TR. Understanding the effects of age, period, and cohort on incidence and mortality rates. *Annu Rev Public Health* 1991; 12:425–57.

Hook EB. Incidence and prevalence as measures of the frequency of birth defects. *Am J Epidemiol* 1982; 116:743–77.

Hook EB, Regal RR. Capture-recapture methods in epidemiology: Methods and limitations. *Epidemiol Rev* 1995; 17:243–64.

Horn JS. *Away With All Pests: An English Surgeon in People's China, 1954–1969*. New York: Monthly Review Press, 1969.

Hunter DJ. The future of molecular epidemiology. *Int J Epidemiol* 1999; 28:S1012–14.

Hyams KC. Developing case definitions for symptom-based conditions: The problem of specificity. *Epidemiol Rev* 1998; 20:148–56.

Idler EL, Binyamini Y. Self-rated health and mortality: A review of 27 community studies. *J Health Soc Behav* 1997; 38:21–37.

Illich I. *Medical Nemesis: The Expropriation of Health*. London: Marion Boyars, 1975.

Illing EM, Kaiserman MJ. Mortality attributable to tobacco use in Canada and its regions 1998. *Can J Public Health* 2004; 95:38–44.

Indian and Northern Affairs Canada. *Aboriginal Women: A Profile from the 1996 Census*. 2nd ed. Ottawa: Public Works and Government Services, 2001. Cat. No. QS-3557-010-BB-A1.

Inhorn MC. Medical anthropology and epidemiology: Divergences or convergences. *Soc Sci Med* 1995; 40:285–90.

Institute of Medicine. *Assessing Medical Technologies*. Washington, DC: National Academy Press, 1985.

Institute of Medicine. *The Future of Public Health*. Washington, DC: National Academy Press, 1988.

International Agency for Research on Cancer. *Tobacco Smoking*. Monographs on the Evaluation of the Carcinogenic Risk of Chemicals to Humans, No. 38. Lyon: IARC, 1986.

Israel RA, Rosenberg HM, Curtin LR. Analytical potential for multiple cause-of-death data. *Am J Epidemiol* 1986; 124:161–79.

Jacobsen M. Against Popperized epidemiology. *Int J Epidemiol* 1976; 5:9–11.

Jacobsen SJ, Bergstralh EJ, Guess HA, Katusic SK, et al. Predictive properties of serum prostate-specific antigen testing in a community-based setting. *Arch Intern Med* 1996; 156:2462–68.

Jacobson D. The cultural context of social support and support network. *Med Anthropol Q* 1987; 1:42–67.

Jadad A. *Randomized Controlled Trials*. London: BMJ Books, 1998.

Jamison DT, Mosley WH, Measham AR, Bobadilla JL (eds.), *Disease Control Priorities in Developing Countries*. New York: Oxford University Press, 1993.

Janes CR, Stall R, Gifford SM (eds.), *Anthropology and Epidemiology: Interdisciplinary Approaches to the Study of Health and Disease*. Dordrecht, Holland: D. Reidel, 1986.

Jarvis M, Tunstall-Pedoe H, Feyerabend C, Vesey C, Saloojee Y. Comparison of tests used to distinguish smokers from non-smokers. *Am J Public Health* 1987; 77:1435–38.

Jasanoff S. Acceptable evidence in a pluralistic society. In: Mayo DG, Hollander RD (eds.), *Acceptable Evidence: Science and Values in Risk Management*. New York: Oxford University Press, 1991:29–47.

Javitt JC, Aiello LP. Cost-effectiveness of detecting and treating diabetic retinopathy. *Ann Intern Med* 1996; 124:164–69.

Jernigan DB, Raghunathan PL, Bell BP, Brechner R, Bresnitz EA, Butler JC, Cetron M, et al. Investigation of bioterrorism-related anthrax, United States, 2001: Epidemiologic findings. *Emerg Infect Dis* 2002; 8:1019–28.

Johnson BB, Covello VT (eds.), *The Social and Cultural Construction of Risk: Essays on Risk Selection and Perception*. Dordrecht, Holland: D. Reidel, 1987.

Judge K. Income distribution and life expectancy: A critical appraisal. *Br Med J* 1995; 311:1282–85.

Kahn HA, Sempos CT. *Statistical Methods in Epidemiology*. New York: Oxford University Press, 1989.

Kannel WB. Clinical misconceptions dispelled by epidemiological research. *Circulation* 1995; 92:3350–60.

Karhausen LR. The poverty of Popperian epidemiology. *Int J Epidemiol* 1995; 24:869–74.

Kark SL. *Community Oriented Primary Care*. New York: Appleton-Century-Croft, 1981.

Karlen A. *Man and Microbes: Disease and Plagues in History and Modern Times*. New York: Simon and Schuster, 1995.

Kars-Marshall C, Spronk-Boon YW, Pollemans MC. National health interview surveys for health care policy. *Soc Sci Med* 1988; 26:223–33.

Karter AJ. Race, genetics, and disease—in search of a middle ground. *Int J Epidemiol* 2002; 32:26–28.

Kasperson RE, Kasperson JX. Hidden hazards. In: Mayo DG, Hollander RD (eds.), *Acceptable Evidence: Science and Values in Risk Management*. New York: Oxford University Press, 1991:9–28.

Kasperson RE, Renn O, Slovic P, Brown HS, Emel J, Goble R, et al. The social amplification of risk: A conceptual framework. *Risk Anal* 1988; 8:177–187.

Katz S, Branch LG, Branson MH, et al. Active life expectancy. *N Engl J Med* 1983; 309:1218–23.

Kawachi I, Kennedy BP, Glass R. Social capital and self-rated health: A contextual analysis. *Am J Public Health* 1999; 89:1187–93.

Kawachi I, Kennedy BP, Lochner K, Prothrow-Stith D. Social capital, income inequality, and mortality. *Am J Public Health* 1997; 87:1491–98.

Kawachi I, Kennedy BP, Wilkinson RG (eds.), *The Society and Population Health Reader: Income Inequality and Health*. New York: New Press, 1999.

Kelly S, Hertzman C, Daniel M. Searching for the biological pathways between stress and health. *Annu Rev Public Health* 1997; 18:437–62.

Kelsey JL, Whittemore AS, Thompson WD, Evans AS. *Methods in Observational Epidemiology*. 2nd ed. New York: Oxford University Press, 1996.

Kendall O, Lipskie T, MacEachern S. Canadian health surveys, 1950–1997. *Chron Dis Can* 1997; 1870–90.

Kennedy BP, Kawachi I, Prothrow-Stith D. Income distribution and mortality: Cross sectional ecological study of the Robin Hood index in the United States. *Br Med J* 1996; 312:1004–7.

Khoury MJ, Burke W, Thomson EJ (eds.), *Genetics and Public Health in the 21st Century Using Genetic Information to Improve Health and Prevent Disease*. New York: Oxford University Press, 2000.

Kindig DA. *Purchasing Population Health: Paying for Results*. Ann Arbor: University of Michigan Press, 1997.

Kindig DA, Stoddart GL. What is population health? *Am J Public Health* 2003; 93:380–83.

King H, Aubert RE, Herman WR. Global burden of diabetes, 1995–2025: Prevalence, numerical estimates, and projections. *Diabetes Care* 1998; 21(9):1414–31.

King RA, Rotter JIR, Motulsky AG (eds.), *The Genetic Basis of Common Diseases*. 2nd ed. New York: Oxford University Press, 2003.

Kirchner T, Nelson J, Burdo H. The autopsy as a measure of accuracy of the death certificate. *N Engl J Med* 1985; 313:1263–69.

Kitzinger J. Introducing focus groups. *Br Med J* 1995; 311:299–302.

Kleinbaum DG. *Logistic Regression: A Self-Learning Text*. New York: Springer-Verlag, 1994.

Kleinbaum DG, Kupper LL, Morgenstern H. *Epidemiologic Research: Principles and Quantitative Methods*. New York, NY: Van Nostrand Reinhold, 1982.

Kleinbaum DG, Kupper LL, Muller KA. *Applied Regression Analysis and Other Multivariable Methods*. 2nd ed. Boston: Duxbury Press, 1987.

Kleinman A. Anthropology and psychiatry: The role of culture in cross-cultural research on illness. *Br J Psychiatry* 1987; 151:447–54.

Kleinman JC. Age-adjusted mortality indexes for small areas: Applications to health planning. *Am J Public Health* 1977; 67:834–40.

Knowler WC, Williams RC, Pettitt DJ, Steinberg AG. Gm 3;5,13,14 and type 2 diabetes mellitus: an association in American Indians with genetic admixture. *Am J Hum Genet* 1988; 43:520–26.

Koopman JS, Longini IM. The ecological effects of individual exposures and nonlinear disease dynamics in populations. *Am J Public Health* 1994; 84:836–42.

Koopman JS, Lynch JW. Individual causal models and population system models in epidemiology. *Am J Public Health* 1999; 89:1170–74.

Koplan JP, Fleming DW. Current and future public health challenges. *JAMA* 2000 284:1696–8.

Kotchick BA, Shaffer A, Forehand R, Miller KS. Adolescent sexual risk behavior: A multi-system perspective. *Clin Psychol Rev* 2001; 21:493–519.

Krahn AD, Manfreda J, Tate RB, Mathewson FAL, Cuddy TE. The natural history of atrial fibrillation: Incidence, risk factors, and prognosis in the Manitoba Follow-Up Study. *Am J Med* 1995; 98:476–84.

Krahn M, Guasparini R, Sherman M, Detsky AS. Costs and cost-effectiveness of a universal, school-based hepatitis B vaccination program. *Am J Public Health* 1998; 88:1638–44.

Krailsheimer AJ (trans and ed.), *Pascal Penseés*. Harmondsworth, UK: Penguin Books, 1966.

Kramer M. *Clinical Epidemiology and Biostatistics*. Berlin: Springer-Verlag, 1988.

Kramer M, Boivin JF. Toward an "unconfounded" classification of epidemiologic research design. *J Chron Dis* 1987; 40:683–88.

Kraut A. Estimates of the extent of morbidity and mortality due to occupational diseases in Canada. *Am J Ind Med* 1994; 25:267–78.

Krieger J, Higgins DL. Housing and health: Time again for public health action. *Am J Public Health* 2002; 92:758–68.

Krieger N. The making of public health data: Paradigms, politics, and policy. *J Public Health Policy* 1992; 13:412–27.

Krieger N. Epidemiology and the web of causation: Has anyone seen the spider? *Soc Sci Med* 1994; 39:887–903.

Krieger N. Questioning epidemiology: Objectivity, advocacy, and socially responsible science. *Am J Public Health* 1999; 89:1151–53.

Krieger N. Epidemiology and social science: Toward a critical re-engagement in the twenty-first century. *Epidemiol Rev* 2000; 22:155–63.

Krieger N. Theories for social epidemiology in the 21st century: An ecosocial perspective. *Int J Epidemiol* 2001; 30:668–77.

Krieger N. Genders, sexes, and health: What are the connections—and why does it matter? *Int J Epidemiol* 2003; 32:652–57.

Krieger N, Williams DR, Moss NE. Measuring social class in U.S. public health research: Concepts, methodologies, and guidelines. *Annu Rev Public Health* 1997; 18:341–78.

Kuh D, Ben-Shlomo Y. *A Life Course Approach to Chronic Disease Epidemiology*. New York: Oxford University Press, 1997.

Kuh D, Hardy R (eds.), *A Life Course Approach to Women*. New York: Oxford University Press, 2002.

Kuhn TS. *The Structure of Scientific Revolutions*. 3rd ed. Chicago: University of Chicago Press, 1996.

Kuller LH. Epidemiology is the study of "epidemics" and their prevention. *Am J Epidemiol* 1991; 134:1051–56.

Ladyman J. *Understanding Philosophy of Science*. London: Routledge, 2002.

Lai D, Hardy RJ. Potential gains in life expectancy or years of potential life lost: Impact of competing risks of death. *Int J Epidemiol* 1999; 28:894–98.

Lamberts H, Wood M. The birth of the International Classification of Primary Care (ICPC). *Fam Pract* 2002; 19:433–35.

Landy D (ed.), *Culture, Disease, and Healing: Studies in Medical Anthropology*. New York: Macmillan, 1977.

Larson CP, Pless B. Risk factors for injury in a three-year-old cohort. *Am J Dis Child* 1988; 142:1052–57.

Lasky T, Stolley PD. Selection of cases and controls. *Epidemiol Rev* 1994; 16: 6–15.

Last JM. What is "clinical epidemiology"? *J Public Health Policy* 1988; 9:159–63.

Last JM. Guidelines on ethics for epidemiologists. *Int J Epidemiol* 1990; 19: 226–29.

Last JM (ed.), *A Dictionary of Epidemiology*. 4th ed. New York: Oxford University Press, 2001.

Lauderdale DS, Furner SE, Miles TP, Goldberg J. Epidemiologic uses of Medicare data. *Epidemiol Rev* 1993; 15:319–27.

Laupacis A, Sackett DL, Roberts RS. An assessment of clinically useful measures of the consequences of treatment. *N Engl J Med* 1988; 318:1728–33.

Lawlor DA, Stone T. Public health and data protection: An inevitable collision or potential for a meeting of minds? *Int J Epidemiol* 2001; 30:1221–25.

Leibson CL, Ballard DJ, Whisnant JP, Melton LJ. The compression of morbidity hypothesis: Promise and pitfalls of using record-linked database to assess secular trends in morbidity and mortality. *Milbank Q* 1992; 70:127–54.

Levin ML, Goldstein H, Gerhardt PR. Cancer and tobacco smoking: A preliminary report. *J Am Med Assoc* 1950; 143:336–38.

Levy BS, Wegman DH (eds.), *Occupational Health: Recognizing and Preventing Work-Related Disease and Injury*. 4th ed. Philadelphia: Lippincott, Williams and Wilkins, 2000.

Liddell FDK. The development of cohort studies in epidemiology: A review. *J Clin Epidemiol* 1988; 41:1217–37.

Lilienfeld D. Definitions of epidemiology. *Am J Epidemiol* 1978; 107:87–90.

Lilienfeld DE. The "greening of epidemiology": Sanitary physicians and the London Epidemiological Society (1830–1870). *Bull Hist Med* 1979; 52: 503–28.

Lilienfeld DE, Black B. The epidemiologist in court: Some comments. *Am J Epidemiol* 1986; 123:961–64.

Lilienfeld AM, Lilienfeld DE. A century of case-control studies: Progress? *J Chron Dis* 1979; 32:5–13.

Lilienfeld DE, Stolley PD. *Foundations of Epidemiology*. 3rd ed. New York: Oxford University Press, 1994.

Lin SS, Kelsey JL. Use of race and ethnicity in epidemiologic research: Concepts, methodological issues, and suggestions for research. *Epidemiol Rev* 2000; 22:187–202.

Livingstone FB. Anthropological implications of sickle-cell gene distribution in West Africa. *Am Anthropologist* 1958; 60:533–62.

Llorca J, Delgado-Rodriguez M. Competing risks analysis using Markov chains: Impact of cerebrovascular and ischemic heart disease in cancer mortality. *Int J Epidemiol* 2001; 30:99–101.

Lloyd SS, Rissing JP. Physician and coding errors in patient records. *J Am Med Assoc* 1985; 254:1330–36.

Lock M. The concept of race: An ideological construct. *Transcult Psychiat Res Rev* 1993; 30:203–27.

Locke FB, King H. Cancer mortality risk among Japanese in the United States. *J Nat Cancer Inst* 1980; 65:1149–56.

Logan S, Spencer N. Smoking and other health related behaviors in the social and environmental context. *Arch Dis Child* 1996; 74:176–79.

Lomas J. Words without action? The production, dissemination, and impact of consensus recommendations. *Annu Rev Public Health* 1991; 12:41–65.

Lowry S. Indoor air quality. *Br Med J* 1989; 299:1388–90.

Lowry S. Noise, space and light. *Br Med J* 1989; 299:1439–42.

Lowry S. Temperature and humidity. *Br Med J* 1989; 299:1326–28.

Lowry S. Sanitation. *Br Med J* 1990; 300:177–79.

Luostarinen T, Hakulinen T, Pukkala E. Cancer risk following a community-based programme to prevent cardiovascular diseases. *Int J Epidemiol* 1995; 24:1094–9.

Macaulay AC, Commanda LE, Freeman WL, Gibson N, McCabe ML, Robbins CM, Twohig PL. Participatory research maximises community and lay involvement. *Brit Med J* 1999; 319:774–78.

Macdonald LA, Sackett DL, Haynes RB, Taylor DW. Labelling in hypertension: A review of the behavioral and psychological consequences. *J Chron Dis* 1984; 37:933–42.

Macfarlane AJ. Infant and perinatal mortality. In: Gail MH, Benichou J (eds.), *Encyclopedia of Epidemiologic Methods*. Chichester: Wiley, 2000: 442–47.

MacIntyre S. The Black Report and beyond: What are the issues? *Soc Sci Med* 1997; 44:723–45.

Mackenbach JP. Public health epidemiology. *J Epidemiol Comm Health* 1995; 49:333–34.

Mackenbach JP. The contribution of medical care to mortality decline: McKeown revisited. *J Clin Epidemiol* 1996; 49:1207–13.

Mackenbach JP. Income inequality and population health: Evidence favouring a negative correlation between income inequality and life expectancy has disappeared. *Br Med J* 2002; 324:1–2.

Mackenbach JP, Gunning-Schepers LJ. How should interventions to reduce inequalities in health be evaluated? *J Epidemiol Community Health* 1997; 51:359–64.

Mackenbach JP, Kunst A. Measuring the magnitude of socioeconomic inequalities in health: An overview of available measures illustrated with two examples from Europe. *Soc Sci Med* 1997; 44:757–71.

Maclure M. Popperian refutation in epidemiology. *Am J Epidemiol* 1985; 121: 343–50.

Maclure M, Willett WC. Misinterpretation and misuse of the kappa statistic. *Am J Epidemiol* 1987; 126:161–69.

MacMahon B, Pugh TF. *Epidemiology: Principles and Methods*. Boston: Little, Brown and Company, 1970.

Maldonado G, Greenland S. Estimating causal effects. *Int J Epidemiol* 2002; 31:422–29.

Manderson L, Aaby P. An epidemic in the field? Rapid assessment procedures and health research. *Soc Sci Med* 1992; 35:834–50.

Mantel H, Haenszel W. Statistical aspects of the analysis of data from retrospective studies of disease. *J Natl Cancer Inst* 1959; 22:719–48.

Markina SS, Maksimova NM, Vitek CR, Bogatyreva EY, Monisov AA. Diphtheria in the Russian Federation in the 1990s. *J Infect Dis* 2000; 181 (Suppl 1):S27–S34.

Marlatt GA. Harm reduction: Come as you are. *Addict Behav* 1996; 21:779–88.

Marmot M, Ryff CD, Bumpass LL, Shipley M, Marks NF. Social inequalities in health: Next questions and converging evidence. *Soc Sci Med* 1997; 44: 901–10.

Marmot M, Wilkinson RG (eds.), *Social Determinants of Health*. Oxford: Oxford University Press, 1999.

Marmot MG, Smith GD, Stansfield S, et al. Health inequalities among British civil servants: The Whitehall II Study. *Lancet* 1991; 337:1387–93.

Marteau TM, Kinmonth AL. Screening for cardiovascular risk: Public health imperative or matter for individual informed choice? *Brit Med J* 2002; 325:78–80.

Martikainen P, Bartley M, Lahelma E. Psychosocial determinants of health in social epidemiology. *Int J Epidemiol* 2002; 31:1091–93.

Martin B. *Scientific Knowledge in Controversy: The Social Dynamics of the Fluoridation Debate*. Albany, NY: SUNY Press, 1991.

Mathers CD, Sadana R, Salomon JA, Murray CJL, Lopez AD. Healthy life expectancy in 191 countries, 1999. *Lancet* 2001; 357:1685–91.

Mayo DG, Hollander RD (eds.), *Acceptable Evidence: Science and Values in Risk Management*. New York: Oxford University Press, 1991.

Mays VM, Ponce NA, Eashington DL, Cochran SD. Classification of race and ethnicity: Implications for public health. *Annu Rev Public Health* 2003; 24:83–110.

Mays N, Pope C (eds.), *Qualitative Research in Health Care*. 2nd ed. London: BMJ Publishing Group, 2000.

McDowell I, Newell C. *Measuring Health: A Guide to Rating Scales and Questionnaires*. 2nd ed. New York: Oxford University Press, 1996.

McDuffie HH, Dosman JA, Semchuk KM, Olenchock SA, Senthilselven A (eds.), *Agricultural Health and Safety: Work-place, Environment, Sustainability*. Boca Raton: CRC Press, 1995.

McElroy A. Biocultural models in studies of human health and adaptation. *Med Anthropol Quarterly* 1990; 4:243–65.

McElroy A, Townsend PK (eds.), *Medical Anthropology in Ecological Perspective*. 3rd ed. Boulder, CO: Westview Press, 1996.

McFarland BH. Comparing period prevalences with application to drug utilization. *J Clin Epidemiol* 1996; 49:473–82.

McHorney CA. Health assessment methods for adults: Past accomplishments and future challenges. *Annu Rev Public Health* 1999; 20:309–35.

McKeown T. *Modern Rise of Population*. London: Edward Arnold, 1976.

McKeown T. *The Role of Medicine: Dream, Mirage or Nemesis.* 2nd ed. Oxford: Basil Blackwell, 1979.

McKeown T. *The Origins of Human Disease.* Oxford: Basil Blackwell, 1988.

McKinlay JB. From "promising report" to "standard procedure": Seven stages in the career of a medical innovation. *Milbank Q* 1981; 59:375–411.

McKinlay JB. The promotion of health through planned sociopolitical change: Challenge for research and policy. *Soc Sci Med* 1993; 36:109–17.

McKinlay J, Marceau L. US public health and the 21st century: Diabetes mellitus. *Lancet* 2000; 356:757–61.

McKinlay JB, McKinlay SM. The questionable effect of medical measures on the decline in mortality in the United States in the twentieth century. *Milbank Q* 1977; 55:405–28.

McKusick VA. *Mendelian Inheritance in Man: A Catalogue of Human Genes and Genetic Disorders.* 12th ed. 3 vols. Baltimore: Johns Hopkins University Press, 1998.

McLeod KS. Our sense of Snow: The myth of John Snow in medical geography. *Soc Sci Med* 2000; 50:923–35.

McMichael AJ. Prisoners of the proximate: Loosening the constraints on epidemiology in an age of change. *Am J Epidemiol* 1999; 149:887–97.

McMichael AJ. *Human Frontiers, Environments and Disease: Past Patterns, Uncertain Futures.* Cambridge: Cambridge University Press, 2001.

McNeil BJ, Pauker SG. Decision analysis for public health: Principles and illustrations. *Annu Rev Public Health* 1984; 5:135–61.

McNeil JM. *Americans with Disabilities 1991–1992: Data from the Survey of Income and Program Participation.* Washington, DC: US Bureau of the Census, 1993.

Meade MS, Earickson RJ. *Medical Geography.* 2nd ed. New York: Guilford Press, 2000.

Mheen H van de, Stronks K, Looman CWN, Mackenbach JP. Does childhood socioeconomic status influence adult health through behavioral factors? *Int J Epidemiol* 1998; 27:431–37.

Michels KB. A renaissance for measurement error. *Int J Epidemiol* 2001; 30:421–22.

Miettinen O. Estimability and estimation in case-referent studies. *Am J Epidemiol* 1976; 103:226–35.

Mill JS. *A System of Logic, Ratiocinative and Inductive, Being a Connected View of the Principles of Evidence and the Methods.* 6th ed. London: Longmans, Green, 1865.

Millar WJ, Last JM. Motor vehicle traffic accident mortality in Canada, 1921–1984. *Am J Prev Med* 1988; 4:220–30.

Miller D. Risk, science and policy: Definitional struggles, information management, the media and BSE. *Soc Sci Med* 1999; 49:1239–55.

Miller MS (ed.), *State of the Peoples: A Global Human Rights Report on Societies in Danger.* Boston: Beacon Press, 1993.

Minkler M, Wallerstein N (eds.), *Community-Based Participatory Research for Health.* San Francisco: Jossey-Bass, 2003.

Molla MT, Wagener DK, Madans JH. Summary measures of population health:

Methods for calculating healthy life expectancy. *Healthy People Statistical Notes*, No. 21. Hyattsville, MD: National Center for Health Statistics, 2001.

Montagu A. *Man's Most Dangerous Myth: The Fallacy of Race.* 6th ed. Walnut Creek, CA: Altamira Press, 1997.

Morgenstern H. Socioeconomic factors: concepts, measurement, and health effects. In: Ostfield AM, Eaker ED (eds.), *Measuring Psychosocial Variables in Epidemiologic Studies of Cardiovascular Disease.* Bethesda, MD: National Institutes of Health, 1985:3–5.

Morgenstern H. Ecologic studies in epidemiology: Concepts, principles, and methods. *Annu Rev Public Health* 1995; 16:61–81.

Morgenstern H, Kleinbaum DG, Kupper LL. Measures of disease incidence used in epidemiologic research. *Int J Epidemiol* 1980; 9:97–104.

Morris JA, Gardner MJ. Calculating confidence intervals for relative risks (odds ratios) and standardised ratios and rates. *Br Med J* 1988; 296:1313–16.

Morris JN. *Uses of Epidemiology.* 3rd ed. Edinburgh: Churchill Livingstone, 1975.

Morrison AS. *Screening in Chronic Disease.* New York: Oxford University Press, 1992.

Morrison HI, Semenciw RM, Mao Y, Wigle DT. Cancer mortality among a group of fluospar miners exposed to radon progeny. *Am J Epidemiol* 1988; 128:1266–75.

Morse JM, Field PA. *Qualitative Research Methods for Health Professionals.* 2nd ed. Thousand Oaks, CA: Sage, 1995.

Morse RM, Flavin DK. The definition of alcoholism. *JAMA* 1992; 268:1012–14.

Mossey JM, Shapiro E. Self-rated health: A predictor of mortality among the elderly. *Am J Public Health* 1982; 72:800–808.

Motulsky AG, Vandepitte J, Fraser GR. Population genetic studies in the Congo. I. Glucose-6-phosphate dehydrogenase deficiency, hemo-globin S, and malaria. *Am J Hum Genet* 1966; 18:514–37.

Moysich KB, Menezes RJ, Michalek AM. Chernobyl-related ionizing radiation exposure and cancer risk: An epidemiological review. *Lancet Oncol* 2002; 3:269–79.

Muecke MA. New paradigms for refugee health problems. *Soc Sci Med* 1992; 35:515–23.

Muñoz N, Bosch FX, Shah KV, Meheus A (eds.), *The Epidemiology of Human Papillomavirus and Cervical Cancer.* Lyon: International Agency for Research on Cancer, 1992 (IARC Sci Pub No. 119).

Murphy S, Egger M. Studies of the social causes of tuberculosis in Germany before the First World War: Extracts from Mosse and Tugendreich's landmark book. *Int J Epidemiol* 2002; 31:742–49.

Murray CJL. Quantifying the burden of disease: The technical basis for disability-adjusted life years. *Bull World Health Organ* 1994; 72:429–45.

Murray CJL, Lopez AD. Global Burden of Disease Study. *Lancet* 1997; 349: 1269–76; 1347–52; 1436–42; 1498–1504.

Murray CJL, Salomon JA, Mathers C. A critical examination of summary measures of population health. *Bull World Health Organ* 2000; 78:981–94.

Murray JJ. *The Prevention of Oral Disease.* 3rd ed. Oxford: Oxford University Press, 1996.

Mustard CA, Frohlich N. Socioeconomic status and the health of the population. *Med Care* 1995; 33:DS43–DS54.

Mustard CA, Roos NP. The relationship of prenatal care and pregnancy complications to birthweight in Winnipeg, Canada. *Am J Public Health* 1994; 84:1450–57.

Mymin D, Mathewson FA, Tate RB, Manfreda J. The natural history of primary first degree atrio-ventricular heart block. *N Engl J Med* 1986; 315: 1183–87.

National Center for Health Statistics. *Healthy People 2000 Final Review.* Hyattsville, MD: Public Health Service, 2001.

National Institute on Alcohol Abuse and Alcoholism. *Tenth Special Report to the U.S. Congress on Alcohol and Health: Highlights from Current Research.* Bethesda, MD: NIAAA, 2000.

National Institutes of Health. *Clinical Guidelines on the Identification, Evaluation, and Treatment of Overweight and Obesity in Adults: The Evidence Report.* Bethesda, MD: NIH, 1998 (NIH Pub No. 98-4083).

National Public Health Laboratory of Finland. *Community Control of Cardiovascular Diseases: The North Karelia Project.* Copenhagen: WHO Regional Office for Europe, 1981.

National Research Council, Commission on Life Sciences. Board on Environmental Studies and Toxicology. *Science and Judgment in Risk Assessment.* Washington, DC: National Academy Press, 1994.

National Research Council, Commission on Life Sciences, Board on Radiation Effects Research. *Health Effects of Exposure to Radon* BEIR-VI. Washington, DC: National Academy Press, 1999.

Nations MK. Epidemiological research on infectious disease: Quantitative rigor or rigor mortis? Insights from ethnomedicine. In: Janes CR, Stall R, Gifford SM (eds.), *Anthropology and Epidemiology: Interdisciplinary Approaches to the Study of Health and Disease.* Dordrecht, Holland: D.Reidel, 1986:3–4.

Naylor CD, Basinski A, Abrams HB, Detsky A. Clinical and population epidemiology: Beyond sibling rivalry? *J Clin Epidemiol* 1990; 43:607–11.

Newcombe HB. *Handbook of Record Linkage: Methods for Health and Statistical Studies, Administration and Business.* Oxford: Oxford University Press, 1988.

Ness RB, Kuller LH (eds.), *Health and Disease among Women: Biological and Environmental Influences.* New York: Oxford University Press, 1998.

Norell SE. *Workbook of Epidemiology.* New York: Oxford University Press, 1995.

Northridge ME. Attributable risk as a link between causality and public health action. *Am J Public Health* 1995; 85:1202–4.

Nuland SB. *The Doctors' Plague: Germs, Childbed Fever, and the Strange Story of Ignac Semmelweis.* New York: W.W. Norton, 2003.

Nutting PA, Wood M, Conner EM. Community-oriented primary care in the United States. *JAMA* 1985; 253:1763–66.

Olshansky SJ, Ault AB. The fourth stage of the epidemiologic transition: The age of delayed degenerative diseases. *Milbank Q* 1986; 64:355–91.

Omran AR. The epidemiological transition: A theory of the epidemiology of population change. *Milbank Q* 1971; 49:509–38.

Oppenheimer GM. Epidemiology and the liberal arts—Toward a new paradigm. *Am J Public Health* 1995; 85:918–20.

Orenstein WA, Bernier RH, Hinman AR. Assessing vaccine efficacy in the field: Further observations. *Epidemiol Rev* 1988; 10:212–41.

Panerai RB, Mohr JP. *Health Technology Assessment: Methodologies for Developing Countries.* Washington DC: Pan American Health Organization, 1989.

Parkin DM, Whelan SL, Ferlay J, Raymond L, Young J (eds.), *Cancer Incidence in Five Continents.* Vol VII. Lyon: International Agency for Research on Cancer, 1997.

Parkinson GHR, ed. *An Encyclopaedia of Philosophy.* London: Routledge, 1988.

Paszol G, Weatherall DJ, Wilson RJM. Cellular mechanisms for the protective effect of haemoglobin S against *P. falciparum* malaria. *Nature* 1978; 274: 701–3.

Patrick DL, Erickson P. *Health Status and Health Policy: Quality of Life in Health Care Evaluation and Resource Allocation.* New York: Oxford University Press, 1993.

Paul BD, ed. *Health, Culture and Community.* New York: Russell Sage, 1955.

Paul BD. The role of beliefs and customs in sanitation programs. *Am J Public Health* 1958; 48:1502–6.

Pearce N. Traditional epidemiology, modern epidemiology, and public health. *Am J Public Health* 1996; 86:678–83.

Pearce N, Crawford-Brown D. Critical discussion in epidemiology: Problems with the Popperian approach. *J Clin Epidemiol* 1989; 42:177–84.

Pearl J. *Causality.* New York: Cambridge University Press, 2000.

Pencheon D, Guest C, Melzer D, Muir Gray JA (eds.), *Oxford Handbook of Public Health Practice.* Oxford: Oxford University Press, 2001.

Petersen W. *Malthus.* Cambridge: Harvard University Press, 1979.

Petitti DB. *Meta-Analysis, Decision Analysis, and Cost-Effectiveness Analysis: Methods for Quantitative Synthesis in Medicine.* 2nd ed. New York: Oxford University Press, 2000.

Petraitis J, Flay BR, Miller TQ. Reviewing theories of adolescent substance use: Organizing pieces in the puzzle. *Psychol Bull* 1995; 117:67–86.

Philippe P. Chaos, population biology, and epidemiology: Some research implications. *Hum Biol* 1993; 65:525–46.

Philippe P, Mansi O. Nonlinearity in the epidemiology of complex health and disease processes. *Theoret Med Bioethics* 1998; 19:591–607.

Phillips DR. Does epidemiological transition have utility for health planners? *Soc Sci Med* 1994; 38:vii–x.

Pidgeon N, Henwood K, Maguire B. Public health communication and the social amplification of risks: present knowledge and future prospects. In: Bennett P, Calman K (eds.), *Risk Communication and Public Health.* New York: Oxford University Press, 1999:65–77.

Pless IB (ed.), *The Epidemiology of Childhood Disorders.* New York: Oxford University Press, 1994.

Poland B, Coburn D, Robertson A, Eakin J. Wealth, equity and health care: A critique of a "population health" perspective on the determinants of health. *Soc Sci Med* 1998; 46:785–98.

Polednak AP. *Racial and Ethnic Differences in Disease*. New York: Oxford University Press, 1989.

Poole C. Ecologic analysis as outlook and method. *Am J Public Health* 1994; 84:715–16.

Pope AM, Tarlov AR (eds.), *Disabilities in America: Toward a National Agenda for Prevention*. Washington, DC: National Academy Press, 1991.

Pope C, Mays N. Reaching the parts other methods cannot reach: An introduction to qualitative methods in health and health services research. *Br Med J* 1995; 311:42–45.

Popper K. *The Logic of Scientific Discovery*. 2nd ed. New York: Harper and Row, 1968.

Potter JD. At the interfaces of epidemiology, genetics and genomics. *Nature Reviews Genetics* 2001; 2:142–47.

Power C, Manor O, Mathews S. The duration and timing of exposure: Effects of socioeconomic environment on adult health. *Am J Public Health* 1999; 89:1059–65.

Power C, Mathew S, Manor O. Inequalities in self rated health in the 1958 birth cohort: Lifetime social circumstances or social mobility. *Br Med J* 1996; 313:449–53.

Preston SH, Heuveline P, Guillot M. *Demography: Measuring and Modeling Population Processes*. Oxford: Blackwell, 2001.

Priestley M. *Disability: A Life Course Approach*. Cambridge: Polity, 2003.

Proctor RN. The Nazi war on tobacco: Ideology, evidence, and possible cancer consequences. *Bull Hist Med* 1997; 71:435–88.

Prothero RM. Forced movements of population and health hazards in tropical Africa. *Int J Epidemiol* 1994; 23:657–64.

Prusiner SB. Prions. *Proc Natl Acad Sci USA* 1998; 95:13363–83.

Psacharopoulos G, Patrinos HA (eds.), *Indigenous People and Poverty in Latin America: An Empirical Analysis*. Washington, DC: World Bank, 1994.

Rabkin SW, Mathewson FA, Tate RB. The relation of blood pressure to stroke prognosis. *Ann Intern Med* 1978; 89:15–20.

Raine A. Biosocial studies of antisocial and violent behavior in children and adults: A review. *J Abnorm Child Psychol* 2002; 30:311–26.

Rehm J. Measuring quantity, frequency and volume of drinking. *Alcohol Clin Exp Res* 1998; 22(Suppl 2):4S–14S.

Rehm J, Ashley MJ, Dubois G. Alcohol and health: Individual and population perspectives. *Addiction* 1997; 92(Suppl 1):S109–S115.

Renton A. Epidemiology and causation: A realist view. *J Epidemiol Comm Health* 1994; 48:79–85.

Rhyne R, Bogue R, Kukulka G, Fulmer H (eds.), *Community Oriented Primary Care: Health Care for the 21st Century*. Washington, DC: American Public Health Association, 1998.

Riboli E, Delendi M. *Autopsy in Epidemiology and Medical Research*. New York: Oxford University Press, 1991.

Rifkin SB, Walt G. Why health improves: Defining the issues concerning "comprehensive primary health care" and "selective primary health care." *Soc Sci Med* 1986; 23:559–66.

Riley JC, Lennon MA, Ellwood RP. The effect of water fluoridation and social inequalities on dental caries in five-year-old children. *Int J Epidemiol* 1999; 28:300–5.

Rimm EB, Williams P, Fosher K, Criqui M, Stampfer M. Moderate alcohol intake and lower risk of coronary heart disease: Meta-analysis of effects on lipids and haemostatic factors. *Br Med J* 1999; 319:1523–28.

Rinaldi RC, Steindles MS, Wilford BB. Classification and standardization of substance abuse terminology. *JAMA* 1988; 259:555–57.

Ringash J. Preventive health care, 2001 update: Screening mammography among women aged 40–49 years at average risk of breast cancer. *Can Med Assoc J* 2001; 164:469–76.

Robbins LC, Hall J. *How to Practice Prospective Medicine*. Indianapolis: Methodist Hospital of Indiana, 1970.

Robertson LS. *Injury Epidemiology*. New York: Oxford University Press, 1992.

Robine JM, Romieu I, Cambois E. Health expectancy indicators. *Bull World Health Organ* 1999; 77:181–85.

Robins J, Greenland S. The probability of causation under a stochastic model for individual risk. *Biometrics* 1989; 45:1125–38.

Robinson JR, Young TK, Roos LL, Gelskey DE. Estimating the burden of disease: Comparing administrative data and self-reports. *Med Care* 1997; 35:932–47.

Roche AM, Evans KR, Stanton WR. Harm reduction: Roads less traveled to the Holy Grail. *Addiction* 1997; 92:1207–12.

Roe DA. *A Plague of Corn: A Social History of Pellagra*. Ithaca, NY: Cornell University Press, 1973.

Roemer MI. Primary care and physician extenders in affluent countries. *Intern J Health Serv* 1977; 7:545–55.

Rogan WJ, Gladen B. Estimating prevalence from the results of a screening test. *Am J Epidemiol* 1978; 107:71–76.

Rogers RG, Hackenberg R. Extending epidemiologic transition theory: A new stage. *Soc Biol* 1987; 34:234–43.

Romeder J-M, McWhinnie JR. Potential years of life lost between ages 1 and 70: An indicator of premature mortality for health planning. *Int J Epidemiol* 1977; 6:143–51.

Romm FJ, Putnam SM. The validity of the medical record. *Med Care* 1981; 19:310–15.

Roos LL, Mustard CA, Nicol JP, McLerran DF, Malenka DJ, Young TK, et al. Registries and administrative data: Organization and accuracy. *Med Care* 1993; 31:201–12.

Roos NP, Havens BJ. Predictors of successful aging: A twelve-year study of Manitoba elderly. *Am J Public Health* 1991; 81:63–68.

Rose G. Sick individuals and sick populations. *Int J Epidemiol* 1985; 14:32–38.

Rose G. *The Strategy of Preventive Medicine*. Oxford: Oxford University Press, 1992.

Rose GA, Blackburn H, Gillum RF, Prineas RJ. *Cardiovascular Survey Methods*. 2nd ed. Geneva: World Health Organization, 1982.

Rosen G. What is social medicine: A genetic analysis of the concept. *Bull Hist Med* 1947; 21:674–733.

Rosen G. *A History of Public Health*. Expanded ed. Baltimore: Johns Hopkins University Press, 1993.

Rosenstock IM. Historical origins of the health belief model. In: Becker MH (ed.), *The Health Belief Model and Personal Health Behavior*. Thorofare, NJ: Charles B. Slack, 1974:1–8.

Ross NA, Wolfson MC, Dunn JR, Berthelot JM, Kaplan GA, Lynch JW. Relation between income inequality and mortality in Canada and in the United States: Cross sectional assessment using census data and vital statistics. *Br Med J* 2000; 320:898–902.

Rossi PH, Wright JD, Anderson AB (eds.), *Handbook of Survey Research*. San Diego, CA: Academic Press, 1983.

Rothman KJ. Causes. *Am J Epidemiol* 1976; 104:587–92.

Rothman KJ (ed.), *Causal Inference*. Chestnut Hill, MA: Epidemiology Resources Inc., 1988.

Rothman KJ. Lessons from John Graunt. *Lancet* 1996; 347:37–39.

Rothman KJ. *Epidemiology: An Introduction*. New York: Oxford University Press, 2002.

Rothman KJ, Adami HO, Trichopoulos D. Should the mission of epidemiology include the eradication of poverty? *Lancet* 1998; 352:810–13.

Rothman KJ, Greenland S. *Modern Epidemiology*. 2nd ed. Philadelphia: Lippincott-Raven, 1998.

Rubel AJ, Garro LC. Social and cultural factors in the successful control of tuberculosis. *Public Health Rep* 1992; 107:626–26.

Russell LB. *Is Prevention Better Than Cure?* Washington DC: The Brookings Institution, 1986.

Sackett DL. Bias in analytic research. *J Chron Dis* 1979; 32:51–63.

Sallis JF, Owen N. *Physical Activity and Behavioral Medicine*. Thousand Oaks, CA: Sage, 1999.

Salonen JT, Tuomilehto J, Nissinen A, Kaplan GA, Puska P. Contribution of risk factor changes to the decline in coronary incidence during the North Karelia Project: A within-community analysis. *Int J Epidemiol* 1989; 18:595–601.

Samet JM. The epidemiology of lung cancer. *Chest* 1993; 103(Suppl 1):20S–9S.

Sanders BS. Measuring community health levels. *Am J Public Health* 1964; 54:1063–70.

Santow G. Social roles and physical health: The case of female disadvantage in poor countries. *Soc Sci Med* 1995; 40:147–61.

Saracci R. The interaction of tobacco smoking and other agents in cancer etiology. *Epidemiol Rev* 1987; 9:175–93.

Saracci R. Epidemiology in progress: Thoughts, tensions, targets. *Int J Epidemiol* 1999; 28:S997–S999.

Sartorius N, Jablensky A, Korten A, Ernberg G, Anker M, Cooper JE, et al. Early manifestations and first-contact incidence of schizophrenia in different cultures. *Psychol Med* 1986; 16:909–28.

Sartwell PE. On the methodology of investigations of etiologic factors in chronic diseases. *J Chron Dis* 1960; 11:61–63.

Saunders RJ, Warford JJ. *Village Water Supply: Economics and Policy in the Developing World*. Baltimore: Johns Hopkins University Press, 1976.

Savitz DA, Poole C, Miller WC. Reassessing the role of epidemiology in public health. *Am J Public Health* 1999; 89:1158–61.

Schaffner KF. Causing harm: Epidemiological and physiological concepts of causation. In: Mayo DG, Hollander RD (eds.), *Acceptable Evidence: Science and Values in Risk Management*. New York: Oxford University Press, 1991:204–17.

Schlesselman JJ. *Case-Control Studies: Design, Conduct, Analysis*. New York: Oxford University Press, 1982.

Schmid TL, Pratt M, Howze E. Policy as intervention: environmental and policy approaches to the prevention of cardiovascular disease. *Am J Public Health* 1995; 85:1207–11.

Schottenfeld D, Fraumeni JF (eds.), *Cancer Epidemiology and Prevention*. 2nd ed. New York: Oxford University Press, 1996.

Schwartz S. The fallacy of the ecologic fallacy: The potential misuses of a concept and the consequences. *Am J Public Health* 1994; 84:819–24.

Segovia J, Bartlett RF, Edwards AC. An empirical analysis of the dimensions of health status measures. *Soc Sci Med* 1989; 29:761–68.

Selby JV. Case-control evaluation of treatment and program efficacy. *Epidemiol Rev* 1994; 16:90–101.

Selik RM, Buehler JW, Karon JM, Chamberland ME, Berkelman RL. Impact of the 1987 revision of the case definition of acquired immune deficiency in the United States. *J Acquir Immune Defic Syndr* 1990; 3:73–82.

Selvin S. *Statistical Analysis of Epidemiologic Data*. 2nd ed. New York: Oxford University Press, 1996.

Semenciw RM, Morrison HI, Mao Y, Johansen H, Davies JW, Wigle DT. Major risk factors for cardiovascular disease mortality in adults: Results from the Nutrition Canada Survey cohort. *Int J Epidemiol* 1988; 17:317–24.

Shaar K, McCarthy M. Definitions and determinants of handicap in people with disabilities. *Epidemiol Rev* 1994; 16:228–42.

Shcherbak YM. Ten years of the Chernobyl era. *Sci Am* 1996; Apr.:44–9.

Shilts R. *And the Band Played On: People, Politics and the AIDS Epidemic*. New York: St. Martin's Press, 1988.

Short JF. The social fabric at risk: Toward the social transformation of risk analysis. *Am Sociol Rev* 1984; 49:711–25.

Shrader-Frechette K. Reductionist approaches to risk. In: Mayo DG, Hollander RD (eds.), *Acceptable Evidence: Science and Values in Risk Management*. New York: Oxford University Press, 1991:218–48.

Shryock HS, Siegel JS. *The Methods and Materials of Demography*. Condensed ed.: Stockwell EG, cond. New York: Academic Press, 1976.

Siem H, Bollini P (eds.), *Migration and Health in the 1990s*. Special issue of *International Migration*, 1992; 30:1–237.

Siemiatycki J. A comparison of mail, telephone, and home interview strategies for household health surveys. *Am J Public Health* 1979; 69:238–45.

Simons RC, Hughes CC (eds.), *The Culture-Bound Syndromes*. Boston: D. Reidel, 1985.

Singh-Manoux A, Clarke P, Marmot M. Multiple measures of socio-economic position and psychosocial health: Proximal and distal measures. *Int J Epidemiol* 2002; 31:1192–99.

Skolbekken JA. The risk epidemic in medical journals. *Soc Sci Med* 1995; 40:291–305.

Skrabanek P. The poverty of epidemiology. *Perspect Biol Med* 1992; 35:182–85.

Slovic P. Perception of risk. *Science* 1987; 236:280–85.

Slovic P. Beyond numbers: A broader perspective on risk perception and risk communication. In: Mayo DG, Hollander RD (eds.), *Acceptable Evidence: Science and Values in Risk Management.* New York: Oxford University Press, 1991:48–65.

Smedley BD, Syme SL (eds.), *Promoting Health: Intervention Strategies from Social and Behavioral Research.* Washington, DC: National Academy Press, 2000.

Smith PJ, Moffatt MEK, Gelskey SC, Hudson S, Kaita K. Are community health interventions evaluated appropriately? A review of six journals. *J Clin Epidemiol* 1997; 50:137–46.

Sontag S. *AIDS and Its Metaphors.* New York: Farrar, Straus, Giroux, 1988.

Soskolne C. Epidemiology: Questions of science, ethics, morality and law. *Am J Epidemiol* 1989; 129:1–8.

Spasoff RA. *Epidemiologic Methods for Health Policy.* New York: Oxford University Press, 1999.

Spasoff RA, McDowell IW. Potential and limitations of data and methods in health risk appraisal: Risk factor selection and measurement. *Health Serv Res* 1987; 22:467–97.

Spitzer WO. The nurse-practitioner revisited: Slow death of a good idea. *N Engl J Med* 1984; 310:1049–51.

Spitzer WO, Sackett DL, Sibley JC, Roberts RS, et al. The Burlington randomized trial of the nurse practitioner. *N Engl J Med* 1974; 290:251–56.

Spitzer WO, Suissa S, Ernst P, Horwitz R, Habbick B, Cockcroft D, et al. The use of β-agonists and the risk of death and near death from asthma. *N Engl J Med* 1992; 326:501–6.

Sreter S. The importance of social intervention in Britain's mortality decline c.1850–1914: A re-interpretation of the role of public health. *Soc Hist Med* 1988; 1:1–38.

Sreter S. The GRO and the public health movement in Britain, 1837–1914. *Soc Hist Med* 1991; 4:435–63.

Sreter S. The population health approach in historical perspective. *Am J Public Health* 2003; 93:421–31.

Stampfer MJ, Willett WC, Colditz GA, Speizer FE, Hennekens CH. A prospective study of past use of oral contraceptive agents and risk of cardiovascular diseases. *N Engl J Med* 1988; 319:1313–17.

Stanton BF, Clemens JD, Aziz KMA, Rahman M. Twenty-four-hour recall, knowledge-attitude-practice questionnaires and direct observation of sanitary practices: A comparative study. *Bull World Health Organ* 1987; 65:217–22.

Stein ZA. HIV prevention: The need for methods women can use. *Am J Public Health* 1990; 80:460–62.

Steiner JF. Talking about treatment: The language of populations and the language of individuals. *Ann Intern Med* 1999; 130:618–22.

Stern MP, Haffner SM. Type II diabetes and its complications in Mexican Americans. *Diabetes Metab Rev* 1990; 6:29–45.

Stevens SS. On the theory of scales of measurement. *Science* 1946; 103:677–80.

Stolley PD, Lasky T. *Investigating Disease Patterns: The Science of Epidemiology.* New York: Scientific American Library, 1995.

Storms DM. *Training and Use of Auxiliary Health Workers: Lessons From Developing Countries.* Monograph No. 3. Washington, DC: American Public Health Association, 1979.

Strauss AL, Corbin J. *Basics of Qualitative Research: Techniques and Procedures for Developing Grounded Theory.* 2nd ed. Thousand Oaks, CA: Sage, 1998.

Stray-Pedersen B, Jenum P. Economic evaluation of preventive programmes against congenital toxoplasmosis. *Scand J Infect Dis* 1992; (Suppl 84): 86–96.

Streiner DL, Norman GR. *Health Measurement Scales: A Practical Guide to Their Development and Use.* 2nd ed. New York: Oxford University Press, 1995.

Stroup DF, Teutsch SM (eds.), *Statistics in Public Health: Quantitative Approaches to Public Health Problems.* New York: Oxford University Press, 1998.

Subramanian SV, Belli P, Kawachi I. The macroeconomic determinants of health. *Annu Rev Public Health* 2002; 23:287–302.

Suerbaum S, Michetti P. *Helicobacter pylori* infection. *N Engl J Med* 2002; 347: 1175–86.

Sullivan DF. A single index of mortality and morbidity. *HSMHA Health Reports* 1971; 86:347–54.

Sundquist J, Malmström M, Johansson SE. Cardiovascular risk factors and the neighbourhood environment: a multilevel analysis. *Int J Epidemiol* 1999; 28:841–45.

Surgeon General. *Smoking and Health: Report of the Advisory Committee to the Surgeon General of the Public Health Service.* Washington, DC: Government Printing Office, 1964. PHS Pub No. 1103.

Surgeon General. *Reducing the Health Consequences of Smoking: 25 Years of Progress: A Report of the Surgeon General.* Bethesda, Md: Department of Health and Human Services, 1989. Report No.: DHHS Pub No. (CDC) 89-8411.

Susser M. Epidemiology in the United States after World War II: The evolution of technique. *Epidemiol Rev* 1985; 7:147–77.

Susser M. The logic of Sir Karl Popper and the practice of epidemiology. *Am J Epidemiol* 1986; 124:711–18.

Susser M. What is a cause and how do we know one? *Am J Epidemiol* 1991; 133:635–48.

Susser M. The trials and tribulations of trials—interventions in communities. *Am J Public Health* 1995; 85:156–58.

Susser M. The longitudinal perspective and cohort analysis. *Int J Epidemiol* 2001; 30:684–87.

Susser M, Susser E. Choosing a future for epidemiology: I. Eras and paradigms. *Am J Public Health* 1996; 86:668–73.

Susser M, Susser E. Choosing a future for epidemiology: II. From black box to Chinese boxes and eco-epidemiology. *Am J Public Health* 1996; 86:674–77.

Susser M, Watson W, Hopper K. *Sociology in Medicine*. 3rd ed. New York: Oxford University Press, 1985.

Swedlund AC, Armelagos GJ (eds.), *Disease in Populations in Transition: Anthropological and Epidemiological Perspectives*. New York: Bergin and Garvey, 1990.

Syme SL, Marmot MG, Kagan A, Kato H, Rhoads G. Epidemiologic studies of coronary heart disease and stroke in Japanese men living in Japan, Hawaii and California: Introduction. *Am J Epidemiol* 1975; 102:477–80.

Szklo M, Nieto FJ. *Epidemiology: Beyond the Basics*. Gaithersburg, MD: Aspen, 2000.

Tallis R, Fillit H, Brocklehurst JC (eds.), *Brocklehurst's Textbook of Geriatric Medicine and Gerontology*. 5th ed. Edinburgh: Churchill Livingston, 1998.

Tate RB, Manfreda J, Krahn AD, Cuddy TE. Tracking of blood pressure over a 40-year period in the University of Manitoba Follow-Up Study, 1948–1988. *Am J Epidemiol* 1995; 142:946–54.

Tarlov AR, St. Peter RF (eds.), *The Society and Population Health Reader. Volume II: A State and Community Perspective*. New York: New Press, 2000.

Taubes G. Epidemiology faces its limits. *Science* 1995; 269:164–69.

Taubes G. The breast-screening brawl. *Science* 1997; 275:1056–59.

Terris M. Newer perspectives on the health of Canadians: Beyond the Lalonde Report. *J Public Health Policy* 1984; 5:327–37.

Terris M. The changing relationships of epidemiology and society. *J Public Health Policy* 1985; 6:15–36.

Tesh S. Disease, causality and politics. *J Health Polit Policy Law* 1981; 6:369–89.

Teutsch SM, Churchill RE (eds.), *Principles and Practice of Public Health Surveillance*. 2nd ed. New York: Oxford University Press, 2000.

Thomas DB, Karagas MR. Migrant studies. In: Schottenfeld D, Fraumeni JF (eds.), *Cancer Epidemiology and Prevention*. 2nd ed. New York: Oxford University Press, 1996:236–54.

Thomlinson R. *Population Dynamics: Causes and Consequences of World Demographic Change*. 2nd ed. New York: Random House, 1976.

Thompson W. Population. *Am J Sociol* 1929; 34:959–75.

Thomsen TF, McGee D, Davidsen M, Jørgensen T. A cross-validation of risk-scores for coronary heart disease mortality based on data from the Glostrup Population Studies and Framingham Heart Study. *Int J Epidemiol* 2002; 31:817–22.

Tilling K. Capture-recapture methods—useful or misleading? *Int J Epidemiol* 2001; 30:12–14.

Tinker A, Daly P, Green C, Saxenian H, Lakshminarayanan R, Gill K. *Women's Health and Nutrition: Making a Difference*. Washington, DC: World Bank, 1994. Discussion Paper 256.

Toniolo P, Boffetta P, Shuker DEG, Rothman N, Hulka B, Pearce N (eds.), *Application of Biomarkers in Cancer Epidemiology*. IARC Publication No. 142. Lyon: International Agency for Research on Cancer, 1997.

Townsend P, Davidson N, Whitehead M (eds.), *Inequalities in Health: The Black*

Report; The Health Divide. New and rev ed. Harmondsworth, England: Penguin Books, 1992.

Trowell HC, Burkitt D (eds.), *Western Diseases: Their Emergence and Prevention.* Cambridge, MA: Harvard University Press, 1981.

Truman BI, Smith-Akin CK, Hinman AR, Gebbie KM, Brownson R, Novick LF, Lawrence RS, Pappaioanou M, Fielding J, Evans CA, Guerra FA, Vogel-Taylor M, Mahan CS, Fullilove M, Zaza S. Developing the Guide to Community Preventive Services—Overview and rationale. *Am J Prev Med* 2000; 18(Suppl 1):18–26.

Tversky A, Kahneman D. Judgement under uncertainty: Heuristics and biases. *Science* 1974; 185:1124–31.

United Nations Scientific Committee on the Effects of Atomic Radiation. *Sources and Effects of Ionizing Radiation.* UNSCEAR 2000 Report to the General Assembly. New York: United Nations, 2000.

U.S. Preventive Services Task Force. *Guide to Clinical Preventive Services.* 2nd ed. Alexandria, VA: International Medical Publishers, 1996.

Vainio H, Boffetta P. Mechanisms of the combined effect of asbestos and smoking in the etiology of lung cancer. *Scand J Work Environ Health* 1994; 20:235–42.

Valente TW. *Evaluating Health Promotion Programs.* New York: Oxford University Press, 2002.

Vandenbroucke JP, Eelkman Rooda HM, Beukers H. Who made John Snow a hero? *Am J Epidemiol* 1991; 133:967–73.

VanLeeuwen JA, Waltner-Yoews D, Abernathy T, Smit B. Evolving models of human health toward an ecosystem context. *Ecosystem Health* 1999; 5:204–19.

Van Os J, Galdos P, Lewis G, Bourgeois M, Mann A. Schizophrenia sans frontièrs: Concepts of schizophrenia among French and British psychiatrists. *Br Med J* 1993; 307:489–92.

Van Willigen J. *Applied Anthropology: An Introduction.* Westport, CT: Bergin and Garvey, 1993.

Vartiainen E, Puska P, Jousilahti P, Korhonen HJ, Pietinen P, Tuomilehto J, Nissinen A. Twenty-year trends in coronary risk factors in North Karelia and in other areas of Finland. *Int J Epidemiol* 1994; 23:495–504.

Veney JE, Kaluzny AD. *Evaluation and Decision Making for Health Services.* 3rd ed. Chicago: Health Administration Press, 1998.

Venters GA. New variant Creutzfeldt-Jakob disease: The epidemic that never was. *Brit Med J* 2001; 323:858–61.

Vernon SW, Buffler PA. The status of status inconsistency. *Epidemiol Rev* 1988; 10: 65–86.

Villarejo D. The health of U.S. hired farm workers. *Annu Rev Public Health* 2003; 24:175–93.

Vineis P, Caporaso N. Tobacco and cancer: Epidemiology and the laboratory. *Environ Health Perspect* 1995; 103:156–60.

Vinicor F. The public health burden of diabetes and the reality of limits. *Diabetes Care* 1998; 21(Suppl 3):C15–8.

Vinten-Johansen P, Brody H, Paneth N, Rachman S, Rip M, Zuck D. *Cholera,*

Chloroform, and the Science of Medicine: A Life of John Snow. New York: Oxford University Press, 2003.

Vitek CR, Wharton M. Diphtheria in the former Soviet Union: Reemergence of a pandemic disease. *Emerg Infect Dis* 1998; 4:539–50.

Vogel VJ. *American Indian Medicine*. Norman: OK: University of Oklahoma Press, 1970.

Wacholder S, McLaughlin JK, Silverman DT, et al. Selection of controls in case-control studies. I. Principles. *Am J Epidemiol* 1992; 135:1019–28.

Wacholder S, Silverman DT, McLaughlin JK, et al. Selection of controls in case-control studies. II. Types of controls. *Am J Epidemiol* 1992; 135: 1029–41.

Wacholder S, Silverman DT, McLaughlin JK, et al. Selection of controls in case-control studies. III. Design options. *Am J Epidemiol* 1992; 135: 1042–50.

Waldram JB, Herring DA, Young TK. *Aboriginal Health in Canada: Historical, Cultural, and Epidemiological Perspectives*. Toronto: University of Toronto, 1995.

Wallace RB, Woolson RF (eds.), *The Epidemiologic Study of the Elderly*. New York: Oxford University Press, 1992.

Waller D, McPherson A (eds.), *Women's Health*. New York: Oxford University Press, 2003.

Walsh JA, Warren KS. Selective primary health care: An interim strategy for disease control in developing countries. *N Engl J Med* 1979; 301:967–74.

Weed DL. On the logic of causal inference. *Am J Epidemiol* 1986; 123:965–79.

Weed DL. Epidemiology, the humanities, and public health. *Am J Public Health* 1995; 85:914–18.

Weed DL. On the use of causal criteria. *Int J Epidemiol* 1997; 26:1137–41.

Weed DL. Interpreting epidemiological evidence: How meta-analysis and causal inference methods are related. *Int J Epidemiol* 2000; 29:387–90.

Weed DL, Hursting SD. Biologic plausibility in causal inference: Current methods and practice. *Am J Epidemiol* 1998; 147:415–25.

Weeks JR. *Population: An Introduction to Concepts and Issues*. 6th ed. Belmont, CA: Wadsworth Publishing Co, 1995.

Weindling P. *Health, Race and German Politics between National Unification and Nazism, 1870–1945*. Cambridge: Cambridge University Press, 1989.

Weinstein M, Hermalin AI, Stoto MA (eds.), *Population Health and Aging: Strengthening the Dialogue Between Epidemiology and Demography*. Baltimore: Johns Hopkins University Press, 2002.

Weiss NS. Application of the case-control method in the evaluation of screening. *Epidemiol Rev* 1994; 16:102–8.

Wellings K, Cleland J. Surveys on sexual health: Recent developments and future directions. *Sex Transm Infect* 2001; 77:238–41.

West P. Rethinking the health selection explanation for health inequalities. *Soc Sci Med* 1991; 32:373–84.

Wildavsky A, Dake K. Theories of risk perception: Who fears what and why? *Daedalus* 1990; 119(4):41–60.

Wilkins R, Adams OB. Health expectancy in Canada, late 1970s: Demographic, regional and social dimensions. *Am J Public Health* 1983; 73:1073–80.

Wilkinson RG. Income distribution and life expectancy. *Br Med J* 1992; 304: 165–68.

Wilkinson RG. *Unhealthy Societies: The Afflictions of Inequality.* London: Routledge, 1996.

Willett WC. *Nutritional Epidemiology.* 2nd ed. New York: Oxford University Press, 1998.

Willett WC. Balancing life-style and genomics research for disease prevention. *Science* 2002; 296:695–98.

Wilson PW, D'Agostino RB, Levy D, Belanger AM, Silbershatz H, Kannel WB. Prediction of coronary heart disease using risk factor categories. *Circulation* 1998; 97:1837–47.

Wilson JMG, Jungner G. *Principles and Practice of Screening for Disease.* Geneva: World Health Organization, 1968.

Wilson R, Crouch EAC. *Risk-Benefit Analysis.* 2nd ed. Cambridge, MA: Center for Risk Analysis, Harvard University, 2001.

Wolfson MC. Health-adjusted life expectancy. *Health Reports* 1996; 8:41–45.

Wolleswinkel-van den Bosch JH, Looman CWN, van Poppel FWA, Mackenbach JP. Cause-specific mortality trends in the Netherlands, 1875–1992: A formal analysis of the epidemiologic transition. *Int J Epidemiol* 1997; 26:772–81.

Wood EW (ed.), *APHA-CDC Recommended Minimum Housing Standards.* Washington, DC: American Public Health Association, 1986.

Woodward M. *Epidemiology: Study Design and Data Analysis.* Boca Raton, FL: Chapman and Hall/CRC, 1999.

Woolf B, Waterhouse J. Studies in infant mortality. Part I. Influence of social conditions in county boroughs of England and Wales. *J Hygiene* 1945; 44:67–98.

World Health Organization. *Health Programme Evaluation: Guiding Principles.* Geneva: WHO, 1981. (Health for All Series No. 6).

World Health Organization. *Diabetes Mellitus: Report of a WHO Study Group.* Geneva: WHO, 1985. Tech Rep Ser 727.

World Health Organization. *Health Principles of Housing.* Geneva: WHO, 1989.

World Health Organization. *Diet, Nutrition, and the Prevention of Chronic Diseases.* Geneva: WHO, 1990. Tech Rep Ser 797.

World Health Organization. Recommended definitions, standards and reporting requirements for ICD-10 related to fetal, perinatal and infant mortality. *World Health Stat Q* 1990; 43:220–27.

World Health Organization. Commission on Health and the Environment. *Our Planet, Our Health.* Geneva: WHO, 1992.

World Health Organization. *International Statistical Classification of Diseases and Related Health Conditions.* 10th rev., vol. 1. Geneva: WHO, 1992.

World Health Organization. *Obesity: Preventing and Managing the Global Epidemic. Report of a WHO Consultation.* Geneva: WHO, 2000. Tech Rep Ser 894.

World Health Organization. *World Health Report 2002.* Geneva: WHO, 2002.

Wright EO. *Class Counts: Comparative Studies in Class Analysis.* New York: Cambridge University Press, 1996.

Wright PWG. Babyhood: The social construction of infant care as a medical problem in England in the years around 1900. In: Lock M, Gordon D (eds.), *Biomedicine Examine.* Dordrecht, Holland: Kluwer Academic Publishers, 1983:299–329.

Wynder EL, Graham EA. Tobacco smoking as a possible etiologic factor in bronchogenic carcinoma: A study of six hundred and eighty-four proved cases. *J Am Med Assoc* 1950; 143:329–36.

Yassi A, Kjellström T, De Kok T, Guidotti T. *Basic Environmental Health.* New York: Oxford University Press, 2001.

Yassi A, Tate R, Fish D. Cancer mortality in workers employed at a transformer manufacturing plant. *Am J Ind Med* 1994; 25:425–37.

Yerushalmy J, Palmer CE. On the methodology of investigations of etiologic factors in chronic diseases. *J Chron Dis* 1959; 10:27–40.

Young TK. *The Health of Native Americans: Towards a Biocultural Epidemiology.* New York: Oxford University Press, 1994.

Young TK, Hershfield ES. A case-control study to evaluate the effectiveness of mass BCG vaccination among Canadian Indians. *Am J Public Health* 1986; 76:783–86.

Young TK, Roos NP, Hammerstrand KM. Estimated burden of diabetes mellitus in Manitoba according to health insurance claims: A pilot study. *Can Med Assoc J* 1991; 144:318–24.

Young TK, Schraer CD, Shubnikov EV, Szathmary EJE, Nikitin YP. Prevalence of diagnosed diabetes in circumpolar indigenous populations. *Int J Epidemiol* 1992; 21:730–36.

Zahm SH, Blair A (eds.), Feasibility of epidemiologic research on migrant and seasonal farmworkers. *Am J Ind Med* 2001; 40(5): special issue.

Zochetti C, Consonni D, Bertazzi PA. Relationship between prevalence rate ratios and odds ratios in cross-sectional studies. *Int J Epidemiol* 1997; 26:220–23.

Zucconi SL, Carson CA. CDC's consensus set of health status indicators: Monitoring and prioritization by state health departments. *Am J Public Health* 1994; 84:1644–46.

Answers to Exercises

CHAPTER 2

EX. 2.1

(a) $34,992/281423 = 0.124 = 12.4\%$
Note: The last three zeros in both the numerator and denominator cancel out and can be deleted prior to the division to save time. This is the *youth dependency ratio*.

(b) $(3,806 + 15,370 + 41,078)/281,423 = 0.214 = 21.4\%$.
Note: This is the *aged dependency ratio*. The *total dependency ratio* is therefore $(12.4\% + 21.4\%) = 33.8\%$.

(c) $(1,949 + 7,862 + 21,044)M : (1,857 + 7,508 + 20,034)F = 30,855M : 29,399F = 100M : (29,399/30,855 \times 100)F = 100M : 95.28F$

(d) $14,410M : 20,582F = (14,410/20,582 \times 100)M : 100F = 70.01M : 100F$

(e) $4,059/281,423 = 0.01442 = 14.42/1,000$

(f) $2,403/281,423 = 0.00854 = 8.54/1,000$

(g) $14.42/1000 - 8.54/1,000 = 5.88/1,000$; alternatively: $(4,059 - 2,403)/281,423 = 0.00588 = 5.88/1,000$

(h) $28,035/4,059,000 = 0.0069 = 6.9/1,000$ live births

(i) $28,035/3,806,000 = 0.0074 = 7.4/1,000$ children aged 0–1
Note: (h) and (i) are similar but not identical; while the numerator is the same, the denominators are different; (i) is hardly ever used as an indicator, compared to (h) which is easier to obtain.

(j) $18,776/4,059,000 = 0.0046 = 4.6/1,000$ live births

(k) $9,259/4,059,000 = 0.0023 = 2.3/1,000$ live births; alternatively: $(6.9/1,000 - 4.6/1,000) = 2.3/1,000$

(l) $1,226,000/143,368,000 = 0.00855 = 8.55/1,000$ women
Note: denominator = all women only, not the total population of men and women

(m) $41,872/143,368,000 = 0.00029 = 0.29/1,000$ women $= 29/100,000$ women

(n) $41,872/1,226,000 = 0.034 = 3.4\%$

EX.2.2

(a) The incidence rate should generally be higher than the mortality rate, since not all cases of cancer are fatal. Note that the mortality rate of cancer in year X refers to the cases that died during that year—not all of whom were also diagnosed in year X and counted in the incidence rate of that year. Even if cancer is 100% fatal, such that all cases diagnosed in year X will eventually die, the mortality rate for year X reflects the incidence in operation in the past, which could be higher or lower than it is in year X. The mortality rate also reflects the successes of available treatments sometime in the past during the variable lifetime of the patients. Other possible, but less important, reasons for the discrepancy between incidence and mortality include inaccurate coding of causes of death and outmigration of cancer patients to seek treatment or live the remainder of their lives outside Canada.

(b) The hospital separation (or discharge) rate for cancer includes multiple separations by the same patients and should thus be higher than the incidence rate, which counts the number of discrete individuals contracting cancer for the first time.

EX. 2.3

The following table summarizes the relevant results:

	Number		Percent		Crude rate (/100,000)	
	Deaths	PYLLs	Deaths	PYLLs	Deaths	PYLLs
All causes	2,403,000	7,709	100.0	100.0	853.9	2.74
Cancer	553,000	1,699	23.0	22.0	196.5	0.60
Heart disease	711,000	1,271	29.6	16.5	252.6	0.45
Unintentional injuries	98,000	1,055	4.1	13.7	34.8	0.37

Population of USA in 2000   281,423,000

(a) Cancer accounts for 23.0%, heart disease 29.6%, and injuries 4.1% of all deaths. The crude death rates for cancer: $553/281,423 = 197/100,000$; heart disease: $711/281,423 = 253/100,000$; and injuries: $98/281,423 = 35/100,000$.

(b) Cancer accounts for 22%, heart disease 16.5% and injuries 13.7% of all PYLLs. Cancer and heart disease affect mainly older people, who are given less "weight" in the computation of PYLL, while injuries kill mostly younger people, who therefore contribute to a higher proportion of PYLLs (13.7% of PYLL, vs. 4.1% of the number of deaths).

EX. 2.4

(a) Crude prevalence of diabetes among Alaskan Indians:
= $(3 + 43 + 156 + 133)/(14{,}840 + 7{,}304 + 3{,}293 + 1{,}234) = 335/26{,}671$
= $0.0126 = 1.26\%$ or $12.6/1{,}000$
Crude prevalence of diabetes among NWT Indians:
= $(9 + 30 + 16 + 9)/(6{,}553 + 2{,}782 + 1{,}307 + 552) = 64/11{,}194 = 0.0057$
= 0.57% or $5.7/1{,}000$

(b) The calculations can best be done on a spreadsheet. While rounded-off figures are shown in the table here, the rounding off is left till the very end in the calculation.

For Alaskan Indians:

Age	N_i	n_i	d_i	r_i	r_iN_i
<25	48,000	14,840	3	0.0002	9.7
25–44	26,000	7,304	43	0.0059	153.1
45–64	19,000	3,293	156	0.0474	900.1
65+	7,000	1,234	133	0.1078	754.5
Total	100,000	26,671	335		1,817.3

The age-standardized prevalence of diabetes $= 1{,}817.3/100{,}000 = 18.2/1{,}000$

For NWT Indians:

Age	N_i	n_i	d_i	r_i	r_iN_i
<25	48,000	6,553	9	0.0014	65.9
25–44	26,000	2,782	30	0.0108	280.4
45–64	19,000	1,307	16	0.0122	232.6
65+	7,000	552	9	0.0163	114.1
Total	100,000	11,194	64		693.0

The age-standardized prevalence of diabetes $= 693/100{,}000 = 6.9/1{,}000$

(c) Direct

(d) To do indirect standardization, one needs the age-specific prevalence of diabetes from a standard (R_i). There is no "world" standard, although one might use an existing data source such as a national survey conducted in the United States or Canada and apply it to the population in each age group among Alaskan Indians and NWT Indians (n_i). The sum of the products (R_in_i) gives the total "expected." Divide the total number of "observed" cases of diabetes (already known: 335 for Alaska and 64 for NWT) by the total "expected." This produces the SMR. Finally multiplying the SMR by the overall prevalence of diabetes in the standard will give the (indirectly) age-standardized prevalence for the two Indian populations.

EX. 2.5

(a)   The graph should look like this:

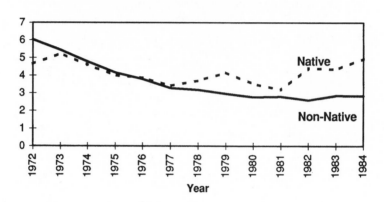

Cholecystectomy Rate among Manitoba Women

Note that the non-Native rate was initially higher, but has been declining steadily. The Native rate has exceeded the non-Native rate since the late 1970s, and shows an upward trend since the early 1980s.

(b)   The graph should look like this:

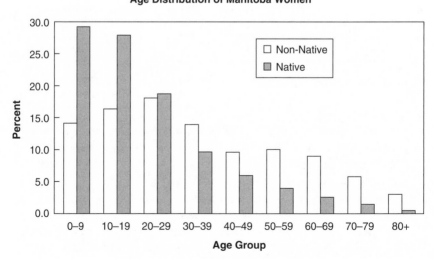

Age Distribution of Manitoba Women

The Native population is "younger," with a higher proportion under the age of 20. The proportion of the elderly, on the other hand, is smaller than in the non-Native population. The different age distributions may affect the trend of crude surgery rates. To account for this difference, a comparison of age-standardized rates is appropriate.

(c)   The graph should look like this:

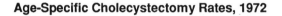

Age-Specific Cholecystectomy Rates, 1972

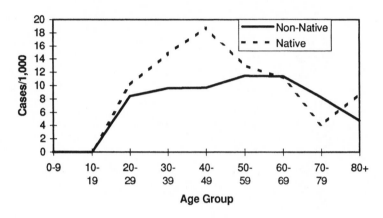

The Native rate is higher than the non-Native rate at most age groups. The peak age group is 40–49 in the Native population, which is earlier than the peak in the non-Native population. The upward turn for Natives aged 80+ is probably a result of the small number of cases and small population involved. When rates for 5 or 10 years are averaged, this peak disappears.

(d)   First, arrange your data in a table:

Age group	N_i	r_i (Non-Native)	r_i (Native)	$r_i N_i$ (Non-Native)	$r_i N_i$ (Native)
0–9	79,913	0	0	0.000	0.000
10–19	91,444	0.00001	0	0.914	0.000
20–29	98,367	0.00841	0.0101	827.266	993.507
30–39	74,994	0.00962	0.01477	721.442	1107.661
40–49	51,823	0.00971	0.0188	503.201	974.272
50–59	53,627	0.01146	0.01301	614.565	697.687
60–69	47,541	0.01139	0.01116	541.492	530.558
70–79	30,854	0.00827	0.00405	255.163	124.959
80+	16,160	0.00473	0.00877	76.437	141.723
Total	544,723			3,540.481	4,570.367

The age-standardized cholecystectomy rate for non-Native women:

$$=3540.481/544{,}723=0.00650=6.5/1{,}000$$

The age-standardized cholecystectomy rate for Native women:

$$=4570.367/544{,}723=0.00839=8.4/1{,}000$$

(e) Again, arrange your data:

Age group	R_i	n_i (Non-Native)	n_i (Native)	$R_i n_i$ (Non-Native)	$R_i n_i$ (Native)
0–9	0.00000	84,354	5,708	0.000	0.000
10–19	0.00000	97,133	4,035	0.000	0.000
20–29	0.00203	77,444	2,178	157.211	4.421
30–39	0.00420	52,885	1,286	222.117	5.401
40–49	0.00461	54,874	851	252.969	3.923
50–59	0.00558	52,007	615	290.199	3.432
60–69	0.00610	37,478	448	228.616	2.733
70–79	0.00452	23,100	247	104.412	1.116
80+	0.00330	13,101	114	43.233	0.376
Total	0.00282	492,376	15,482	1,298.758	21.403

The results are:

	Non-Native	Native
Total Observed	2,970	72
Total Expected	1,298.758	21.403
SMR	2,970/1,298.758 = 2.287	72/21.403 = 3.364
Standardized rate	2.287 × 0.00282 = 0.00645	3.364 × 0.00282 = 0.00949
	= 6.5/1,000	= 9.5/1,000

CHAPTER 3

EX. 3.1

The following 2 × 2 table can be constructed from the information provided:

Survey self-report	Physician/hospital claim Diabetes	Physician/hospital claim No diabetes	Total
Diabetes	133	60	193
No diabetes	41	2,485	2,526
Total	174	2,545	2,719

(a) The sensitivity of survey self-report as a means of detecting diabetes =133/174 =76.4%

(b) Specificity in this situation is defined as the proportion of respondents who report not having any diabetes among those who do not have a physician/hospital claim for diabetes; i.e., 2,485/2,545 =97.6%

(c) 133/193 =68.9%

(d) Positive predictive value

(e) A "linkage study" links two databases electronically using some common identifiers. Actual names would be ideal, but confidentiality rules usually demand the deletion of names prior to data linkage. Some unique personal number (e.g., health insurance or social security number), provided it is recorded and retained in both databases, can usually be used. It can be supplemented by data of birth, sex, and/or residence code to improve the proportion of successful match.

EX. 3.2

The following 2×2 table can be constructed from the information provided:

Private physicians	Indian health service		
	Reported	Missed	Total
Reported	8	5	13
Missed	37	?	?
Total	45	?	N

(a) $N = [(13 + 1)(45 + 1)/(8 + 1)] - 1 = 70.6$ (with the correction factor), or $N = (13)(45)/8 = 73.1$ (without the correction factor)

(b) The rate for private physicians is $13/70.6 = 18.4\%$ (with the correction factor) or $13/73.1 = 17.8\%$ (without the correction factor); the rate for IHS is $45/70.6 = 63.7\%$ (with the correction factor) or $45/73.1 = 61.6\%$ without the correction factor.

(c) The birth prevalence of FAS based on private physicians only = $13/19,914 = 0.07\%$
The birth prevalence of FAS based on IHS data only $= 45/19,914 = 0.23\%$

(d) The ascertainment-adjusted prevalence of FAS $= 70.6/19,914 = 0.35\%$ (with the correction factor); and $73.1/19,914 = 0.37\%$ (without the correction factor)

EX. 3.3

Create a spreadsheet with the data necessary to do the graphs requested:

PSA level	Sen (TP)	Spec (TN)	1-Spec (FP)
1.0	0.99	0.43	0.57
1.5	0.97	0.62	0.38
2.0	0.94	0.75	0.25
2.5	0.92	0.81	0.19
3.0	0.90	0.84	0.16
3.5	0.87	0.89	0.11
4.0	0.85	0.91	0.09
4.5	0.82	0.93	0.07
5.0	0.80	0.95	0.05
6.0	0.73	0.97	0.03
7.0	0.66	0.98	0.02

(a) The ROC curve, with sensitivity against (1-specificity), should look like this:

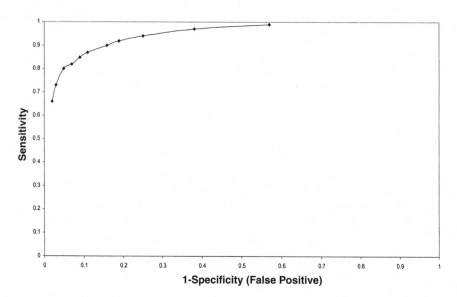

(b) With sensitivity against specificity, the graph should look like this, which is the mirror image of (a):

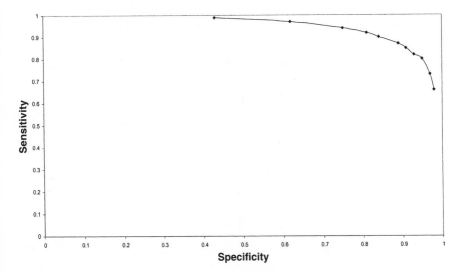

(c) A PSA cutoff point around 3.5 appears to provide the best trade-off.

EX. 3.4

$$p = (p' + \beta - 1)/(\alpha + \beta - 1)$$
$$= (0.208 + 0.93 - 1)/(0.76 + 0.93 - 1)$$
$$= 0.138/0.69$$
$$= 0.20$$

Having taken into account the sensitivity and specificity of verbal autopsy, the proportion of all deaths due to TB/AIDS is only marginally changed, from 20.8% to 20.0%.

EX. 3.5

Based on the information provided,

(a)   The epidemic curve should look something like this:

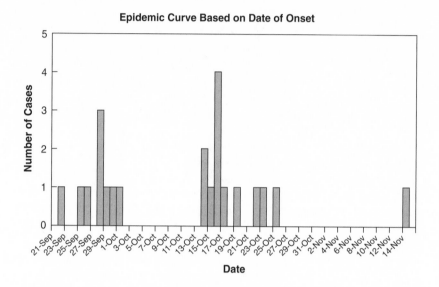

Epidemic Curve Based on Date of Onset

There were two clusters, the first (consisting of nine cases) occurring in late September, and the second (12 cases) in mid-October. All but two cases in the first cluster were from New York City and New Jersey. All five cases from the Washington, D.C., metropolitan area (listed under Virginia and Maryland in the table) are found in the second cluster.

(b)   The median age of the victims was 46 years. *Median* is preferable to *mean* in this situation because of two extreme outliers (one aged 0.6 years and one aged 94 years), resulting in the wide range of the ages. It indicates that it is mostly middle-aged adults in the working age who were affected.

(c)   The case–fatality ratio = 5/22 = 22.7%

(d)   In terms of occupation, all but four cases (category C) were mail handlers and media company employees who worked at sites where potentially contaminated mail was received or processed. It was likely that the bioterrorist(s) used the mail to disseminate anthrax spores.

CHAPTER 4

EX. 4.1

(a) In every region of the country, there is a gradation from social class I to V, with I having the lowest and V the highest IMR.

(b) In general, IMR increases as one moves from south to north. The difference is not evident for those in social class I but is most marked in social class V.

(c) One can conclude that SES has a marked impact on IMR. Social class as measured by the Registrar-General in England and Wales is based on the occupational category of the head of household. Geographical region also tends to reflect SES, with the north generally more depressed economically. However, alternative explanations are possible, as geographical regions may reflect other potential determinants; e.g., access to medical care, climate, population density, and many others. The data provided are not sufficient to decide on which ones are responsible for the observed pattern.

(d) The graph should look like this. This is an example where a 3-D graph is needed to show the relationships between three variables:

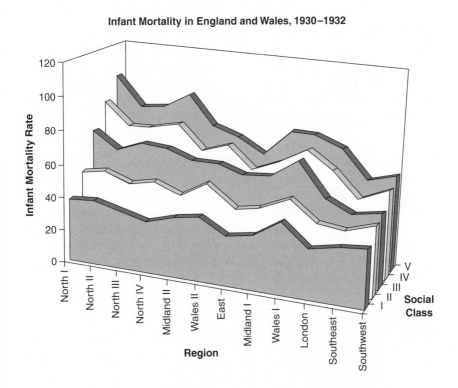

Infant Mortality in England and Wales, 1930–1932

EX. 4.2

(a) SMRs for all causes ($445/369.9 = 1.20$); infectious diseases ($16/7.9 = 2.01$); all cancers ($185/85.3 = 2.17$); cancer of buccal cavity/pharynx ($6/2.2 = 2.74$); cancer of trachea/bronchus/lung ($113/21.5 = 5.25$); silicosis ($6/0.1 = 64.0$); injuries ($43/33.8 = 1.27$).

(b) From the evidence provided, yes. It might be difficult to determine the biological mechanism that increases the risk of infectious diseases. Interested students should consult the original paper, which also provides 95% confidence intervals for the SMRs, all of which, with the exception of injuries, have 95%CI exceeding unity.

(c) The SMR increases as the cumulative WLM increases, suggestive of a dose–response relationship (see Chapter 5), as shown in this graph:

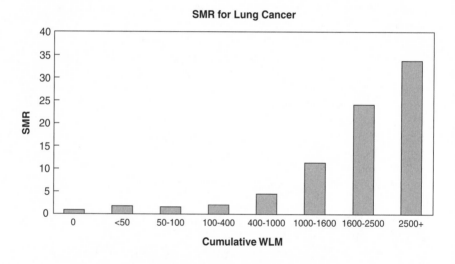

SMR for Lung Cancer

(d) The relationship could have been confounded by other factors that were not measured; for example, smoking (see Chapter 6). However, it would be difficult to argue that the dose–response relationship between radiation exposure and cancer is due to the fact that those with more radiation exposure smoked more.

EX. 4.3

(a) Individuals whose birth weight was $\leq 3.0\,\text{kg}$ and who are the most overweight at age 11.

(b) The lower the birth weight the higher the risk of adult diabetes; the more overweight at age 11, the higher the risk of adult diabetes.

(c)

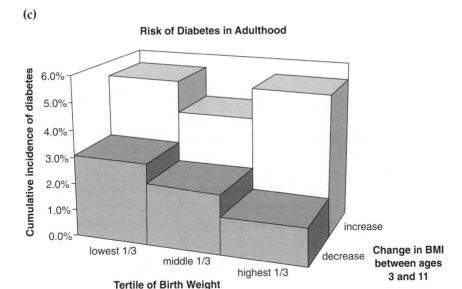

Risk of Diabetes in Adulthood

(d)   Low birth weight, overweight at any age, and increase in BMI are risk factors for diabetes.

CHAPTER 5

EX. 5.1

Comparing smoking and cholesterol, one would tend to favor interventions directed at smoking, which is associated with a higher PAR. Comparing men and women, women are associated with higher PARs for both risk factors. It should be noted that the PAR, while helpful, is not the exclusive indicator of need or priority for interventions. In the "real world," it may well be effective and efficient to organize health promotion programs directed at more than just one risk factor or more than one target group (see Chapter 7).

EX. 5.2

(a)   RR $= 43.1/11 = 3.92$

(b)   Nurse A: the on-duty death rate is $31/1{,}278$ person-hours $=$ $24.26/1{,}000$ person-hours; the off-duty death rate is $2/5{,}323$ person-hours $= 0.38/1{,}000$ person-hours.
Nurse D: the on-duty death rate is $18/1{,}204$ person-hours $= 14.95/1{,}000$ person-hours; the off-duty death rate is $15/5{,}397$ person-hours $= 2.78/1{,}000$ person-hours.

(c)   RR =0.02426/0.0038 =64
(d)   RR =0.02426/0.01495 =1.6

EX. 5.3

(a)   Strength of association. Note that a relative risk of 2.8 is considered "strong," although there is no hard-and-fast rule about the value above which an RR is labeled as "strong."
(b)   Biological gradient or dose–response relationship
(c)   Consistency
(d)   Temporality
(e)   HPV appears to be necessary, as viral DNA can be demonstrated in almost all cases of cervical cancer. By itself HPV is not sufficient to cause cancer as other factors may be needed for the infection to progress to cancer.
(f)   While HPV DNA can be identified in cancer specimens, the virus cannot be "isolated" and "inoculated" into experimental animals to produce the cancer, thus a critical condition of Koch's postulate will not be met.

EX. 5.4

(a)   *H. pylori* can be found in almost all cases of gastritis; therefore, it is necessary. One could perhaps argue whether "almost all" constitutes "all."
(b)   That *H. pylori* alone can cause gastritis is supported by experiments with mice and human volunteers. Koch's third postulate is thus satisfied. However, that as much as one-third of the population can harbor the organism and yet show no signs of the disease means that infection does not always result in disease, indicating that *H. pylori* is not sufficient.
(c)   *H. pylori* can cause more than one disease: gastritis, ulcers, and stomach cancer. However, specificity still holds if one considers these as different stages of a disease. One can also say that *H. pylori* causes only one type of disease in the stomach and no other disease elsewhere in the body, and is thus specific.
(d)   Yes, one can explain it in terms of the infection triggering off an immune response, which affects the secretion of gastric acids and mucus.
(e)   Yes, there have been experiments involving human volunteers and laboratory mice. Also, antibiotics trials have been shown to eradicate the disease.

CHAPTER 6

EX. 6.1

(a) Crude odds ratio = $(35 \times 50) / (163 \times 36) = 0.30$
(b) Mantel-Haenszel summary OR =

$$\frac{[(23 \times 33) / (52 + 93)] + [(12 \times 17) / (19 + 120)]}{[(29 \times 60) / (52 + 93)] + [(7 \times 103) / (19 + 120)]} = 0.39$$

EX. 6.2

(a) The various relative risks can be arranged in a 2×2 table:

	No asbestos	Asbestos
No smoking	1.0	$RR_A = 58.4/11.3 = 5.2$
Smoking	$RR_S = 122.6/11.3 = 10.8$	$RR_{AS} = 601.6/11.3 = 53.2$

(b) RR of lung cancer from asbestos exposure among smokers = $601.6/122.6 = 4.9$
(c) In an additive model, if there were no interaction, one would expect: $RR_{AS} = (RR_A + RR_S - 1)$
From the above table, $RR_{AS} = 53.2$, which exceeds $(RR_A + RR_S - 1)$, which is 15.0. One can conclude that there is interaction, and the effect is synergistic.
(d) In a multiplicative model, if there were no interaction, one would expect:
$RR_{AS} = RR_A \times RR_S$
From the above table, $RR_{AS} = 53.2$, whereas $(RR_A \times RR_S) = 56.2$. One can conclude that there is interaction if one considers the two to be sufficiently different. However, if one accepts that 53.2 and 56.2 are more or less the same, then there is no interaction.

EX. 6.3

(a) Yes, all three conditions are satisfied: smoking is associated with oral cancer; smoking is associated with use of mouthwash; smoking is not a consequence of using mouthwash.
(b) No, two conditions are not satisfied: yellow teeth are not associated with cancer; yellow teeth are a consequence of smoking.
(c) Yes, all three conditions are satisfied: smoking is associated with heart disease; smoking is associated with periodontal disease; smoking is not a consequence of periodontal disease.

CHAPTER 8

EX. 8.1

(a) CBA. An alternative to expressing efficiency as benefit-to-cost ratio is in terms of net economic benefit (i.e., benefit minus cost)

(b) This study encompasses both CEA and CUA, the former when "person-years of sight saved" is used as the measure of health effect and the latter when "QALY saved" is used. While there are no specific alternatives being studied, the implied comparison is "no screening." Also, a list of cost–utility ratios for other procedures totally unrelated to diabetes obtained from the literature is presented for comparison.

(c) This is cost analysis, comparing alternative treatments for the same disease. Effectiveness is not assessed or compared.

(d) The study as described contains a cost analysis, a cost-effectiveness analysis, and a sensitivity analysis.

(e) The study assesses only effectiveness, as no estimation of costs is involved.

Index

Biological gradient, 178, 185–86
Biological monitoring, 131
Biological oxygen demand (BOD), 130
Biomarkers, 131, 141
Bioterrorism, 6, 98, 113
Birth cohort, 157, 247
Birth rate, crude, 35, 62. *See also* Fertility rate
Birth weight, low, 39, 156, 175–76, 269
Black box, 11, 152
Black Death, 9
Black Report, 152
Blinding, 229–30
Blood pressure. *See* Hypertension
Bovine spongiform encephalopathy (BSE), 201–4
Bradford Hill's criteria of causation. *See* Hill, Austin Bradford
BRCA1, BRCA2 genes, 124, 192
Breast feeding, 264, 270
British Columbia Health Status Registry, 119
Broad Street pump. *See* Snow, John

Canada Communicable Diseases Report, 73
Canada Fitness Survey, Health Survey, 75
Canada's Health Promotion Survey, 75
Canadian Community Health Survey, 76
Canadian Health and Disability Survey, 75
Canadian Institute of Health Information, 68, 74
Canadian Institutes of Health Research, 4
Canadian Mortality Database, 71, 210
Canadian National Breast Screening Study, 289
Canadian Sickness Survey, 75
Canadian Task Force on the Periodic Health Examination (Preventive Health Care), 273, 281, 290

Cancer, 12, 51, 52, 55–58, 62, 74, 103, 112, 121, 124, 138, 141, 144, 154, 175, 192, 195, 204, 212, 252–55, 261–62, 269, 274, 288–90
Cancer Incidence in Five Continents, 47, 54
Cancer Prevention Study, 138
Cancer registries. *See* Disease registries
Capture-recapture method, 79–80, 112
Carcinogens, 126, 138, 255
Cardiovascular diseases, 11–13, 51, 53, 63, 103, 122, 124, 133, 138, 142, 143, 144, 156, 182, 196, 204, 210, 254–57, 269, 274, 275, 277, 290–93
Case-control study, 123, 220, 222, 224–27, 229, 252, 273, 303
nested, 229
Case-fatality ratio, 29, 268
Cassel, John, 149
Category fallacy, 106
Causation, concepts of, 181–88
Cause
necessary, sufficient, 181, 184, 187, 212–13
remote, proximate, 178, 182
Censoring, 26
Census, 31, 33, 34, 62, 79, 154, 217, 244
Centers for Disease Control, 13, 68, 73, 74, 77, 85, 144, 288
Chadwick, Edwin, 148
Chemoprophylaxis, chemoprevention, 267, 270, 271
Chernobyl, 163–66
Childbed fever. *See* Puerperal fever
Chlamydia, 73
Chloracne, 127
Chlorofluorocarbons (CFC), 128
Cholecystectomy. *See* Gallbladder disease
Cholera, 13, 15–16
Cholesterol, 11, 122, 159, 161, 178, 211, 272, 274, 277, 291–92
Chromosomal disorders, 118, 120
Chronic diseases, 11, 51, 182, 184